Association of Physical Fitness and Motor Competence with Health and Well-Being in Children and Adolescents

Association of Physical Fitness and Motor Competence with Health and Well-Being in Children and Adolescents

Editors

Clemens Drenowatz
Klaus Greier

MDPI • Basel • Beijing • Wuhan • Barcelona • Belgrade • Manchester • Tokyo • Cluj • Tianjin

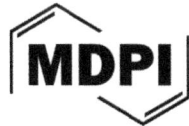

Editors

Clemens Drenowatz
Division of Sport Physical
Activity and Health
University of Education
Upper Austria
Linz
Austria

Klaus Greier
Division of Physical
Education and Sports
University of Education
Stams - KPH-ES
Stams
Austria

Editorial Office
MDPI
St. Alban-Anlage 66
4052 Basel, Switzerland

This is a reprint of articles from the Special Issue published online in the open access journal *International Journal of Environmental Research and Public Health* (ISSN 1660-4601) (available at: www.mdpi.com/journal/ijerph/special_issues/physical_fitness_motor_competence).

For citation purposes, cite each article independently as indicated on the article page online and as indicated below:

LastName, A.A.; LastName, B.B.; LastName, C.C. Article Title. *Journal Name* **Year**, *Volume Number*, Page Range.

ISBN 978-3-0365-7049-5 (Hbk)
ISBN 978-3-0365-7048-8 (PDF)

© 2023 by the authors. Articles in this book are Open Access and distributed under the Creative Commons Attribution (CC BY) license, which allows users to download, copy and build upon published articles, as long as the author and publisher are properly credited, which ensures maximum dissemination and a wider impact of our publications.

The book as a whole is distributed by MDPI under the terms and conditions of the Creative Commons license CC BY-NC-ND.

Contents

Preface to "Association of Physical Fitness and Motor Competence with Health and Well-Being in Children and Adolescents" vii

Wesley O'Brien, Zeinab Khodaverdi, Lisa Bolger, Orla Murphy, Conor Philpott and Philip E. Kearney
Exploring Recommendations for Child and Adolescent Fundamental Movement Skills Development: A Narrative Review
Reprinted from: *Int. J. Environ. Res. Public Health* **2023**, *20*, 3278, doi:10.3390/ijerph20043278 . . . 1

Nina Eisenburger, David Friesen, Fabiola Haas, Marlen Klaudius, Lisa Schmidt and Susanne Vandeven et al.
Predicting Psychosocial Health of Children and Adolescents with Obesity in Germany: The Underappreciated Role of Physical Fitness
Reprinted from: *Int. J. Environ. Res. Public Health* **2021**, *18*, 11188, doi:10.3390/ijerph182111188 . 15

Kathrin Bretz, Harald Seelig, Ilaria Ferrari, Roger Keller, Jürgen Kühnis and Simone Storni et al.
Basic Motor Competencies of (Pre)School Children: The Role of Social Integration and Health-Related Quality of Life
Reprinted from: *Int. J. Environ. Res. Public Health* **2022**, *19*, 14537, doi:10.3390/ijerph192114537 . 27

Yunfei Zheng, Weibing Ye, Mallikarjuna Korivi, Yubo Liu and Feng Hong
Gender Differences in Fundamental Motor Skills Proficiency in Children Aged 3–6 Years: A Systematic Review and Meta-Analysis
Reprinted from: *Int. J. Environ. Res. Public Health* **2022**, *19*, 8318, doi:10.3390/ijerph19148318 . . . 41

Clemens Drenowatz, Si-Tong Chen, Armando Cocca, Gerson Ferrari, Gerhard Ruedl and Klaus Greier
Association of Body Weight and Physical Fitness during the Elementary School Years
Reprinted from: *Int. J. Environ. Res. Public Health* **2022**, *19*, 3441, doi:10.3390/ijerph19063441 . . . 55

Wonseok Choi and Wonjae Jeon
A Study on the Subjectivity of Parents Regarding "0th-Period Physical Education Class" of Middle Schools in Korea Using Q-Methodology
Reprinted from: *Int. J. Environ. Res. Public Health* **2022**, *19*, 7760, doi:10.3390/ijerph19137760 . . . 67

Armando Cocca, Martin Niedermeier, Vera Prünster, Katharina Wirnitzer, Clemens Drenowatz and Klaus Greier et al.
Self-Rated Health Status of Upper Secondary School Pupils and Its Associations with Multiple Health-Related Factors
Reprinted from: *Int. J. Environ. Res. Public Health* **2022**, *19*, 6947, doi:10.3390/ijerph19116947 . . . 79

Mohamed Alaeddine Guembri, Ghazi Racil, Mohamed-Ali Dhouibi, Jeremy Coquart and Nizar Souissi
Evaluation of Age Based-Sleep Quality and Fitness in Adolescent Female Handball Players
Reprinted from: *Int. J. Environ. Res. Public Health* **2022**, *20*, 330, doi:10.3390/ijerph20010330 . . . 89

Tanja Eberhardt, Klaus Bös and Claudia Niessner
Changes in Physical Fitness during the COVID-19 Pandemic in German Children
Reprinted from: *Int. J. Environ. Res. Public Health* **2022**, *19*, 9504, doi:10.3390/ijerph19159504 . . . 101

Sabrina Demarie, Emanuele Chirico, Cecilia Bratta and Cristina Cortis
Puberal and Adolescent Horse Riders' Fitness during the COVID-19 Pandemic: The Effects of Training Restrictions on Health-Related and Functional Motor Abilities
Reprinted from: *Int. J. Environ. Res. Public Health* **2022**, *19*, 6394, doi:10.3390/ijerph19116394 . . . **115**

Yanlong Guo, Xueqing Ma, Denghang Chen and Han Zhang
Factors Influencing Use of Fitness Apps by Adults under Influence of COVID-19
Reprinted from: *Int. J. Environ. Res. Public Health* **2022**, *19*, 15460, doi:10.3390/ijerph192315460 . **129**

Preface to "Association of Physical Fitness and Motor Competence with Health and Well-Being in Children and Adolescents"

Available research has indicated a decline in physical fitness and motor competence over the last several decades. Movement restrictions and policies that have emphasized social distancing, due to the recent COVID-19 pandemic, may have further increased the prevalence of youth with insufficient physical fitness and motor competence. As physical fitness and motor competence are critical contributors to an active and healthy lifestyle, it is important to re-emphasize their role in the general health and development of children and adolescents and, accordingly, future public health. Particularly with the re-opening of schools, sports clubs, and public parks, the promotion of activities that enhance physical fitness and motor competence in children and adolescents is warranted. This reprint highlights the importance of physical fitness and motor competence for the health and well-being of children and adolescents, by providing an interdisciplinary platform for research addressing this topic.

Clemens Drenowatz and Klaus Greier
Editors

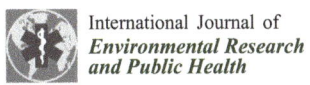

Review

Exploring Recommendations for Child and Adolescent Fundamental Movement Skills Development: A Narrative Review

Wesley O'Brien [1,*], Zeinab Khodaverdi [2], Lisa Bolger [3], Orla Murphy [1], Conor Philpott [1] and Philip E. Kearney [4]

1. Sports Studies and Physical Education Programme, School of Education, University College Cork, 2 Lucan Place, Western Road, T12 K8AF Cork, Ireland
2. Department of Biobehavioral Studies, Teachers College, Columbia University, New York, NY 10027, USA
3. Department of Sport, Leisure and Childhood Studies, Munster Technological University (Cork Campus), T12 P928 Cork, Ireland
4. Sport & Human Performance Research Centre, Department of Physical Education and Sport Sciences, University of Limerick, V94 T9PX Limerick, Ireland
* Correspondence: wesley.obrien@ucc.ie

Abstract: Fundamental movement skills (FMS) are frequently referred to as the *"building blocks"* of movement for children and adolescents in their lifelong physical activity journey. It is critical, however, that FMS are developed within Physical Education learning environments and other sport-related settings, specifically as these building blocks of movement require appropriate teaching and practice opportunities. While FMS are well-established as an *"important focus"* for children and adolescents, to the authors' knowledge, there appears to be no standardized FMS development guidelines existent within the literature. This paper will examine whether the frequency, intensity, time, and type (FITT) principle could be transferable to interventions focusing on FMS development, and if so, whether sufficient consistency of findings exists to guide practitioners in their session design. Applying the FITT principle in this way may help to facilitate the comparison of FMS-related intervention studies, which may contribute to the future development of practical FMS-related guidelines for children and adolescents.

Keywords: motor skills; school; physical education; teaching; coaching; youth

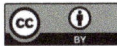

1. Introduction

Fundamental movement skills (FMS) are common motor activities with a general goal [1], which involve the use of large muscle groups within the body [2,3]. In terms of their categorical distinction, FMS are often differentiated into three subsets: (1) locomotor skills (e.g., running and skipping); object-control/ball skills (e.g., throwing and catching); and (3) stability skills (e.g., balancing and twisting) [2]. As an important component of the motor-development domain, FMS facilitate participation in physical activity and contribute to the holistic development of children and adolescents [1–3]. Previous evidence suggests that the development of FMS proficiency in children and adolescents can serve as the foundational building blocks for future lifelong daily activities [4]. FMS proficiency increases the likelihood of children and adolescents developing specialized movement sequences for participating effectively across a variety of organized and unorganized physical activities [2].

FMS are commonly viewed as a central tenet and developmental stage within the motor-skills domain [2,5]. In terms of Physical Education (PE), physical activity (PA), and sport settings, FMS have a critical role in both promoting and maintaining healthy developmental trajectories in children and adolescents [6]. In terms of empirical health-related research associations, positive relationships have been consistently found between FMS and PA, physical fitness, body composition, self-belief, and executive functioning [7,8].

While these positive associations between FMS and health have been observed quite frequently within the literature, children and adolescents do not solely acquire these motor skills as a result of the maturation process [9,10]. The development of FMS proficiency in children and adolescents is often dependent on the quality of the instructional environment and the provision of practice-based opportunities [2,11], augmenting the importance of key stakeholders, such as PE teachers, sport pedagogues, coaches, and researchers, within this process.

Research and practice have consistently highlighted how FMS interventions are successful in promoting skills and physical health [12–14]; however, the specific parameters for FMS-related recommendations have not been systematically investigated in PE, PA, and sport settings. The evidence to date has identified various strategies for measuring FMS-training exposure (e.g., types of FMS interventions) in children and adolescents; however, the general concepts for quantifying the frequency, duration (time), and intensity of FMS-related training [15] is less known among PE teachers, coaches, and sport practitioners. Together, the combined frequency, intensity, time, and type (FITT) product [16] has the potential to yield an evidence-informed FMS-related training dose for children and adolescents. The well-established FITT principle has been traditionally used to characterise recommended guidelines for PA and exercise [17].

Despite the growing number of FMS-related interventions in PE, PA, and sport settings, there appears to be an inconsistency as to *"what works"* in terms of an appropriate FMS-related training dosage [13]. The development of FMS in children and adolescents was empirically and correctly established as *"an important focus"* in 2016 [11]. Now, what remains for PE teachers, coaches, sport pedagogues, and researchers is the implementation of evidence-informed FMS-related recommendations. The FITT training principle may be one such way of providing this implementation guidance for practitioners, particularly once sufficient evidence is identified across studies to develop appropriate recommendations. Indeed, other health-and-exercise-related fields have previously used the FITT principle to categorise successful intervention features and provide subsequent recommendations for practitioners [18,19]. This paper, therefore, seeks to examine whether FMS interventions present sufficient consistency to be summarised and modified using the FITT principle, with the overall aim of providing evidence-informed and practical FMS-related recommendations for practitioners.

2. Methods Section

As part of this narrative review, a search was conducted using seven databases, including PubMed, MEDLINE, SPORTDiscus, CINAHL, Scopus, Web of Science, and EMBASE, without any date restriction for articles pertaining to motor skills interventions in typically developing children and adolescents from all socioeconomic backgrounds.

The main search group terms were: "fundamental motor skills" OR "FMS" OR "motor skill" OR "movement skill" OR "motor development" OR "motor performance" OR "balance" OR "stability" OR "motor ability" AND "children" OR "adolescent" OR "youth", OR "preschooler" AND "intervention" OR "program" OR "study" OR "trial". To exclude studies that specifically examined youth participants with disorders/disabilities, the following terms were used: AND NOT "disability" OR "disorder" OR "autism" OR "impairment" OR "cerebral palsy".

The criteria used to include a study in this narrative were as follows:

(1) The study needed to measure motor skill performance as an outcome and include pre- or post-timepoint intervention assessments, or both. It is important to note that neither the type of motor skill battery assessment tool nor the measurement approach was a determining factor in either including or excluding a study;

(2) Only articles published in English and in peer-reviewed journals were considered. All books, reviews, theses, dissertations, commentaries, qualitative studies, and case studies were excluded from the review process as part of this narrative review.

Section 3 below provides information as part of this narrative review on the included FITT components of the motor skill intervention studies that have been reviewed.

3. Components of FITT Principle

3.1. Frequency

The "F" within the FITT principle stands for frequency and relates to how often a person participates in exercise-related training sessions [15]. To determine the frequency of FMS-related training sessions or interventions, a specific priority in this research was placed towards published randomized controlled trials (RCTs) in FMS, specifically as they are the most likely research designs to provide impartial information on the frequency variable [20]. As part of this specifically tailored narrative research search, a total of 36 RCTs were retrieved across a 25-year timeline (1997–2022), with 88% of the published research reporting on frequency-related FMS data. From the critical review of this RCT research, Table 1 documents the frequency of FMS-related training sessions and interventions, with the existing frequency evidence ranging from one to five FMS sessions a week. Interestingly, Table 1 further highlights that 8 of the existing 40 RCTs do not appear to report the frequency of their associated FMS-related training sessions or interventions.

Outside of this specific RCT search in FMS, other systematic review evidence has further attempted to synthesize the effectiveness of FMS-related interventions (RCTs and non-RCTs) on motor skill development [12,13,21–23]. Aligned to the data reported above in Table 1, the findings from Wick et al. (2017) similarly reported a frequency range of one to five FMS sessions a week for children and adolescents [13].

Table 1. The reported frequencies of FMS-related training sessions/interventions from randomized controlled trial evidence from 1997 to 2022.

No. FMS Sessions/Week	1 × FMS Session/Week	2 × FMS Sessions/Week	3 × FMS Sessions/Week	4 × FMS Sessions/Week	5 × FMS Sessions/Week	Frequency Not Reported
	6 studies Cliff et al. (2011) [24] Foulkes et al. (2017) [25] Johnson et al. (2019) [26] McGrane et al. (2018) [27] Pesce et al. (2016) [28] Smyth & O'Keeffe (1998) [29]	16 studies Derri et al. (2001) [30] Donath et al. (2015) [31] Gallotta et al. (2017) [32] Goodway & Branta, (2003) [33] Goodway et al. (2003) [34] Hamilton et al. (1999) [35] Iivonen et al. (2011) [36] Johnson et al. (2019) [26] Marshall & Bouffard, (1997) [37] Palmer et al. (2019) [38] Roach & Keats (2018) [39] Robinson & Goodway (2009) [40] Robinson et al. (2017) [41] Veldman et al. (2017) [42] Zask et al. (2012) [43] Berleze & Valentini (2022) [44]	3 studies Hashemi et al. (2015) [45] Jones et al. (2011) [46] Robinson et al. (2022) [47]	2 studies De Oliveira et al. (2019) [48] Hestbaek et al. (2021) [49]	5 studies Alhassan et al. (2012) [50] Engel et al. (2018) [51] Roth et al. (2015) [52] Webster et al. (2020) [53] Staiano et al. (2022) [54]	8 studies Chan et al. (2019) [55] Cohen et al. (2015) [56] Lander et al. (2017) [57] McKenzie et al. (2002) [58] Miller et al. (2015) [59] Salmon et al. (2008) [60] Trost & Brookes (2021) [61] van Beurden et al. (2003) [62]

Note: No. = number; sessions/week = sessions a week; FMS = fundamental movement (motor) skills.

Overall, the evidence presented above suggests that a frequency of 2 days per week for FMS-related activities appears to be somewhat prevalent and commonly reported in many studies [13,20]. Furthermore, researchers and practitioners ought to consider if there is an optimal FMS-related frequency focus per week, which might result in maximal skill acquisition outcomes in children and adolescents. At this point, it seems to be unclear as to whether the interaction of FMS-related frequencies with the other FITT components (intensity, time, and type) may impact the quality of FMS acquisition. While some studies report having a varying number of FMS-related training sessions or interventions per week, other research illustrates the total volume time (minutes) of FMS-related activities per week, irrespective of the frequency variable [61]. In this sense, therefore, the important debate of frequency versus time for FMS needs more clarification and guidance for those working with children and adolescents in a physically active setting.

3.2. Intensity

The "I" within the FITT principle stands for "intensity". Within the context of PA, intensity refers to the energy expended during a given time period [63]. In the context of

FMS session design, however, another interpretation of intensity might also be considered as the number of skill executions within a given time period. Children's practice of FMS, whether in the context of a PE lesson or a coaching session, will ideally achieve the dual objectives of reaching moderate-to-vigorous levels of PA for immediate health benefits while also promoting quality skill development [62]. With appropriate activity design and monitoring of intensity, both of these objectives can be met within the same session.

For children and adolescents between the ages of 5 and 17 years old, the World Health Organisation (WHO) recommend 60 min of moderate-to-vigorous physical activity (MVPA) daily [64]. There are five categories of well-established PA-related exercise intensities, beginning with *sedentary*, which typically refers to sitting or other stationary activities, requiring minimal energy and low levels of movement [65]. *Light-intensity* activity refers to activities that can be easily sustained for 60 min without incurring a noticeable change in breathing rate, and often, these activities require less than three times the resting energy expenditure [65]. *Moderate intensity* refers to using between 3 and 6 times more energy than a resting state, while *vigorous intensity* refers to using 6 to 9 times more energy when compared to a resting state [65]. *High-intensity* activity, however, refers to expending energy in excess of 9 times the amount used at rest.

Monitoring PA intensity is a critical component for evaluating cardiorespiratory fitness, and consistent participation at higher-intensity PA has the potential to positively impact other health markers, such as blood glucose and blood lipid levels [66]. The consistent associations found between FMS and PA indicate that a high level of motor competence can contribute to long-term PA engagement [67]. Minimal research, however, exists pertaining to the intensity of activity accrued during the performance of FMS activities [68] or the associated quality of skill execution.

Recent studies with populations of children and adolescents have examined energy expenditure during the performance of object-control skills (kick, throw, strike) [68,69]. The Sacko et al. (2019) study (n = 42; 22 males; mean age = 8.1 ± 0.8 years) reported that the practice of kicking, throwing, and striking at a rate of two maximal-effort attempts per minute appears to meet the threshold for moderate-intensity PA as it surpasses the 4.0 metabolic equivalent (METs) [69]. Further research among children (n = 30; 16 males; (9.4 ± 1.4 years) has suggested a slow cadence (i.e., kicking a football in a passing motion every 6 s but not at maximal effort), results in a light intensity of activity between 1.5 and 2.9 METs [70]. Notably, these studies differ in the effort applied from participants; the Sacko et al. (2019) study sought maximal effort from participants, whereas the Duncan et al. (2020) study referred to a short passing motion with a football at a slow tempo [69,71]. Such tempo and light-energy expenditure may be common within physical education or coaching during isolated task practices [69,71]. To achieve a *vigorous PA intensity* threshold, 10 attempts per minute at a maximal effort for FMS-related practices were deemed to be needed [69], whereas 20 attempts of short-range kicking were required to reach moderate intensity [71]. Thus, depending upon the effort required and rate of attempts, the practice of individual FMS may produce light, moderate, or vigorous levels of PA.

In contrast to the aforementioned studies on energy expenditure when performing individual FMS [69,71], FMS practice sessions will often include activities in which multiple FMS are performed within the context of a game [72]. According to the compendium of physical activities for children and adolescents, various forms of game play commonly result in levels of vigorous intensity being attained [73]. Several examples of organised games (i.e., basketball, soccer, tennis), in addition to less formal playground and active locomotor play (i.e., hopscotch, freeze tag, sharks and minnows) typically allow children and adolescents to meet the vigorous-intensity threshold across 4 identified age ranges (6 to 9 years old, 10 to 12 years old, 13 to 15 years old, and 16 to 18 years old) [73]. Thus, provided that games are appropriately designed (i.e., number of participants, size of playing area, etc.), it appears that such activities are a viable means of meeting the PA objective of FMS sessions [59].

In relation to skill development, extensive research has shown that practicing FMS in isolation, coupled with appropriate instruction and feedback, can develop children's skill levels [33,40,74,75]. While the overall time spent in activities is typically reported in these studies, the number of skill executions within that time period is not. Interventions with a larger emphasis on the use of games to enhance FMS have also proved successful [59,71,76,77]. As with interventions based upon practicing skills in isolation, specific information on the rate of skill executions within these games is typically not provided either. Additional information on the rate of skill executions per unit time would prove valuable for practitioners in their design of practice sessions, and potentially to researchers seeking to understand the mechanisms underpinning effective interventions.

Skill development is an individual process that demands a tailored approach due to varying environmental constraints and the interactions between the task and the individual themselves [5]. Game-based approaches, such as Teaching Games for Understanding [78,79], propose that the teacher or coach draw upon both game forms and more isolated activities as required to meet their individual learners' needs. Practitioners need to understand how their choice of activity (isolated task or game form; maximum or submaximal effort; etc.) will influence both PA levels and skill development. As such, a singular definitive recommendation regarding which intensity to utilise in a physically active setting to develop FMS is not advisable from the current evidence presented. Instead, Physical Education teachers, sport pedagogues, coaches, and researchers should acknowledge and justify their selections of individual activities and combinations of activities within a session/lesson plan so as to meet learners' PA and skill development needs [68,69].

3.3. Time

When considering recommended FMS guidelines for children and adolescents, the variable of "time" under the FITT acronym can refer to either (1) the duration of time devoted to motor skill instruction and practice across a complete intervention [22,75] or (2) the duration in minutes of motor skill instruction and practice in a singular FMS session of intervention [13].

A previous meta-analysis by Logan et al. (2012), which specifically examined motor skill interventions in children, found that no significant relationship existed between the duration in minutes of the FMS intervention dose and the subsequent effect size of participant FMS improvements post intervention (the intervention–dose response). Many interventions for FMS identified within this meta-analysis were noted as lasting from between 6 and 15 weeks in length, and ranged from 480 to 1440 min (8 to 24 h) total in duration [22]. More recently, Robinson et al. (2017) suggested that 600 min (10 h) of high-quality instruction for pre-schoolers could significantly improve children's motor competence, and the authors reported similar improvements for children's FMS performances, regardless of whether participants had received a 660 min (n = 27, 13 males, 14 females, mean age = 4.4 years, SD = 0.6 years), 720 min (n = 23, 11 males, 12 females, mean age = 4.4 years, SD = 0.4 years), or 900 min (n = 25, 13 males, 12 females, mean age = 4.5 years, SD = 0.5 years) dose of FMS instruction as part of the Children's Health Activity Motor Program (CHAMP) intervention across a 12-week period [75]. In other studies of younger children aged between 2 and 6 years old, evidence would suggest that interventions with a shorter duration (ranging from 1 month to 5 months) have demonstrated significantly higher effect sizes for FMS proficiency when compared with studies of longer durations (6 months or longer) [13]. It has been theorised that the activities provided in the intervention may, over time, become repetitive and monotonous to the children, leading participants to disengage from the intervention and its associated activities [22].

Tompsett et al. (2017) in their updated systematic review of pedagogical approaches used in FMS interventions reported that individual FMS session durations vary widely across the FMS-related literature for children and adolescents, with session durations of: 20 min, 30 min, 40 min, 45 min, 60 min, and 90+ min being reported. Findings from this systematic review observed that both the session duration and the number of sessions per week (frequency) were not associated with FMS proficiency outcomes in participants aged 5–18 years [80]. Many evidence-informed FMS studies with children and adolescents in sport and PE settings have cited that the implementation of two sessions a week appears to promote positive changes in FMS competence, with total session time across the week equalling approximately 60 min [40,74,81,82].

The use, however, of one session a week in the 30–60 min range has also been found to be effective in promoting enhanced skill growth and motor development among children and adolescents [83–85]. Aligned to the FITT principle, no clear guidelines for the suggested FMS session(s) time exists in child and adolescent FMS-related research. Existing evidence from above, however, suggests that somewhere between 30 and 60 min per session would appear appropriate for FMS-related skill development. Notwithstanding the relationship between the individual, the task, and the environment in which the motor skill task is performed [86–88], the time available for FMS devotion will likely depend on the intervention setting, be that a community-based sports club, or in a school environment through Physical Education classes, for example.

Overall, while no specific FMS guidelines for time have been consistently set within the literature for increased FMS competence in children and adolescents, some impactful research has reported that successful FMS-related interventions appear to comprise at least 600 min of quality instruction time, with effective FMS session durations lasting somewhere between 30 and 60 min per week and being no longer than 6 months overall in duration (particularly when training those in early childhood). Future research regarding the FMS training of children and adolescents is needed, by specifically examining dose–response relationships for meaningful FMS-related intervention guidelines [13,75,80].

3.4. Type

FMS development is influenced not just by the frequency, intensity, and time engaged in practice; practitioners must also select the type of practice. In a recent systematic review of the pedagogical approaches used in FMS interventions for children and adolescents [80], it was revealed that FMS interventions are indeed effective at improving FMS proficiency (27 of 29 included studies). Central to the success of these interventions are the deliberate decisions that trained and/or experienced practitioners make when designing and delivering developmentally appropriate activities [2]. This culminating section on the FITT principle's relationship with FMS will focus on three decisions that practitioners may need to make in relation to type of practice: (i) the nature of guidance, (ii) the level of autonomy afforded to learners, and (iii) the extent to which the FMS are performed in isolation or in the context of a game form (Table 2).

Table 2. Dimensions of practice type to enhance fundamental movement skills.

Dimension			
Nature of Guidance	**Direct instruction:** movement solution specified through some combination of demonstration, instruction, physical guidance, and/or prescriptive feedback.	⟺	**Indirect instruction:** manipulation of constraints (e.g., distance from target; object to be thrown) to encourage alternative behaviour/exploration.
Learner Autonomy	**Teacher selects** content, sequence, and duration of practice activities.	⟺	**Learner selects** content, sequence, and duration of practice activities.
Skill Context	**Isolated** technical practice (exercise), often with task decomposition.	⟺	**Contextualised** skill practice (game), often with simplification and/or exaggeration.

3.4.1. Nature of Guidance

High-quality instruction, practice, and feedback are essential factors for the development of FMS proficiency in children and adolescents [2]. While unstructured, minimally supervised "free play" interventions do appear to lead to improvements in FMS (e.g., [46,89,90]), these improvements are less than those observed in peer groups that receive additional guidance. While some form of additional guidance can enhance learning, this quality instruction may be delivered in different ways [2,91]. For example, direct instruction is where a movement solution is prescribed for the learner by the practitioner. This prescription may be provided in the form of demonstrations, cue words, and/or targeted feedback, all of which is designed to help a child modify their action towards a more proficient pattern (e.g., [74,75]). In contrast, indirect instruction refers to manipulations of the task, equipment, or playing space to elicit behavioural responses from the learner (e.g., [92,93]). For example, instructions to throw "as far as you can" or the use of distant targets may be used to encourage a stepping action and additional trunk rotation within the overarm throw. Importantly, effective indirect instruction does not force a learner towards a single, specific solution, but rather encourages the exploration of alternative movement solutions [94].

One proposed advantage of indirect instruction is that it encourages a learner to become sensitive to the demands of any movement situation, and to adjust their movement accordingly [72]. However, limited research has directly compared direct and indirect instruction while controlling for other variables [93,95], and this research has produced equivocal findings in relation to movement competence, with direct instruction enhancing the development of certain movement components, and indirect instruction enhancing the development of others. The impact of these differing instructional approaches on broader benefits (e.g., intrinsic motivation, creativity) have not been investigated [96]. In addition, many FMS interventions (e.g., SKIP–[97]) utilise both direct and indirect instruction in combination. Effective teachers and coaches can and do use both direct and indirect instruction, often within the same session [91], with the decision depending upon the aim of the activity, and the specific characteristics of the learner and teacher.

3.4.2. Learner Autonomy

The ideal FMS session is one which supports children to become proficient movers while also enhancing their motivation to partake in PA [98]. According to self-determination theory [99,100], an autonomy-supporting learning environment enhances motivation. Within the context of FMS development, autonomy refers to viewing learners as individuals who are deserving of understanding and, within appropriate limits, of choosing the direction of their development [101]. In practical terms, an autonomy-supporting environment is one in which learners are provided with a rationale for activities, their feelings are taken into consideration, and they are provided with as much choice and opportunities for independent action as appropriate in the context [101]. While the provision of a rationale for activities and consideration of learner's feelings should be present within all FMS sessions, the instructor should determine the appropriate degree of choice to be provided to learners.

Within low-autonomy FMS sessions, the teacher/coach selects the content, duration, and order of activities to be practiced [74,102]. In contrast, during high-autonomy FMS sessions, the learner has a degree of choice about which activities to engage in, which variations of each skill to engage with (e.g., which target to throw at, which object to throw with), how long to spend on each task, and whether they would like feedback on any particular effort [103,104].

Multiple studies have demonstrated the benefits of incorporating learner autonomy within an FMS intervention (e.g., [104,105]). However, in many studies on learner autonomy, the interventions differ on both the level of autonomy provided and on the nature and/or quantity of the instruction provided. Valentini and Goodway (2004b) found benefits for a high-autonomy group relative to a low-autonomy group in terms of heightened variable practice conditions, however the group also differed in the use of private rather than public feedback [105]. The most focused test of autonomy was provided by Robinson and Goodway (2009) [40], who provided highly individualised feedback to participants in both a low-autonomy (the teacher made all decisions about what to practice and when based on their professional judgement) and a high-autonomy group (the learner made all decisions); the groups did not differ in relation to improvements in FMS levels. Taken as a whole, these studies suggest that incorporating learner autonomy is beneficial for FMS development (or at least, does not reduce learning), and may have additional motivational benefits. However, the level of autonomy will vary depending upon the aim of the activity, as well as on learner and teacher characteristics [91]. For example, where an instructor has developed children's ability to self-direct their play appropriately, higher levels of autonomy can be provided. Furthermore, within a single session, different levels of autonomy may be deemed appropriate for different activities; for example, low autonomy might be appropriate when the priority is to assess children's performances on a novel activity.

3.4.3. Skill Context

Another decision for practitioners in relation to type of practice relates to the extent to which skills are practiced in the context of games or in isolation. Practicing individual FMS in a station-based structure [33,75] provides children and adolescents with the opportunity to perform numerous practice attempts across a wide range of FMS. Such an approach can prove both engaging and enjoyable as long as a suitable range of activities and variations are provided [85]. In contrast, contextualised skill practices see learners perform multiple FMS in a game context [72,77] applied to achieve a higher-order objective. Such games can be simplified or have elements exaggerated in order to provide an appropriate challenge for learners.

There is a concern that isolated technical exercises may show limited opportunities for transfer to game forms, especially from an ecological dynamics theoretical perspective, where the movement a child demonstrates arises from the specific constraints of the situation [86,106]. In addition, practice in the context of game forms is thought to provide young learners with greater opportunities to demonstrate creativity, problem solving and, decision making [72]. However, for many skills, there are common principles of effective and safe movement which may be best appreciated initially in isolation. Furthermore, the flow of information which guides movement is not just in the external world (e.g., location of target for a throw, intervening obstacles) but also internal to the body in the form of kinaesthetic information from muscles and joints (e.g., absence of knee valgus when landing). Exploring movements in isolation, alongside the implementation of established elements of game-based approaches [107], may facilitate the learner to tune into this kinaesthetic information flow.

Research comparing technical exercises against games skills have reported mixed results. For example, Jarani et al. (2016) reported that 8-year-old Albanian children showed superior improvements in a range of motor skills tests if they performed exercises as individuals (e.g., gait exercises to improve running speed) rather than as small groups (e.g., tag games to improve running speed) [108]. In contrast, Miller et al. (2015) reported that 10-year-old Australian children showed significant improvements in throwing and catching following a games-based intervention compared with lessons featuring a higher proportion of isolated technical training [59]. Thus, as with learner autonomy, it appears that the question facing instructors is not whether isolated or contextualised activities are most effective but rather how and when each type of practice should be applied in order to maximise learning. Indeed, many interventions incorporate both isolated and contextualised activities [24,109,110]. An implication for researchers is to report the degree to which isolated and contextualised skill practices are present within their sessions (e.g., [59]).

This section reviewed three key dimensions of the type of practice and instruction: the nature of guidance, learner autonomy, and the skill context. Each dimension represents a spectrum of activity and instructional design that a teacher or coach can select from depending upon their aims and the needs of the learners. For researchers, additional clarity and consistency is required in the reporting of each dimension of practice type.

4. Conclusions

In exploring recommendations for child and adolescent FMS development, an outline of the range of guidelines identified in this narrative review are summarised in Table 3 below using the FITT principle. As a means of equipping practitioners with evidence-based recommendations for child and adolescent FMS development, the use of the FITT principle could be a promising, "user-friendly" strategic approach. As explored in this narrative review, however, a lack of sufficient consistency across published FMS interventions appears to exist across the different studies in terms of intervention frequency, intensity, time, and type. As such, regarding the FITT principle, the evidence is insufficient to provide robust recommendations for practitioners. For these reasons, the guideline ranges presented in Table 3 are therefore not intended to represent robust recommendations but rather to provide a summary of the different findings reported within the available evidence.

Table 3. The FITT formula: identified guideline ranges for the FMS development of children and adolescents.

	Fundamental Movement Skills
F	**Frequency:** At a minimum 2 times per week (unknown if higher dosages of FMS-related frequencies per week bring about additional motor competence and/or motor skill development).
I	**Intensity:** Moderate-to-vigorous thresholds, with a priority towards object-control skills. Desired FMS intensities can be reached through direct and indirect instructional practice pedagogies.
T	**Time:** Aim for between 30 to 60 minutes of FMS-related activities per week, striving for at least 600 minutes of total intervention or overall program dosage time.
T	**Type:** Avail of FMS teacher/coach expertise, supported by parents/guardians. Practice FMS regularly in structured (games, stations) and unstructured activities (free play).

It is recommended, rather, that the FITT principle may be used to structure future investigations of child and adolescent FMS interventions, whereby future researchers might report their FMS intervention study designs, in accordance with the FITT principle, to facilitate commonality and comparisons between studies. Such improved reporting and clarity between FMS intervention study designs would strongly contribute to the quality of studies seeking to evaluate the impact of the FITT principle. The authors of the current study, however, strongly suggest that some clear elements need to be considered if seeking to promote quality FMS research in children and adolescents when using the FITT principle.

Reporting the frequency (i.e., dosage) of FMS sessions is a clear necessity for future research. Many FMS intervention studies are evaluated within physical education settings. The duration of such classes and the number of taught classes per week typically vary across countries and continents. Outlining a consistent approach for the frequency of FMS-related physical education lessons may be necessary to examine how the frequency variable could be operationalised in diverse education (or community sport settings). Regarding intensity, some FMS-related research has assessed this variable using portable gas analysers, which evaluate oxygen consumption on a breath-by-breath basis both prior to and during exercise. For FMS practitioners in the field, given that cost is often a prohibitive factor within measurement studies, the use of heart rate monitors or smart watch devices may be considered reasonable alternative measurement devices to gauge exercise intensity during FMS sessions. Future research studies should clearly outline time recommendations when reporting on the FMS-related prescription of intervention studies, with the findings of the current narrative review suggesting that a range of between 30 and 60 min of FMS-specific work per week might be appropriate for the motor development of children and adolescents. Within a school or community sport setting, practitioners are encouraged to target this 30 to 60 min time threshold through allocated classroom or sport-related session times. Clearer specifications on the type of activities used to improve FMS in children and adolescents should be clarified within future research studies as a strategy to identify replicable trends that can be adapted for use within and across countries. It is very important to note that in research and practical settings, the type of instructional offering for promoting individual autonomy within FMS may vary. Such instructional climates may be dependent on the context of the skill, the mode of delivery, and whether additional elements, such as decision making, motivation, etc., may also need to be targeted.

It is recommended by this authorship team that future prospective studies seeking to evaluate the "FITT" principle within FMS environments should provide a clear outline of the frequency (dosage) and time (duration) of the sessions undertaken and specify the instructional methods implemented, with a supportive rationale on the types of activities offered, in addition to measuring intensity. Such consistency in the reporting of FMS interventions for children and adolescents may allow for the future provision of evidence-informed, FMS-related recommendations for use by practitioners, including Physical Education teachers, sport pedagogues, coaches, parents, guardians, and researchers.

Author Contributions: All members of the authorship team wrote differing sections of the current manuscript. W.O. initiated the original conceptual idea and led the manuscript write-up, with P.E.K. assisting the direction of this paper from a critical skill acquisition perspective. Z.K. expertly assisted the team with methodological input, search strategy techniques and referencing. C.P., O.M. and L.B. assisted specific writing tasks relating to the sections on intensity, time and type. All authors have read and agreed to the published version of the manuscript.

Funding: This research received no external funding.

Institutional Review Board Statement: Not applicable.

Informed Consent Statement: Not applicable.

Data Availability Statement: Not applicable.

Acknowledgments: The authors acknowledge all cited scholars within this manuscript for allowing the team to access the required published data and specific FMS-related study findings that crucially informed the direction of this manuscript's write-up.

Conflicts of Interest: There are no conflict of interest to report from any of the authorship team.

References

1. Wickstrom, R.L. *Fundamental Movement Patterns*, 2nd ed.; Lea & Febiger: Philadelphia, PA, USA, 1977.
2. Goodway, J.D.; Ozmun, J.C.; Gallahue, D.L. *Understanding Motor Development: Infants, Children, Adolescents, Adults*, 8th ed.; Jones & Bartlett Learning: Burlington, MA, USA, 2019.
3. Payne, V.G.; Isaacs, L.D. *Human Motor Development: A Lifespan Approach*; Routledge: Abingdon-on-Thames, UK, 2017.
4. Logan, S.W.; Ross, S.M.; Chee, K.; Stodden, D.F.; Robinson, L.E. Fundamental motor skills: A systematic review of terminology. *J. Sport. Sci.* **2018**, *36*, 781–796. [CrossRef] [PubMed]
5. Newell, K.M. What are Fundamental Motor Skills and What is Fundamental About Them? *J. Mot. Learn. Dev.* **2020**, *8*, 280–314. [CrossRef]
6. Stodden, D.F.; Goodway, J.D.; Langendorfer, S.J.; Roberton, M.A.; Rudisill, M.E.; Garcia, C.; Garcia, L.E. A Developmental Perspective on the Role of Motor Skill Competence in Physical Activity: An Emergent Relationship. *Quest* **2008**, *60*, 290–306. [CrossRef]
7. Bremer, E.; Cairney, J. Fundamental Movement Skills and Health-Related Outcomes: A Narrative Review of Longitudinal and Intervention Studies Targeting Typically Developing Children. *Am. J. Lifestyle Med.* **2016**, *12*, 148–159. [CrossRef]
8. Lubans, D.R.; Morgan, P.J.; Cliff, D.P.; Barnett, L.M.; Okely, A.D. Fundamental movement skills in children and adolescents: Review of associated health benefits. *Sport. Med. (Auckl. N. Z.)* **2010**, *40*, 1019–1035. [CrossRef] [PubMed]
9. O'Brien, W.; Belton, S.; Issartel, J. Fundamental movement skill proficiency amongst adolescent youth. *Phys. Educ. Sport Pedagog.* **2016**, *21*, 557–571. [CrossRef]

10. O'Brien, W.; Duncan, M.J.; Farmer, O.; Lester, D. Do Irish Adolescents Have Adequate Functional Movement Skill and Confidence? *J. Mot. Learn. Dev.* **2018**, *6*, S301–S319. [CrossRef]
11. Barnett, L.M.; Stodden, D.; Cohen, K.E.; Smith, J.J.; Lubans, D.R.; Lenoir, M.; Iivonen, S.; Miller, A.D.; Laukkanen, A.; Dudley, D.; et al. Fundamental Movement Skills: An Important Focus. *J. Teach. Phys. Educ.* **2016**, *35*, 219–225. [CrossRef]
12. Morgan, P.J.; Barnett, L.M.; Cliff, D.P.; Okely, A.D.; Scott, H.A.; Cohen, K.E.; Lubans, D.R. Fundamental movement skill interventions in youth: A systematic review and meta-analysis. *Pediatrics* **2013**, *132*, e1361–e1383. [CrossRef] [PubMed]
13. Wick, K.; Leeger-Aschmann, C.S.; Monn, N.D.; Radtke, T.; Ott, L.V.; Rebholz, C.E.; Cruz, S.; Gerber, N.; Schmutz, E.A.; Puder, J.J.; et al. Interventions to Promote Fundamental Movement Skills in Childcare and Kindergarten: A Systematic Review and Meta-Analysis. *Sport. Med. (Auckl. N. Z.)* **2017**, *47*, 2045–2068. [CrossRef] [PubMed]
14. Bolger, L.E.; Bolger, L.A.; O'Neill, C.; Coughlan, E.; O'Brien, W.; Lacey, S.; Burns, C.; Bardid, F. Global levels of fundamental motor skills in children: A systematic review. *J. Sport. Sci.* **2021**, *39*, 717–753. [CrossRef]
15. Wasfy, M.M.; Baggish, A.L. Exercise Dose in Clinical Practice. *Circulation* **2016**, *133*, 2297–2313. [CrossRef]
16. Barisic, A.; Leatherdale, S.T.; Kreiger, N. Importance of frequency, intensity, time and type (FITT) in physical activity assessment for epidemiological research. *Can. J. Public Health Rev. Can. De Sante Publique* **2011**, *102*, 174–175. [CrossRef]
17. Burnet, K.; Kelsch, E.; Zieff, G.; Moore, J.B.; Stoner, L. How fitting is F.I.T.T.?: A perspective on a transition from the sole use of frequency, intensity, time, and type in exercise prescription. *Physiol. Behav.* **2019**, *199*, 33–34. [CrossRef]
18. Billinger, S.A.; Boyne, P.; Coughenour, E.; Dunning, K.; Mattlage, A. Does aerobic exercise and the FITT principle fit into stroke recovery? *Curr. Neurol. Neurosci. Rep.* **2015**, *15*, 519. [CrossRef] [PubMed]
19. Power, V.; Clifford, A.M. Characteristics of optimum falls prevention exercise programmes for community-dwelling older adults using the FITT principle. *Eur. Rev. Aging Phys. Act.* **2013**, *10*, 95–106. [CrossRef]
20. Khodaverdi, Z.; O'Brien, W.; Clark, C.C.; Duncan, M. Motor Competence Interventions in Children and Adolescents - Theoretical and Atheoretical Approaches: A Systematic Review. *J. Sport. Sci.* **2022**, 1–13. [CrossRef] [PubMed]
21. Van Capelle, A.; Broderick, C.R.; van Doorn, N.; Ward, R.E.; Parmenter, B.J. Interventions to improve fundamental motor skills in pre-school aged children: A systematic review and meta-analysis. *J. Sci. Med. Sport* **2017**, *20*, 658–666. [CrossRef] [PubMed]
22. Logan, S.W.; Robinson, L.E.; Wilson, A.E.; Lucas, W.A. Getting the fundamentals of movement: A meta-analysis of the effectiveness of motor skill interventions in children. *Child Care Health Dev.* **2012**, *38*, 305–315. [CrossRef]
23. Eddy, L.H.; Wood, M.L.; Shire, K.A.; Bingham, D.D.; Bonnick, E.; Creaser, A.; Mon-Williams, M.; Hill, L.J.B. A systematic review of randomized and case-controlled trials investigating the effectiveness of school-based motor skill interventions in 3- to 12-year-old children. *Child Care Health Dev.* **2019**, *45*, 773–790. [CrossRef]
24. Cliff, D.P.; Okely, A.D.; Morgan, P.J.; Steele, J.R.; Jones, R.A.; Colyvass, K.; Baur, L.A. Movement Skills and Physical Activity in Obese Children: Randomized Controlled Trial. *Med. Sci. Sport. Exerc.* **2011**, *43*, 90–100. [CrossRef] [PubMed]
25. Foulkes, J.D.; Knowles, Z.; Fairclough, S.J.; Stratton, G.; O'Dwyer, M.; Ridgers, N.D.; Foweather, L. Effect of a 6-Week Active Play Intervention on Fundamental Movement Skill Competence of Preschool Children. *Percept. Mot. Ski.* **2017**, *124*, 393–412. [CrossRef] [PubMed]
26. Johnson, J.L.; Rudisill, M.E.; Hastie, P.; Wadsworth, D.; Strunk, K.; Venezia, A.; Sassi, J.; Morris, M.; Merritt, M. Changes in Fundamental Motor-Skill Performance Following a Nine-Month Mastery Motivational Climate Intervention. *Res. Q. Exerc. Sport* **2019**, *90*, 517–526. [CrossRef] [PubMed]
27. McGrane, B.; Belton, S.; Fairclough, S.J.; Powell, D.; Issartel, J. Outcomes of the Y-PATH Randomized Controlled Trial: Can a School-Based Intervention Improve Fundamental Movement Skill Proficiency in Adolescent Youth? *J. Phys. Act. Health* **2018**, *15*, 89–98. [CrossRef]
28. Pesce, C.; Masci, I.; Marchetti, R.; Vazou, S.; Sääkslahti, A.; Tomporowski, P.D. Deliberate Play and Preparation Jointly Benefit Motor and Cognitive Development: Mediated and Moderated Effects. *Front. Psychol.* **2016**, *7*, 349. [CrossRef]
29. Smyth, P.; Q'Keeffe, S.n.L. Fundamental motor skills: The effects of teaching intervention programmes. *Ir. J. Psychol.* **1998**, *19*, 532–539. [CrossRef]
30. Derri, V.; Tsapakidou, A.; Zachopoulou, E.; Kioumourtzoglou, E. Effect of a Music and Movement Programme on Development of Locomotor Skills by Children 4 to 6 Years of Age. *Eur. J. Phys. Educ.* **2001**, *6*, 16–25. [CrossRef]
31. Donath, L.; Faude, O.; Hagmann, S.; Roth, R.; Zahner, L. Fundamental movement skills in preschoolers: A randomized controlled trial targeting object control proficiency. *Child Care Health Dev.* **2015**, *41*, 1179–1187. [CrossRef]
32. Gallotta, M.C.; Emerenziani, G.P.; Iazzoni, S.; Iasevoli, L.; Guidetti, L.; Baldari, C. Effects of different physical education programmes on children's skill-and health-related outcomes: A pilot randomised controlled trial. *J Sport. Sci* **2017**, *35*, 1547–1555. [CrossRef]
33. Goodway, J.D.; Branta, C.F. Influence of a motor skill intervention on fundamental motor skill development of disadvantaged preschool children. *Res. Q. Exerc. Sport* **2003**, *74*, 36–46. [CrossRef]
34. Goodway, J.D.; Crowe, H.; Ward, P. Effects of motor skill instruction on fundamental motor skill development. *Adapt. Phys. Act. Q.* **2003**, *20*, 298–314. [CrossRef]
35. Hamilton, M.; Goodway, J.D.; Haubenstricker, J. Parent-Assisted Instruction in a Motor Skill Program for At-Risk Preschool Children. *Adapt. Phys. Act. Q.* **1999**, *16*, 415–426. [CrossRef]
36. Iivonen, S.; Sääkslahti, A.; Nissinen, K. The development of fundamental motor skills of four-to five-year-old preschool children and the effects of a preschool physical education curriculum. *Early Child Dev. Care* **2011**, *181*, 335–343. [CrossRef]

37. Marshall, J.D.; Bouffard, M. The Effects of Quality Daily Physical Education on Movement Competency in Obese versus Nonobese Children. *Adapt. Phys. Act. Q.* **1997**, *14*, 222. [CrossRef]
38. Palmer, K.K.; Chinn, K.M.; Robinson, L.E. The effect of the CHAMP intervention on fundamental motor skills and outdoor physical activity in preschoolers. *J. Sport Health Sci.* **2019**, *8*, 98–105. [CrossRef]
39. Roach, L.; Keats, M. Skill-Based and Planned Active Play Versus Free-Play Effects on Fundamental Movement Skills in Preschoolers. *Percept. Mot. Ski.* **2018**, *125*, 651–668. [CrossRef]
40. Robinson, L.E.; Goodway, J.D. Instructional climates in preschool children who are at-risk. Part I: Object-control skill development. *Res. Q. Exerc. Sport* **2009**, *80*, 533–542. [CrossRef]
41. Robinson, L.E.; Veldman, S.L.C.; Palmer, K.K.; Okely, A.D. A Ball Skills Intervention in Preschoolers: The CHAMP Randomized Controlled Trial. *Med. Sci. Sport. Exerc.* **2017**, *49*, 2234–2239. [CrossRef]
42. Veldman, S.L.; Palmer, K.K.; Okely, A.D.; Robinson, L.E. Promoting ball skills in preschool-age girls. *J. Sci. Med. Sport* **2017**, *20*, 50–54. [CrossRef]
43. Zask, A.; Barnett, L.M.; Rose, L.; Brooks, L.O.; Molyneux, M.; Hughes, D.; Adams, J.; Salmon, J. Three year follow-up of an early childhood intervention: Is movement skill sustained? *Int. J. Behav. Nutr. Phys. Act.* **2012**, *9*, 127. [CrossRef]
44. Berleze, A.; Valentini, N.C. Intervention for Children with Obesity and Overweight and Motor Delays from Low-Income Families: Fostering Engagement, Motor Development, Self-Perceptions, and Playtime. *Int. J. Environ. Res. Public Health* **2022**, *19*, 2545. [CrossRef] [PubMed]
45. Hashemi, M.; Khameneh, N.N.; Salehian, M.H. Effect of selected games on the development of manipulative skills in 4–6 year-old preschool girls. *Med. Dello Sport* **2015**, *68*, 49–55.
46. Jones, R.A.; Riethmuller, A.; Hesketh, K.; Trezise, J.; Batterham, M.; Okely, A.D. Promoting Fundamental Movement Skill Development and Physical Activity in Early Childhood Settings: A Cluster Randomized Controlled Trial. *Pediatr. Exerc. Sci.* **2011**, *23*, 600–615. [CrossRef] [PubMed]
47. Robinson, L.E.; Palmer, K.K.; Santiago-Rodríguez, M.E.; Myers, N.D.; Wang, L.; Pfeiffer, K.A. Protocol for a multicenter-cluster randomized clinical trial of a motor skills intervention to promote physical activity and health in children: The CHAMP afterschool program study. *BMC Public Health* **2022**, *22*, 1544. [CrossRef]
48. De Oliveira, J.A.; Rigoli, D.; Kane, R.; McLaren, S.; Goulardins, J.B.; Straker, L.M.; Dender, A.; Rooney, R.; Piek, J.P. Does 'Animal Fun' improve aiming and catching, and balance skills in young children? *Res. Dev. Disabil.* **2019**, *84*, 122–130. [CrossRef]
49. Hestbaek, L.; Vach, W.; Andersen, S.T.; Lauridsen, H.H. The Effect of a Structured Intervention to Improve Motor Skills in Preschool Children: Results of a Randomized Controlled Trial Nested in a Cohort Study of Danish Preschool Children, the MiPS Study. *Int. J. Env. Res. Public Health* **2021**, *18*, 12272. [CrossRef]
50. Alhassan, S.; Nwaokelemeh, O.; Ghazarian, M.; Roberts, J.; Mendoza, A.; Shitole, S. Effects of locomotor skill program on minority preschoolers' physical activity levels. *Pediatr. Exerc. Sci.* **2012**, *24*, 435–449. [CrossRef]
51. Engel, A.; Broderick, C.; Ward, R.; Parmenter, B. Study Protocol: The Effect of a Fundamental Motor Skills Intervention in a Preschool Setting on Fundamental Motor Skills and Physical Activity: A Cluster Randomized Controlled Trial. *Clin. Pediatr.* **2018**, *3*, 1. [CrossRef]
52. Roth, K.; Kriemler, S.; Lehmacher, W.; Ruf, K.C.; Graf, C.; Hebestreit, H. Effects of a Physical Activity Intervention in Preschool Children. *Med. Sci. Sport. Exerc.* **2015**, *47*, 2542–2551. [CrossRef]
53. Webster, E.K.; Kracht, C.L.; Newton, R.L., Jr.; Beyl, R.A.; Staiano, A.E. Intervention to Improve Preschool Children's Fundamental Motor Skills: Protocol for a Parent-Focused, Mobile App–Based Comparative Effectiveness Trial. *JMIR Res. Protoc.* **2020**, *9*, e19943. [CrossRef]
54. Staiano, A.E.; Newton, R.L.; Beyl, R.A.; Kracht, C.L.; Hendrick, C.A.; Viverito, M.; Webster, E.K. mHealth Intervention for Motor Skills: A Randomized Controlled Trial. *Pediatrics* **2022**, *149*, e2021053362. [CrossRef] [PubMed]
55. Chan, C.H.S.; Ha, A.S.C.; Ng, J.Y.Y.; Lubans, D.R. The A+FMS cluster randomized controlled trial: An assessment-based intervention on fundamental movement skills and psychosocial outcomes in primary schoolchildren. *J. Sci. Med. Sport* **2019**, *22*, 935–940. [CrossRef] [PubMed]
56. Cohen, K.E.; Morgan, P.J.; Plotnikoff, R.C.; Callister, R.; Lubans, D.R. Physical activity and skills intervention: SCORES cluster randomized controlled trial. *Med. Sci. Sport. Exerc.* **2015**, *47*, 765–774. [CrossRef] [PubMed]
57. Lander, N.; Morgan, P.J.; Salmon, J.O.; Barnett, L.M. Improving Early Adolescent Girls' Motor Skill: A Cluster Randomized Controlled Trial. *Med. Sci. Sport. Exerc.* **2017**, *49*, 2498–2505. [CrossRef] [PubMed]
58. McKenzie, T.L.; Sallis, J.F.; Broyles, S.L.; Zive, M.M.; Nader, P.R.; Berry, C.C.; Brennan, J.J. Childhood movement skills: Predictors of physical activity in Anglo American and Mexican American adolescents? *Res. Q. Exerc. Sport* **2002**, *73*, 238–244. [CrossRef] [PubMed]
59. Miller, A.; Christensen, E.M.; Eather, N.; Sproule, J.; Annis-Brown, L.; Lubans, D.R. The PLUNGE randomized controlled trial: Evaluation of a games-based physical activity professional learning program in primary school physical education. *Prev. Med.* **2015**, *74*, 1–8. [CrossRef] [PubMed]
60. Salmon, J.; Ball, K.; Hume, C.; Booth, M.; Crawford, D. Outcomes of a group-randomized trial to prevent excess weight gain, reduce screen behaviours and promote physical activity in 10-year-old children: Switch-play. *Int. J. Obes. (2005)* **2008**, *32*, 601–612. [CrossRef] [PubMed]

61. Trost, S.G.; Brookes, D.S.K. Effectiveness of a novel digital application to promote fundamental movement skills in 3- to 6-year-old children: A randomized controlled trial. *J Sport. Sci* **2021**, *39*, 453–459. [CrossRef] [PubMed]
62. van Beurden, E.; Barnett, L.M.; Zask, A.; Dietrich, U.C.; Brooks, L.O.; Beard, J. Can we skill and activate children through primary school physical education lessons? "Move it Groove it"–a collaborative health promotion intervention. *Prev. Med.* **2003**, *36*, 493–501. [CrossRef]
63. Ainsworth, B.E.; Haskell, W.L.; Herrmann, S.D.; Meckes, N.; Bassett, D.R., Jr.; Tudor-Locke, C.; Greer, J.L.; Vezina, J.; Whitt-Glover, M.C.; Leon, A.S. 2011 Compendium of Physical Activities: A second update of codes and MET values. *Med. Sci. Sport. Exerc.* **2011**, *43*, 1575–1581. [CrossRef] [PubMed]
64. World Health Organization (WHO). *WHO Guidelines on Physical Activity and Sedentary Behaviour: At A Glance*; World Health Organization: Geneva, Switzerland, 2020.
65. Norton, K.; Norton, L.; Sadgrove, D. Position statement on physical activity and exercise intensity terminology. *J. Sci. Med. Sport* **2010**, *13*, 496–502. [CrossRef] [PubMed]
66. Farooq, A.; Martin, A.; Janssen, X.; Wilson, M.G.; Gibson, A.M.; Hughes, A.; Reilly, J.J. Longitudinal changes in moderate-to-vigorous-intensity physical activity in children and adolescents: A systematic review and meta-analysis. *Obes. Rev. Off. J. Int. Assoc. Study Obes.* **2020**, *21*, e12953. [CrossRef]
67. Engel, A.C.; Broderick, C.R.; van Doorn, N.; Hardy, L.L.; Parmenter, B.J. Exploring the Relationship Between Fundamental Motor Skill Interventions and Physical Activity Levels in Children: A Systematic Review and Meta-analysis. *Sport. Med. (Auckl. N. Z.)* **2018**, *48*, 1845–1857. [CrossRef]
68. Sacko, R.S.; Utesch, T.; Bardid, F.; Stodden, D.F. The impact of motor competence on energy expenditure during object control skill performance in children and young adults. *Braz. J. Mot. Behav.* **2021**, *15*, 91–106. [CrossRef]
69. Sacko, R.S.; Nesbitt, D.; McIver, K.; Brian, A.; Bardid, F.; Stodden, D.F. Children's metabolic expenditure during object projection skill performance: New insight for activity intensity relativity. *J. Sport. Sci.* **2019**, *37*, 1755–1761. [CrossRef] [PubMed]
70. Duncan, M.J.; Dobell, A.; Noon, M.; Clark, C.C.T.; Roscoe, C.M.P.; Faghy, M.A.; Stodden, D.; Sacko, R.; Eyre, E.L.J. Calibration and Cross-Validation of Accelerometery for Estimating Movement Skills in Children Aged 8-12 Years. *Sensors* **2020**, *20*, 2776. [CrossRef] [PubMed]
71. Duncan, M.J.; Noon, M.; Lawson, C.; Hurst, J.; Eyre, E.L.J. The Effectiveness of a Primary School Based Badminton Intervention on Children's Fundamental Movement Skills. *Sports* **2020**, *8*, 11. [CrossRef] [PubMed]
72. Smith, W.; Ovens, A.; Philpot, R. Games-based movement education: Developing a sense of self, belonging, and community through games. *Phys. Educ. Sport Pedagog.* **2021**, *26*, 242–254. [CrossRef]
73. Butte, N.F.; Watson, K.B.; Ridley, K.; Zakeri, I.F.; McMurray, R.G.; Pfeiffer, K.A.; Crouter, S.E.; Herrmann, S.D.; Bassett, D.R.; Long, A.; et al. A Youth Compendium of Physical Activities: Activity Codes and Metabolic Intensities. *Med. Sci. Sport. Exerc.* **2018**, *50*, 246–256. [CrossRef]
74. Brian, A.; Taunton, S. Effectiveness of motor skill intervention varies based on implementation strategy. *Phys. Educ. Sport Pedagog.* **2018**, *23*, 222–233. [CrossRef]
75. Robinson, L.E.; Palmer, K.K.; Meehan, S.K. Dose–Response Relationship: The Effect of Motor Skill Intervention Duration on Motor Performance. *J. Mot. Learn. Dev.* **2017**, *5*, 280–290. [CrossRef]
76. Costello, K.; Warne, J. A four-week fundamental motor skill intervention improves motor skills in eight to 10-year-old Irish primary school children. *Cogent Soc. Sci.* **2020**, *6*, 1724065. [CrossRef]
77. Miller, A.; Christensen, E.; Eather, N.; Gray, S.; Sproule, J.; Keay, J.; Lubans, D. Can physical education and physical activity outcomes be developed simultaneously using a game-centered approach? *Eur. Phys. Educ. Rev.* **2016**, *22*, 113–133. [CrossRef]
78. Kirk, D.; MacPhail, A. Teaching Games for Understanding and Situated Learning: Rethinking the Bunker-Thorpe Model. *J. Teach. Phys. Educ.* **2002**, *21*, 177–192. [CrossRef]
79. O'Leary, N. Learning informally to use the 'full version' of teaching games for understanding. *Eur. Phys. Educ. Rev.* **2016**, *22*, 3–22. [CrossRef]
80. Tompsett, C.; Sanders, R.; Taylor, C.; Cobley, S. Pedagogical Approaches to and Effects of Fundamental Movement Skill Interventions on Health Outcomes: A Systematic Review. *Sport. Med. (Auckl. N. Z.)* **2017**, *47*, 1795–1819. [CrossRef] [PubMed]
81. Kelly, L.; O'Connor, S.; Harrison, A.J.; Ní Chéilleachair, N.J. Effects of an 8-week school-based intervention programme on Irish school children's fundamental movement skills. *Phys. Educ. Sport Pedagog.* **2021**, *26*, 593–612. [CrossRef]
82. Vernadakis, N.; Papastergiou, M.; Zetou, E.; Antoniou, P. The impact of an exergame-based intervention on children's fundamental motor skills. *Comput. Educ.* **2015**, *83*, 90–102. [CrossRef]
83. Bryant, E.S.; Duncan, M.J.; Birch, S.L.; James, R.S. Can Fundamental Movement Skill Mastery Be Increased via a Six Week Physical Activity Intervention to Have Positive Effects on Physical Activity and Physical Self-Perception? *Sports* **2016**, *4*, 10. [CrossRef]
84. Eyre, E.L.J.; Clark, C.C.T.; Tallis, J.; Hodson, D.; Lowton-Smith, S.; Nelson, C.; Noon, M.; Duncan, M.J. The Effects of Combined Movement and Storytelling Intervention on Motor Skills in South Asian and White Children Aged 5–6 Years Living in the United Kingdom. *Int. J. Environ. Res. Public. Health* **2020**, *17*, 3391. [CrossRef]
85. Farmer, O.; Cahill, K.; O'Brien, W. Gaelic4Girls-The Effectiveness of a 10-Week Multicomponent Community Sports-Based Physical Activity Intervention for 8 to 12-Year-Old Girls. *Int. J. Environ. Res. Public Health* **2020**, *17*, 6928. [CrossRef] [PubMed]
86. Rudd, J.R.; Woods, C.; Correia, V.; Seifert, L.; Davids, K. An ecological dynamics conceptualisation of physical 'education': Where we have been and where we could go next. *Phys. Educ. Sport Pedagog.* **2021**, *26*, 293–306. [CrossRef]

87. Newell, K.M. *Motor Development in Children: Aspects of Coordination and Control in Constraints on the Development of Coordination*; Wade, K.H., Whiting, H.T.A., Eds.; Martinus Nijhoff Publishers: Leiden, The Netherlands, 1986.
88. Davids, K.; Araújo, D.; Hristovski, R.; Passos, P.; Chow, J.Y. Ecological Dynamics and Motor Learning Design in Sport. In *Skill Acquisition in Sport: Research, Theory and Practice*, 2nd ed.; Routledge: Abingdon-on-Thames, UK, 2012; pp. 112–130.
89. Miedema, S.T.; Brian, A.; Pennell, A.; Lieberman, L.; True, L.; Webster, C.; Stodden, D. The Effects of an Integrative, Universally Designed Motor Skill Intervention for Young Children With and Without Disabilities. *Adapt. Phys. Act. Q. APAQ* **2022**, *39*, 179–196. [CrossRef] [PubMed]
90. Palmer, K.K.; Miller, A.L.; Meehan, S.K.; Robinson, L.E. The Motor skills At Playtime intervention improves children's locomotor skills: A feasibility study. *Child Care Health Dev.* **2020**, *46*, 599–606. [CrossRef] [PubMed]
91. Rink, J. *Teaching Physical Education for Learning*, 7th ed.; McGraw-Hill: New York, NY, USA, 2014.
92. Buszard, T.; Reid, M.; Masters, R.; Farrow, D. Scaling the Equipment and Play Area in Children's Sport to improve Motor Skill Acquisition: A Systematic Review. *Sport. Med. (Auckl. N. Z.)* **2016**, *46*, 829–843. [CrossRef]
93. Sweeting, T.; Rink, J.E. Effects of Direct Instruction and Environmentally Designed Instruction on the Process and Product Characteristics of a Fundamental Skill. *J. Teach. Phys. Educ.* **1999**, *18*, 216–233. [CrossRef]
94. Roberts, W.M.; Newcombe, D.J.; Davids, K. Application of a Constraints-Led Approach to pedagogy in schools: Embarking on a journey to nurture Physical Literacy in primary physical education. *Phys. Educ. Sport Pedagog.* **2019**, *24*, 162–175. [CrossRef]
95. Lorson, K.M.; Goodway, J.D. Influence of Critical Cues and Task Constraints on Overarm Throwing Performance in Elementary Age Children. *Percept. Mot. Ski.* **2007**, *105*, 753–767. [CrossRef]
96. Rudd, J.R.; Crotti, M.; Fitton-Davies, K.; O'Callaghan, L.; Bardid, F.; Utesch, T.; Roberts, S.; Boddy, L.M.; Cronin, C.J.; Knowles, Z.; et al. Skill Acquisition Methods Fostering Physical Literacy in Early-Physical Education (SAMPLE-PE): Rationale and Study Protocol for a Cluster Randomized Controlled Trial in 5–6-Year-Old Children From Deprived Areas of North West England. *Front. Psychol.* **2020**, *11*, 1228. [CrossRef]
97. Altunsöz, I.H.; Goodway, J.D. SKIPing to motor competence: The influence of project successful kinesthetic instruction for preschoolers on motor competence of disadvantaged preschoolers. *Phys. Educ. Sport Pedagog.* **2016**, *21*, 366–385. [CrossRef]
98. Fitton Davies, K.; Foweather, L.; Watson, P.M.; Bardid, F.; Roberts, S.J.; Davids, K.; O'Callaghan, L.; Crotti, M.; Rudd, J.R. Assessing the motivational climates in early physical education curricula underpinned by motor learning theory: SAMPLE-PE. *Phys. Educ. Sport Pedagog.* **2021**, *15*, 1–28. [CrossRef]
99. Deci, E.L.; Ryan, R.M. *Intrinsic Motivation and Self-Determination in Human Behavior*; Springer Science & Business Media: Berlin, Germany, 1985.
100. Ryan, R.M.; Deci, E.L. *Self-determination Theory: Basic Psychological Needs in Motivation, Development, and Wellness*; The Guilford Press: New York, NY, USA, 2017; p. xii, 756.
101. Mageau, G.A.; Vallerand, R.J. The coach–athlete relationship: A motivational model. *J. Sport. Sci.* **2003**, *21*, 883–904. [CrossRef]
102. Goodway, J.; Rudisill, M.E.; Valentini, N.C. The influence of instruction on catching: A developmental approach. *Res. Q. Exerc. Sport* **1999**, *70*, A67–A68.
103. Rudisill, M.E.; Johnson, J.L. Mastery Motivational Climates in Early Childhood Physical Education: What Have We Learned over the Years? *J. Phys. Educ. Recreat. Danc.* **2018**, *89*, 26–32. [CrossRef]
104. Valentini, N.C.; Rudisill, M.E. An Inclusive Mastery Climate Intervention and the Motor Skill Development of Children with and Without Disabilities. *Adapt. Phys. Act. Q.* **2004**, *21*, 330–347. [CrossRef]
105. Valentini, N.C.; Rudisill, M.E. Motivational Climate, Motor-Skill Development, and Perceived Competence: Two Studies of Developmentally Delayed Kindergarten Children. *J. Teach. Phys. Educ.* **2004**, *23*, 216–234. [CrossRef]
106. Oslin, J.L.; Mitchell, S.A. Form Follows Function. *J. Phys. Educ. Recreat. Danc.* **1998**, *69*, 46–49. [CrossRef]
107. Launder, A.G.; Piltz, W. *Play Practice: Engaging and Developing Skilled Players from Beginner to Elite*; Human Kinetics: Champaign, IL, USA, 2013.
108. Jarani, J.; Grøntved, A.; Muca, F.; Spahi, A.; Qefalia, D.; Ushtelenca, K.; Kasa, A.; Caporossi, D.; Gallotta, M.C. Effects of two physical education programmes on health- and skill-related physical fitness of Albanian children. *J. Sport. Sci.* **2016**, *34*, 35–46. [CrossRef]
109. Foweather, L.; McWhannell, N.; Henaghan, J.; Lees, A.; Stratton, G.; Batterham, A.M. Effect of a 9-Wk. after-School Multiskills Club on Fundamental Movement Skill Proficiency in 8- to 9-Yr.-Old Children: An Exploratory Trial. *Percept. Mot. Ski.* **2008**, *106*, 745–754. [CrossRef]
110. Mitchell, B.; McLennan, S.; Latimer, K.; Graham, D.; Gilmore, J.; Rush, E. Improvement of fundamental movement skills through support and mentorship of class room teachers. *Obes. Res. Clin. Pract.* **2013**, *7*, e230–e234. [CrossRef]

Disclaimer/Publisher's Note: The statements, opinions and data contained in all publications are solely those of the individual author(s) and contributor(s) and not of MDPI and/or the editor(s). MDPI and/or the editor(s) disclaim responsibility for any injury to people or property resulting from any ideas, methods, instructions or products referred to in the content.

Article

Predicting Psychosocial Health of Children and Adolescents with Obesity in Germany: The Underappreciated Role of Physical Fitness

Nina Eisenburger *[ID], David Friesen, Fabiola Haas, Marlen Klaudius, Lisa Schmidt, Susanne Vandeven and Christine Joisten [ID]

Department for Physical Activity in Public Health, Institute of Movement and Neurosciences, German Sport University Cologne, Am Sportpark Müngersdorf 6, 50933 Cologne, Germany; d.friesen@dshs-koeln.de (D.F.); f.haas@dshs-koeln.de (F.H.); m.klaudius@dshs-koeln.de (M.K.); ernaehrungschmidt@gmail.com (L.S.); canollo@web.de (S.V.); c.joisten@dshs-koeln.de (C.J.)
* Correspondence: ninaeisen@gmail.com

Abstract: *Background*: The aim of this study was to analyze the inhibitory and promotive factors of psychosocial health in the context of childhood obesity, incorporating physical fitness as an additional, potentially relevant predictor. *Methods*: The sample comprised cross-sectional data of 241 children and adolescents with obesity and overweight from the German Children's Health InterventionaL TriaL III program (12.5 ± 2.1 years; 51.9% girls). Demographics and lifestyle patterns were assessed via parent reports. Anthropometric data and physical fitness in relation to body weight (W/kg) were measured. Children and adolescents completed standardized questionnaires (GW-LQ-KJ, FSK-K) to assess health-related quality of life (HRQOL) and five dimensions of self-concept (scholastic, social, physical, behavioral, and self-worth). *Results*: Multiple linear regression analysis showed that HRQOL was significantly related to relative physical fitness (W/kg; $\beta = 0.216$, $p = 0.011$) as were scholastic ($\beta = 0.228$, $p = 0.008$) and social self-concept ($\beta = 0.197$, $p = 0.023$). Increasing body mass index (BMI) Z-scores, age, physical activity (hours/day), low parental educational levels, and/or migration background were negatively associated with three subdomains of self-concept (physical, behavioral, self-worth; all $p < 0.05$). *Conclusion*: The results emphasize BMI Z-scores, age, physical activity, migration background, and parents' educational level as relevant predictors of psychosocial health in the context of childhood obesity. Additionally, this study adds physical fitness as a key determinant of HRQOL and self-concept. To enable the development of more effective weight management, therapeutic strategies should therefore consider addressing these aspects and improving physical fitness in particular not only for weight loss but also to strengthen psychosocial health.

Keywords: childhood obesity; health-related quality of life; self-concept; self-perception; physical fitness; psychosocial health

1. Introduction

Childhood and adolescent obesity is a globally recognized public-health concern [1]. In addition to physical comorbidities, such as the increased risk of developing metabolic syndrome, type 2 diabetes, cardiovascular diseases, orthopedic complications, or increased rates of cancer, among others, a growing body of research has documented the psychosocial burden in affected children and adolescents [2]. Psychosocial impairments, such as a poor self-esteem, a negative self-perception or self-concept, can result in a vicious circle of weight gain [3–6]. Besides this, a negative self-concept has been found to mediate the inverse relationship between high body mass index (BMI) and health-related quality of life (HRQOL) [7], a multidimensional construct aggregating individuals' physical and psychological health, emotional state, and social functioning [8]. Already in 2014, Buttitta et al. concluded in a review of HRQOL in children and adolescents with obesity, that scientific findings regarding the obesity-related impairment in all dimensions of HRQOL of children and youth were mostly congruent [9].

Consequently, in addition to weight reduction/stagnation and lifestyle counseling, improving mental health, including HRQOL and self-concept, plays a central role in weight management programs [4,10]. To target therapeutic strategies accordingly, the identification of potential inhibitory and promotive obesity-relevant factors for psychosocial health has become a research priority [8–11]. In this regard, evidence suggests that sex, age, socioeconomic status, and migration background not only affect the prevalence of obesity in children and adolescents but also their HRQOL and self-concept [8,12–14]. Further key determinants of both weight status and psychosocial health are lifestyle patterns, such as level of physical inactivity or sedentary behavior, which is characterized by energy expenditure ≤ 1.5 metabolic equivalents and predominantly involves prolonged sitting and/or laying (e.g., screen-viewing activities, passive transportation) [15,16]. An objective measure of physical activity levels and sedentary behavior is physical fitness [15]. Thus, prior research indicates that it is important to also include physical fitness in the analysis of psychosocial health [17]. Studies with non-overweight children have yielded promising results in terms of psychosocial improvements associated with increased fitness [18–20]. Knowing that physical fitness is a mediator in the relationship between childhood and adolescent obesity and self-concept [21,22] and HRQOL [15,23,24], supports the need to further investigate its predictive potential for the psychosocial health of affected children and adolescents. Therefore, the aim of this cross-sectional analysis was to examine determinants of weight-specific HRQOL and subdomains of self-concept in the context of obesity in childhood and adolescence, while considering physical fitness as an additional potentially relevant predictor. Given the vicious cycle between mental health and weight gain, identifying the factors underlying this dynamic may contribute to the development of more effective weight management strategies and recommendations for improved care.

2. Materials and Methods

2.1. Sample Description

The data for this cross-sectional analysis came from the Children's Health InterventionaL TriaL (CHILT) III. CHILT III is an 11-month, family-based, multi-component program for obesity prevention and therapy, registered in the German Clinical Trials Register under ID DRKS00026785. It was launched in 2003 at the German Sport University, Cologne. The target groups were children and adolescents aged 8–16 years with obesity or overweight if displaying cardiovascular risk factors, such as arterial hypertension or hyperlipoproteinemia [25].

The minimum criteria for inclusion in this study were participation in the CHILT III program between 2003 and 2020; complete height, weight, age, and body fat percentage data at baseline; and fully completed HRQOL and/or self-concept questionnaires. After excluding extreme values, a final data set of 241 children and adolescents (51.9% girls) and their parents (n = 459: 236 mothers, 223 fathers) remained (see Figure 1).

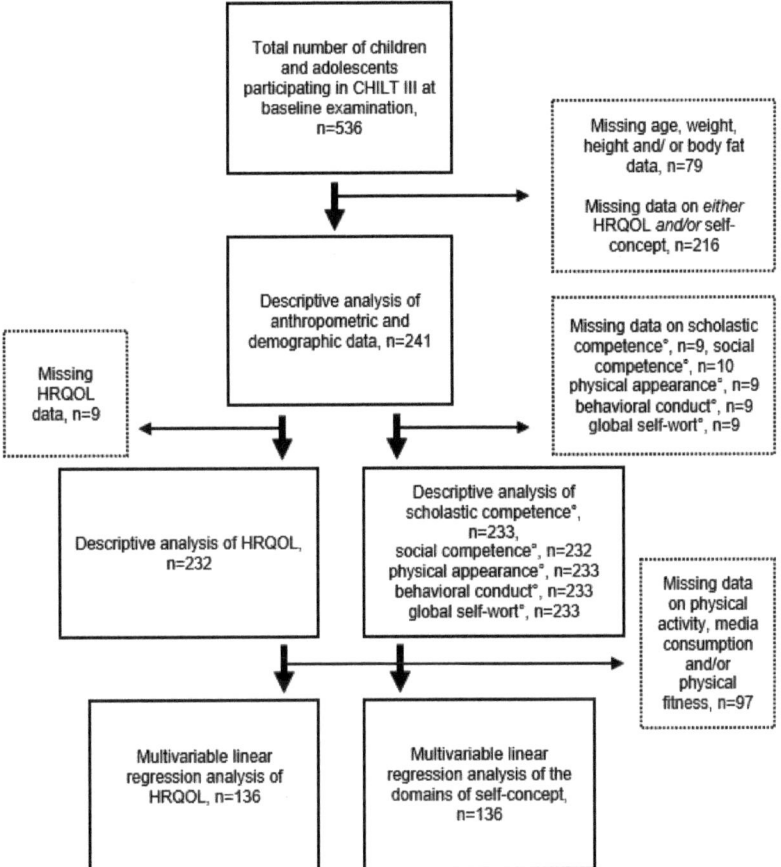

Figure 1. Flow Chart of Number of Participants in the Study; HRQOL, Health-Related Quality of Life; CHILT, Children's Health InterventionaL Trial; ° subdomains of self-concept; vertical arrows, stepwise procedure of the study; horizontal arrows, stepwise exclusion criteria.

2.2. Anthropometric Data

Standard calibrated scales and stadiometers were used to measure and weigh each child. Height and weight were measured with the child barefoot. Weight included clothing, such as light sportswear. BMI (weight (kg)/height^2 (m^2)) was assessed and sex- and age-specific weight-for-height BMI Z-scores were calculated according to the German percentile graphs of Kromeyer-Hauschild et al. [26] using the following equation:

$$(BMI/M(t))L(t)-1)/(L(t) \times S(t)),$$

where M(t), L(t) and S(t) reflect age- and gender-specific parameters of the child. Children were then categorized as overweight (>90th percentile and ≤97th percentile) or obese (>97th percentile). Body composition was determined by measuring skin-fold thickness to the nearest 0.2 mm in triplicate at the triceps (tric) and subscapula (subs) with a body fat caliper (Harpender Skinfold Caliper HSK-BI, British Indicators, West Sussex, England) following a standardized protocol [27]. The mean of the three measures was considered the final value. When tric+subsc was >35 mm (n = 230) the following sex- and age-specific equations by Slaughter (1988) [28] were used to compute the body fat percentage, as these had also been used during previous studies on similar populations [29]:

$$\text{Girls, \%fat} = 0.546 \times (\text{sum of tric and subs}) + 9.7$$

$$\text{Boys, \%fat} = 0.783 \times (\text{sum of tric and subs}) - 1.7$$

When tric + subsc was ≤35 mm ($n = 11$), Slaughter's fat-percentage equations were used according to Rodrígez et al. 2005 [30].

2.3. Demographics and Lifestyle Patterns

At the beginning of the program, parents completed standardized questionnaires assessing the demographics and lifestyle patterns of both themselves and their children [25]. Demographic variables selected for inclusion in the study were children's sex, age, migration background, and parent's educational background. Time spent in physical activity and on media consumption, which is often used to reflect sedentary behavior, were included to examine lifestyle patterns [31]. Parents' educational background was dichotomized into two categories: "high", when both parents had completed secondary school ("Abitur/Fachabitur"), and "low", when neither parent had an educational degree, a different one other than secondary school, or only one parent had completed secondary school [32]. The migration background of the child was treated as a dichotomous variable assessed by the language spoken at home (German/non-German) [33].

Regarding the child's level of physical activity, parents were asked if and for how many minutes per week their child was physically active apart from time spent at school. Media consumption was assessed by asking parents to provide the total number of minutes spent by their child per day watching TV, playing a game console, using the computer/Internet, listening to music, and/or using their mobile phone. For this study, media consumption and physical activity were summed and transformed into continuous variables measured in hours per day.

2.4. Physical Fitness

Physical fitness was measured in peak mechanical power (PMP (W)) and peak oxygen consumption (VO_2max (mL/min), data not shown) using a bicycle ergometer (Ergoline Ergometrics 900) on which the children and adolescents exercised until exhaustion. Prior to testing, participants were familiarized with the test procedure and the bicycle ergometer was adjusted individually (height of seat and handlebar position). Testing began with a workload of 25 W and increased by 25 W every 2 min [25]. Throughout the testing session, the participant was verbally encouraged by staff to achieve maximal effort. Due to the comparably larger sample size, peak mechanical power ($n = 238$) was used as a proxy for physical fitness instead of VO_2max ($n = 228$). Test results were related to body weight as W/kg.

2.5. Health-Related Quality of Life

The weight-specific quality-of-life questionnaire for children and adolescents with overweight and obesity ("Fragebogen zur gewichtsbezogenen Lebensqualität für übergewichtige und adipöse Kinder und Jugendliche" (GW-LQ-KJ)) by Warschburger and Fromme (2004) [34] is a self-assessment tool specifically designed to assess the HRQOL of children and adolescents with obesity and overweight. In this study, we used version B of the GW-LQ-KJ which consists of 11 items (e.g., "Because of my weight, I was reluctant to go to the public swimming pool"). The children and adolescents were asked to evaluate the statements by estimating the frequency of occurrence in the last 2 weeks on a five-point Likert scale (ranging from "always" to "never"). The results were recoded so that high values indicated high HRQOL. A summed score was calculated and adjusted to be within a range of 0–100. Dividing the mean individual values by the number of completed questionnaires provided the relative mean.

For reliability analysis, Cronbach's α was calculated. The internal consistency of the HRQOL score of the present sample (n = 226) was satisfying, with α = 0.82.

2.6. Self-Concept

The FSK-K ("Fragebogen zur Erfassung von Selbst—und Kompetenzeinschätzungen bei Kindern") is a German version of Harter's Self-Perception Profile for Children [35] and has been used in previous studies in the context of childhood obesity [36]. It is a 30-item self-report to assess the multidimensional self-concept of children. Each item is scored on a scale of 1–4 in an alternative-statement format, with a positive statement on one side (e.g., "I want to stay the way I am") and a negative statement on the other side (e.g., "I would like to be someone else"). The child decided which side of the description was "sort of true" or "really true" for him/her.

The FSK-K integrates five scales for assessing perceived domain-specific self-concept: scholastic competence, social competence, physical appearance, behavioral conduct, and global self-worth. After recoding, the highest domain-specific competence was defined as a mean score of 100. Internal consistency of the domains of self-concept was α = 0.79 for scholastic competence (n = 231), α = 0.82 for social competence (n = 223), α = 0.76 for physical appearance (n = 215), α = 0.77 for behavioral conduct (n = 228), and α = 0.71 for global self-worth (n = 215).

2.7. Statistical Analysis

Descriptive statistics for anthropometric data, demographics, lifestyle patterns, and physical fitness are provided. Continuous variables are shown as means ± standard deviation (SD), minimum (min), and maximum (max), and categorical variables as frequencies and percentages. The association between the selected determinants, HRQOL, and the dimensions of self-concept were explored by backward stepwise multiple linear regression analysis, with p > 0.05 designating the removal of variables. The dependent variables were the HRQOL score and the score of each of the five domains of self-concept. One model was used for each domain. Predictors included in the baseline model were age, sex, BMI Z-score, body fat (%), physical fitness (W/kg), physical activity (hours per day), media consumption (hours per day), migration background (German (yes/no)), and parental educational background (High (yes/no)). A squared term for age was also included as a covariate given that the relationship between HRQOL/(physical) self-concept and age is non-linear [37]. Significance was set at p < 0.05. All analyses were performed using IBM SPSS Statistics Version 27.0.

3. Results

The average BMI Z-score of the sample was 2.45 ± 0.46, with 212 participants classified as obese (88%) and 29 (12%) considered overweight. For a more detailed description of the sample characteristics, see Table 1.

For reference, the six baseline multiple linear regression models explaining HRQOL and the dimensions of self-concept (scholastic competence, social competence, physical appearance, behavioral conduct, and global self-worth) adjusting for all independent variables are shown in Table S1 in the supplementary material. Table 2 summarizes the resulting final models after the removal of all insignificant variables using backward stepwise multiple regression analysis.

Table 1. Descriptive Sample Characteristics.

Variable		n (%)	Mean (SD)	Min	Max
Sex	Female	125 (51.9%)			
	Male	116 (48.1%)			
Percentile	Obese	212 (88.0%)			
	Overweight	29 (12.0%)			
Migration Background	Yes/German	209 (86.7%)			
	No/Non-German	32 (13.3%)			
Parent's Educational Degree [1]	High	57 (23.7%)			
	Low	184 (76.3%)			
Physical Variables	Age (years)	241	12.5 (2.07)	7.3	17.1
	Height (m)	241	1.58 (0.11)	1.23	1.89
	Weight (kg)	241	76.7 (19.9)	37.4	148.4
	BMI (kg/m^2)	241	30.9 (4.8)	20.5	56.6
	BMI Z-score	241	2.45 (0.46)	1.43	3.80
	Body fat (%)	241	42.1 (9.0)	26.1	83.2
	Relative Physical fitness (W/kg)	241	1.7 (0.4)	0.9	3.3
Lifestyle Variables	Physical Activity (hours/day)	162	0.7 (0.6)	0	2.9
	Media Consumption (hours/day)	190	2.5 (1.8)	0	8.5
Psychosocial Variables	HRQOL	232	77.7 (14.3)	29.1	100.0
	Scholastic Competence °	233	75.6 (16.7)	25.0	100.0
	Social Competence °	232	76.0 (18.6)	25.0	100.0
	Physical Appearance °	233	54.1 (15.6)	25.0	100.0
	Behavioral Conduct °	232	74.1 (16.4)	29.2	100.0
	Global Self-Worth °	233	72.3 (16.3)	25.0	100.0

[1] High, both parents have completed secondary school; Low, only one parent/neither mother nor father have completed secondary school; HRQOL, Health-Related Quality of Life; n, number of participants; SD, Standard Deviation; Min, Minimum; Max, Maximum; ° Subdomains of Self-Concept; Psychosocial variables are based on scores ranging from 0 (lowest) to 100 (highest).

Table 2. Final Models from Backard Stepwise Multivariable Linear Regression Analysis.

Model	Final Predictor/s *	β (s.e.)	p-Value of Coefficient	R^2	Adj. R^2 (p-Value of Final Model)
HRQOL (n = 136)	Relative Physical fitness (W/kg)	0.216 (3.128)	0.011	0.047	0.040 (0.011)
Scholastic Competence ° (n = 136)	Relative Physical fitness (W/kg)	0.228 (3.289)	0.008	0.052	0.045 (0.008)
Social Competence ° (n = 136)	Relative Physical fitness (W/kg)	0.197 (3.786)	0.023	0.038	0.031 (0.023)
Physical Appearance ° (n = 136)	Age (years)	−0.276 (0.641)	0.001	0.190	0.171 (<0.001)
	BMI Z-score	−0.334 (2.726)	<0.001		
	Physical Activity (hours/week)	−0.164 (0.301)	0.040		
Behavioral Conduct ° (n = 136)	High Parental Educational Level [a]	0.204 (2.942)	0.016	0.071	0.057 (0.008)
	German/No Migration Background [b]	0.169 (4.442)	0.045		
Global Self-Worth ° (n = 136)	Age (years)	−0.186 (0.719)	0.028	0.077	0.063 (0.005)
	High Parental Educational Level [a]	0.224 (3.005)	0.008		

* After removal of all insignificant variables. Significance was set at p < 0.05; HRQOL, Health-Related Quality of Life; β, Standardized Coeffecient Beta; s.e., Standard Error; Adj, Adjusted; ° Subdomain of Self-Concept; Reference Categories: [a] low parental educational level (only one parent/neither mother nor father have completed secondary school/Abitur), [b] Non-German.

After all other factors had been accounted for in the final models explaining HRQOL, scholastic competence, and social competence, relative physical fitness remained the only significant predictor. Participants with high levels of relative physical fitness (W/kg) showed higher HRQOL ($\beta = 0.216$, $p = 0.011$; Adj. $R^2 = 0.040$, $p = 0.011$) and perceived scholastic ($\beta = 0.228$, $p = 0.008$; Adj. $R^2 = 0.045$, $p = 0.008$) and social competence ($\beta = 0.197$, $p = 0.023$; Adj. $R^2 = 0.031$, $p = 0.023$). Relative physical fitness explained approximately 3.1–4.75% of total variability in each of these first three models.

We found BMI Z-score and physical activity to be significantly associated with only one of the dependent variables investigated. More precisely, BMI Z-score ($\beta = -0.334$, $p < 0.001$) and self-reported physical activity ($\beta = -0.164$, $p = 0.040$) significantly predicted physical appearance. Jointly with age ($\beta = -0.276$, $p = 0.001$), the three predictors accounted for approximately 17% of the total variability in the final physical appearance model (Adj. $R^2 = 0.171$, $p < 0.001$).

In the fifth model explaining behavioral conduct, high parental educational levels ($\beta = 0.204$, $p = 0.016$) and migration background (No/German; $\beta = 0.169$, $p = 0.045$) showed a positive association to this subdomain of self-concept and explained a significant proportion of variance (Adj. $R^2 = 0.057$, $p = 0.008$). Higher parental education was also positively associated with global self-worth ($\beta = 0.224$, $p = 0.008$), and together with age ($\beta = -0.186$, $p = 0.028$) accounted for approximately 6% of total variability in the final global self-worth model (Adj. $R^2 = 0.063$, $p = 0.005$).

4. Discussion

Childhood and adolescent obesity impacts various dimensions of psychosocial health, including health-related quality of life (HRQOL) and personal self-concept [3]. Thus, a comprehensive understanding of the dynamics and possible influencing factors between weight and mental health is a key step toward improving weight management programs. In this context, our results confirmed previous findings on the negative association between increasing age, high BMI Z-scores, migration background, low parental education, and psychosocial health [12,13,32]. In addition, the results revealed that relative physical fitness was a major predictor of HRQOL, and of the social and scholastic self-concept of children and adolescents with overweight and obesity.

4.1. Anthropometric and Demographic Determinants of Psychosocial Health of Children and Adolescents with Obesity

Consistently with the literature, we identified the physical self-concept to be most affected by high BMI Z-scores [9]. The higher the Z-score, the more dissatisfied participants were with their physical appearance in our sample. Many studies have concluded that girls with overweight or obesity are especially susceptible to body dissatisfaction [5]; however, other studies have not yielded results containing differences between the sexes [2]. While we did not find differences related to sex between any dimension of self-concept or HRQOL, we did find age to be a significant predictor in our study. These results are not surprising when considered in the context of the effects of puberty. Pubescent individuals are particularly vulnerable to low self-esteem and negative body image [5,37]. Our findings thus support those of earlier research, which suggested that addressing body image should be included as a highly relevant issue in obesity-treatment agendas to improve patients' self-esteem, particularly in adolescence [10].

Migration background and low socioeconomic status have been identified as key determinants of obesity and are also associated with determinants of psychosocial health [12,32]. Several researchers have recommended interventions at an early stage in childhood to address children who—due to their familial background—are particularly at risk of developing obesity and psychosocial impairments [4]. In line with this, our findings indicate that children and adolescents with obesity and overweight who have a migration background or whose parents had comparatively low education assessed their behavioral conduct and global self-worth as worse than their German counterparts. Considering the observed age effect in our study, the need for early action becomes especially evident. Besides this, the strong influence of familial background and behavior-specific family variables (e.g., lifestyle patterns and nutrition) in the context of both obesity and the subdomains of self-concept underpin the need for parental involvement in intervention strategies [13].

4.2. Associations between Physical Fitness, Physical Activity, and Psychosocial Health of Children and Adolescents with Obesity

In weight management programs, most participating families focus on weight loss as the key determinant of program success [24]. However, when considering the underlying causal relationships between weight gain, active lifestyle, and psychosocial health, the latter should be regarded as equally important outcome measures [9,34,35]. In this regard, our results demonstrate that physical fitness may be an important contributor to achieving program goals beyond mere weight loss. While its positive effect on physical health and weight management is undisputed, this study, on the one hand, identifies the importance of physical fitness for the personal self-concept and, on the other hand, reemphasizes the relevance of physical fitness for HRQOL in childhood [20], adolescence [19,24], and in the context of obesity [23]. Because it is associated with both physical and psychosocial dimensions [18,21,22], our results hence suggest that a focus on improving fitness could lead to more sustainable therapy outcomes than short-term weight loss [17].

It is important to note that objectively measured fitness played a greater role for the selected markers of psychosocial health than subjectively measured physical activity or self-reported media consumption in our sample. In comparison to physical fitness, self-reported media consumption was not a significant predictor in the present analysis. Physical activity was negatively associated solely with perceived physical appearance. The observed negative relationship between physical activity and appearance was not consistent with previous studies [18,22] which may be explained by the fact that engaging in physical activity may reveal fundamental movement-skill difficulties compared to non-overweight peers, leading to an impairment of physical self-concept [14]. Therefore, our results indicate that—in addition to physical fitness improvements—motor skill development in children and adolescents with overweight and obesity may be critical in intervention strategies [14].

4.3. Strengths and Limitations

A major strength of our study is that physical fitness, body height, weight, and fat percentage were objectively measured by trained staff according to standardized methods. In addition to the large sample and the number of determinants analyzed, further strength is the utilization of a weight-specific HRQOL-measurement tool that has been shown to have good psychometric properties.

The primary limitation of our study is the cross-sectional design, which does not allow any conclusions to be drawn regarding the causal direction of the relationship between the observed variables. Furthermore, several obesity-relevant factors were not included due to incomplete data such as dietary habits, type of school, single parenting, and parents' BMI. The inclusion of these limited data would have resulted in too great a sample size restriction. As such, there may be additional factors that could confound the association between the independent variables. Selection bias, information bias, and social desirability bias, that is, in self-reports on physical activity and media consumption, are further limitations. As a treatment-seeking population, the participants potentially shared characteristics, such as motivation, that distinguished them from other groups. Besides this, as some data were self-reported, the study is not free from information bias.

5. Conclusions

This study adds to the existing body of research by identifying inhibitory and promotive factors for HRQOL and self-concept in the context of childhood obesity, with implications for therapy and care. The results identify physical fitness as a key predictor of weight-specific HRQOL and subdomains of self-concept of children and adolescents with obesity. These findings suggest that improvements in physical fitness may hold even more promise for positive psychosocial health outcomes in weight management programs than weight loss or participation in physical activity alone. In addition, addressing at-risk children from lower socioeconomic or migration backgrounds at an early stage might be crucial not only to prevent obesity but also to improve mental health. Our findings furthermore indicate that strategies to promote body satisfaction and motor abilities could be critical especially in adolescence to improve the physical self-concept of adolescents with overweight and obesity but future longitudinal studies are required to investigate the robustness and causality of our findings.

Supplementary Materials: The following materials are available online at https://www.mdpi.com/article/10.3390/ijerph182111188/s1, Table S1: Baseline Multivariable Linear Regression Models.

Author Contributions: N.E. analyzed the data and wrote the manuscript. C.J. supervised the analysis, provided methodological guidance, and revised the manuscript. D.F., M.K. and F.H. (who work as sports scientists in the program) and L.S. and S.V. (who are responsible for the areas of nutrition and psychology in the program) conducted the medical tests and gathered the data. C.J. is the leader of the CHILT III program and created the study design. All authors have read and agreed to the published version of the manuscript.

Funding: This research did not receive any financial support from funding agencies in the public, commercial, or not-for-profit sectors.

Institutional Review Board Statement: The study was conducted according to the guidelines of the Declaration of Helsinki, and approved by the Ethics Committee Ethics of the German Sport University Cologne for the ethic request with the number 107/2014 which was updated on 17 May 2021 ("Children's Health InterventionaL Trial III—ein ambulantes, multimodales, familienbasiertes Schulungsprorgamm zur Therapie von Ubergewicht und Adipositas im Kindes- und Jugendalter").

Informed Consent Statement: Informed consent was obtained from the participants' parents.

Data Availability Statement: The data used and analyzed during the current study involve sensitive patient information and indirect identifiers. As a result, the datasets are available from the corresponding author only on reasonable request.

Acknowledgments: We gratefully acknowledge all CHILT III participants and their parents. We would also like to thank Hidayet Oruc and Jonas Juretzko for their support during the program and Selina Müller for her help in researching and calculating the HROQL scores.

Conflicts of Interest: The authors declare no conflict of interest.

References

1. Di Cesare, M.; Sorić, M.; Bovet, P.; Miranda, J.J.; Bhutta, Z.; Stevens, G.A.; Laxmaiah, A.; Kengne, A.-P.; Bentham, J. The epidemiological burden of obesity in childhood: A worldwide epidemic requiring urgent action. *BMC Med.* **2019**, *17*, 212. [CrossRef]
2. Rankin, J.; Matthews, L.; Cobley, S.; Han, A.; Sanders, R.; Wiltshire, H.D.; Baker, J.S. Psychological consequences of childhood obesity: Psychiatric comorbidity and prevention. *Adolesc. Health Med. Ther.* **2016**, *7*, 125–146. [CrossRef] [PubMed]
3. Buttitta, M.; Rousseau, A.; Guerrien, A. A New Understanding of Quality of Life in Children and Adolescents with Obesity: Contribution of the Self-determination Theory. *Curr. Obes. Rep.* **2017**, *6*, 432–437. [CrossRef]
4. Fonvig, C.E.; Hamann, S.A.; Nielsen, T.R.H.; Johansen, M.Ø.; Grønbæk, H.N.; Mollerup, P.M.; Holm, J.-C. Subjective evaluation of psychosocial well-being in children and youths with overweight or obesity: The impact of multidisciplinary obesity treatment. *Qual. Life Res.* **2017**, *26*, 3279–3288. [CrossRef]
5. Sánchez-Miguel, P.A.; González, J.J.P.; Sánchez-Oliva, D.; Alonso, D.A.; Leo, F.M. The importance of body satisfaction to physical self-concept and body mass index in Spanish adolescents. *Int. J. Psychol.* **2019**, *54*, 521–529. [CrossRef]
6. Sánchez-Miguel, P.A.; León-Guereño, P.; Tapia-Serrano, M.A.; Hortigüela-Alcalá, D.; López-Gajardo, M.A.; Vaquero-Solís, M. The Mediating Role of the Self-Concept between the Relationship of the Body Satisfaction and the Intention to Be Physically Active in Primary School Students. *Front. Public Health* **2020**, *8*, 113. [CrossRef]
7. Wallander, J.L.; Taylor, W.C.; Grunbaum, J.A.; Franklin, F.A.; Harrison, G.G.; Kelder, S.H.; Schuster, M.A. Weight status, quality of life, and self-concept in African American, Hispanic, and white fifth-grade children. *Obesity* **2009**, *17*, 1363–1368. [CrossRef]
8. Meixner, L.; Cohrdes, C.; Schienkiewitz, A.; Mensink, G.B.M. Health-related quality of life in children and adolescents with overweight and obesity: Results from the German KIGGS survey. *BMC Public Health* **2020**, *20*, 1722. [CrossRef]
9. Buttitta, M.; Iliescu, C.; Rousseau, A.; Guerrien, A. Quality of life in overweight and obese children and adolescents: A literature review. *Qual. Life Res.* **2014**, *23*, 1117–1139. [CrossRef] [PubMed]

10. Gow, M.L.; Tee, M.S.Y.; Garnett, S.P.; Baur, L.A.; Aldwell, K.; Thomas, S.; Lister, N.B.; Paxton, S.J.; Jebeile, H. Pediatric obesity treatment, self-esteem, and body image: A systematic review with meta-analysis. *Pediatr. Obes.* **2020**, *15*, e12600. [CrossRef] [PubMed]
11. Perez-Sousa, M.A.; Olivares, P.R.; Garcia-Hermoso, A.; Gusi, N. Does anthropometric and fitness parameters mediate the effect of exercise on the HRQoL of overweight and obese children/adolescents? *Qual. Life Res.* **2018**, *27*, 2305–2312. [CrossRef]
12. Reiss, F.; Meyrose, A.-K.; Otto, C.; Lampert, T.; Klasen, F.; Ravens-Sieberer, U. Socioeconomic status, stressful life situations and mental health problems in children and adolescents: Results of the German BELLA cohort-study. *PLoS ONE* **2019**, *14*, e0213700. [CrossRef]
13. Cislak, A.; Safron, M.; Pratt, M.; Gaspar, T.; Luszczynska, A. Family-related predictors of body weight and weight-related behaviours among children and adolescents: A systematic umbrella review. *Child Care Health Dev.* **2012**, *38*, 321–331. [CrossRef]
14. Poulsen, A.A.; Desha, L.; Ziviani, J.; Griffiths, L.; Heaslop, A.; Khan, A.; Leong, G.M. Fundamental movement skills and self-concept of children who are overweight. *Int. J. Pediatr. Obes.* **2011**, *6*, e464–e471. [CrossRef]
15. Eddolls, W.T.B.; McNarry, M.A.; Lester, L.; Winn, C.O.N.; Stratton, G.; Mackintosh, K.A. The association between physical activity, fitness and body mass index on mental well-being and quality of life in adolescents. *Qual. Life Res.* **2018**, *27*, 2313–2320. [CrossRef] [PubMed]
16. Barnett, T.A.; Contreras, G.; Ghenadenik, A.E.; Zawaly, K.; van Hulst, A.; Mathieu, M.-È.; Henderson, M. Identifying risk profiles for excess sedentary behaviour in youth using individual, family and neighbourhood characteristics. *Prev. Med. Rep.* **2021**, *24*, 101535. [CrossRef]
17. Rodriguez-Ayllon, M.; Cadenas-Sanchez, C.; Esteban-Cornejo, I.; Migueles, J.H.; Mora-Gonzalez, J.; Henriksson, P.; Martín-Matillas, M.; Mena-Molina, A.; Molina-García, P.; Estévez-López, F.; et al. Physical fitness and psychological health in overweight/obese children: A cross-sectional study from the ActiveBrains project. *J. Sci. Med. Sport* **2018**, *21*, 179–184. [CrossRef]
18. Vedul-Kjelsås, V.; Sigmundsson, H.; Stensdotter, A.-K.; Haga, M. The relationship between motor competence, physical fitness and self-perception in children. *Child Care Health Dev.* **2012**, *38*, 394–402. [CrossRef]
19. Evaristo, O.S.; Moreira, C.; Lopes, L.; Abreu, S.; Agostinis-Sobrinho, C.; Oliveira-Santos, J.; Oliveira, A.; Mota, J.; Santos, R. Cardiorespiratory fitness and health-related quality of life in adolescents: A longitudinal analysis from the LabMed Physical Activity Study. *Am. J. Hum. Biol.* **2019**, *31*, e23304. [CrossRef]
20. Bermejo-Cantarero, A.; Álvarez-Bueno, C.; Martínez-Vizcaino, V.; Redondo-Tébar, A.; Pozuelo-Carrascosa, D.P.; Sánchez-López, M. Relationship between both cardiorespiratory and muscular fitness and health-related quality of life in children and adolescents: A systematic review and meta-analysis of observational studies. *Health Qual. Life Outcomes* **2021**, *19*, 127. [CrossRef]
21. Mitchell, N.G.; Moore, J.B.; Bibeau, W.S.; Rudasill, K.M. Cardiovascular fitness moderates the relations between estimates of obesity and physical self-perceptions in rural elementary school students. *J. Phys. Act. Health* **2012**, *9*, 288–294. [CrossRef]
22. Babic, M.J.; Morgan, P.J.; Plotnikoff, R.C.; Lonsdale, C.; White, R.L.; Lubans, D.R. Physical activity and physical self-concept in youth: Systematic review and meta-analysis. *Sports Med.* **2014**, *44*, 1589–1601. [CrossRef]
23. Perez-Sousa, M.A.; Olivares, P.R.; Escobar-Alvarez, J.A.; Parraça, J.A.; Gusi, N. Fitness as mediator between weight status and dimensions of health-related quality of life. *Health Qual. Life Outcomes* **2018**, *16*, 155. [CrossRef]
24. Marques, A.; Mota, J.; Gaspar, T.; de Matos, M.G. Associations between self-reported fitness and self-rated health, life-satisfaction and health-related quality of life among adolescents. *J. Exerc. Sci. Fit.* **2017**, *15*, 8–11. [CrossRef]
25. Lier, L.M.; Breuer, C.; Ferrari, N.; Friesen, D.; Maisonave, F.; Schmidt, N.; Graf, C. Individual Physical Activity Behaviour and Group Composition as Determinants of the Effectiveness of a Childhood Obesity Intervention Program. *Obes. Facts* **2021**, *14*, 100–107. [CrossRef]
26. Kromeyer-Hauschild, K.; Wabitsch, M.; Kunze, D.; Geller, F.; Geiß, H.C.; Hesse, V.; von Hippel, A.; Jaeger, U.; Johnsen, D.; Korte, W.; et al. Perzentile für den Body-mass-Index für das Kindes- und Jugendalter unter Heranziehung verschiedener deutscher Stichproben. *Mon. Kinderheilkd.* **2001**, *149*, 807–818. [CrossRef]
27. Lohman, T.G.; Roche, A.F.; Martorell, R. *Anthropometric Standardization Reference Manual*; Human Kinetics Books: Champaign, IL, USA, 1988; ISBN 9780873221214.
28. Slaughter, M.H.; Lohman, T.G.; Boileau, R.; Horswill, C.A.; Stillman, R.J.; Van Loan, M.D.; Bemben, D.A. Skinfold equations for estimation of body fatness in children and youth. *Hum. Biol.* **1988**, *60*, 709–723.
29. Chan, D.F.Y.; Li, A.M.; So, H.K.; Yin, J.; Nelson, E.A.S. New Skinfold-thickness Equation for Predicting Percentage Body Fat in Chinese Obese Children. *Hong Kong J. Paediatr.* **2008**, *14*, 96–102.
30. Rodríguez, G.; Moreno, L.A.; Blay, M.G.; Blay, V.A.; Fleta, J.; Sarría, A.; Bueno, M. Body fat measurement in adolescents: Comparison of skinfold thickness equations with dual-energy X-ray absorptiometry. *Eur. J. Clin. Nutr.* **2005**, *59*, 1158–1166. [CrossRef]
31. Wu, X.Y.; Han, L.H.; Zhang, J.H.; Luo, S.; Hu, J.W.; Sun, K. The influence of physical activity, sedentary behavior on health-related quality of life among the general population of children and adolescents: A systematic review. *PLoS ONE* **2017**, *12*, e0187668. [CrossRef]
32. Plachta-Danielzik, S.; Müller, M.J. Socio-Economic Aspects. In *Metabolic Syndrome and Obesity in Childhood and Adolescence*; Kiess, W., Wabitsch, M., Maffeis, C., Sharma, A.M., Eds.; S. KARGER AG: Basel, Switzerland, 2015; pp. 68–74. ISBN 978-3-318-02798-3.
33. Bau, A.-M.; Sannemann, J.; Ernert, A.; Babitsch, B. Einflussfaktoren auf die gesundheitsbezogene Lebensqualität von 10- bis 15-jährigen Mädchen in Berlin. *Gesundheitswesen* **2011**, *73*, 273–279. [CrossRef] [PubMed]

34. Warschburger, P.; Fromme, C.; Petermann, F. Konzeption und Analyse eines gewichtsspezifischen Lebensqualitätsfragebogens für übergewichtige und adipöse Kinder und Jugendliche (GW-LQ-KJ). *Z. Klin. Psychol. Psychiatr. Psychother.* **2005**, *4*, 356–369.
35. Wünsche, P.; Schneewind, K.A. Entwicklung eines Fragebogens zur Erfassung von Selbst- und Kompetenzeinschätzungen bei Kindern (FSK-K). *Diagnostica* **1989**, *35*, 217–235.
36. Reinehr, T.; Kersting, M.; Wollenhaupt, A.; Alexy, U.; Kling, B.; Ströbele, K.; Andler, W. Evaluation der Schulung "OBELDICKS" für adipöse Kinder und Jugendliche. *Klin. Padiatr.* **2005**, *217*, 1–8. [CrossRef]
37. Harrist, A.W.; Swindle, T.M.; Hubbs-Tait, L.; Topham, G.L.; Shriver, L.H.; Page, M.C. The Social and Emotional Lives of Overweight, Obese, and Severely Obese Children. *Child Dev.* **2016**, *87*, 1564–1580. [CrossRef] [PubMed]

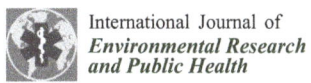

International Journal of
Environmental Research and Public Health

Article

Basic Motor Competencies of (Pre)School Children: The Role of Social Integration and Health-Related Quality of Life

Kathrin Bretz [1,*], Harald Seelig [2], Ilaria Ferrari [1], Roger Keller [3], Jürgen Kühnis [4], Simone Storni [5] and Christian Herrmann [1]

1. Physical Education Research Group, Zurich University of Teacher Education, 8090 Zurich, Switzerland
2. Department of Sport, Exercise and Health, University of Basel, 4052 Basel, Switzerland
3. Centre for Inclusion and Health in Schools, Zurich University of Teacher Education, 8090 Zurich, Switzerland
4. Expert Group Physical Education, Schwyz University of Teacher Education, 6410 Goldau, Switzerland
5. Didactics of Physical Education, University of Applied Sciences and Arts of Southern Switzerland, 6600 Locarno, Switzerland
* Correspondence: kathrin.bretz@phzh.ch; Tel.: +41-43-305-50-38

Abstract: In (pre)school, children acquire and deepen their basic motor competencies (BMCs) and interact with peers and friends. BMCs are a central developmental goal in childhood and the prerequisite for participation in sportive aspects of social life. Both motor competencies and social integration are linked to children's health-related quality of life (HRQoL). The aim of the present study was to describe the connection between BMCs, social relationships, and aspects of HRQoL in (pre)school children. In this study, the BMCs of N = 1163 preschool children (M = 5.7 years, SD = 0.57, 52% boys) and N = 880 first and second graders (M = 7.5 years, SD = 0.58, 51% boys) were tested. The children's social integration was assessed by the teachers; the HRQoL was recorded from the parents' perspective. In both preschool and primary school, children with better BMCs also showed higher values in their social integration. Moreover, the results indicated a connection between BMCs and general HRQoL in primary school and BMCs and physical well-being in preschool. As BMCs, social integration, and HRQoL seem to be connected in (pre)school, this should be considered both from developmental and health-oriented perspectives, as well as for physical education (PE) lessons.

Keywords: kindergarten; sport; health; motor skills; physical education; well-being

Citation: Bretz, K.; Seelig, H.; Ferrari, I.; Keller, R.; Kühnis, J.; Storni, S.; Herrmann, C. Basic Motor Competencies of (Pre)School Children: The Role of Social Integration and Health-Related Quality of Life. *Int. J. Environ. Res. Public Health* 2022, 19, 14537. https://doi.org/10.3390/ijerph192114537

Academic Editors: Clemens Drenowatz and Klaus Greier

Received: 20 September 2022
Accepted: 4 November 2022
Published: 5 November 2022

Publisher's Note: MDPI stays neutral with regard to jurisdictional claims in published maps and institutional affiliations.

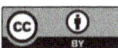

Copyright: © 2022 by the authors. Licensee MDPI, Basel, Switzerland. This article is an open access article distributed under the terms and conditions of the Creative Commons Attribution (CC BY) license (https://creativecommons.org/licenses/by/4.0/).

1. Introduction

Throughout childhood, children develop and extend their basic motor repertoire in contexts of social interaction (e.g., (pre)school, interactions with peers, sport clubs). Basic motor competencies (BMCs) are necessary for participation in the culture of sport and exercise [1,2]. They facilitate a basic capacity for the development of higher competency levels and further participation in sports and exercise [2]. BMCs are also the prerequisite for acquisition of sport-specific motor skills and positively influence a physically active lifestyle over an individual's lifespan [2]. BMCs further lead to the development of a large repertoire of movement skills [3]. This process is strongly influenced by opportunities for practice [4]. Preschools and primary schools should offer situations in which children can extend their BMCs [5]. Physical education (PE) classes with various movement situations are particularly suitable, as all children participate in them in contrast to extracurricular activities. The development of BMCs is a core development task in preschool and primary school and is also addressed in PE curricula [5].

For all children, school is an expanded social environment with new tasks and challenges [6]. Interpersonal relationship skills are addressed in the curricula and defined as a central life skill by the World Health Organization (WHO) [6,7]. Interpersonal relationship skills help children to relate to the people around them in a positive way. Moreover, they are acquired in contexts involving social interaction and are important for making friends and getting involved in peer groups [6,8]. Social interactions and peer relationships are central to healthy child development [9,10]. Friendships are associated with a variety of positive psychological and behavioral outcomes for children, which continue into early adulthood [11]. Children choose friends and peers by participating in similar activities (e.g., sports, music, art) or interacting with those who behave similarly [12]. In early childhood, children are more likely to choose same-gender friendships and different genders show different play behavior, which can already be observed at preschool age [13]. While boys more often engage in physically active games, girls desire friendly closeness and cohesion more than boys [13]. Girls exert a lot of effort establishing and maintaining positive social relationships and spend time in smaller groups with closer friends [12,14].

In order to ensure adequate learning opportunities for every child, it is important to promote social integration in the class in addition to subject-specific competencies in PE [15]. This is particularly important in the context of sport and play situations, as this can only happen in the interplay between BMCs and social integration [9].

Positive associations between BMCs and social relationships have been found in preschool-aged children [16]. In addition, 9 to 12 year old children with poorer motor competencies have been found to be less preferred by their peers in both play and classroom settings [17]. Children with developmental coordination disorder, in particular, have been found to be less socially integrated and more likely to experience exclusion in class [18].

Integration with peers and interactions with friends are highly important for children's quality of life, as well as their well-being [19]. Health-related quality of life (HRQoL) is a multidimensional and complex construct described as an individual's perception of his or her position in life [20]. It includes physical, emotional, mental, social, and behavioral components of well-being and functioning from the subjective perspective [20]. The assessment of HRQoL in children has increasingly become the focus of health research [21]. An assessment of HRQoL can be used to identify subgroups or individuals who are at higher risk of health problems [22]. Therefore, HRQoL is especially examined in children with special needs or diseases, such as developmental coordination disorder or chronic illness [23,24].

Both BMCs and social integration have a positive influence on children's mental and physical health [25,26]. Studies investigating the determinants of HRQoL in (pre)school children show that children with higher motor competencies have better HRQoL levels [24,26–28]. Moreover, children with low motor competencies show a higher risk of negative interpersonal (peer problems) and intrapersonal (low self-assessment) consequences at the psychosocial level, which can result in worse mental health and well-being [18,29,30]. Integration with peers and interactions with friends are highly important for quality of life, as positive relationships with friends have a strong effect on children's subjective well-being [25,28].

However, little research has been conducted on the connections between (basic) motor competencies, social integration, and HRQoL in children, especially in preschoolers [26,31]. As previous studies have investigated the relationship between motor competencies and HRQoL mainly in children with DCD or special needs, there is a need to investigate this relationship in normally developing children as well. What should be taken into account in particular is the idea of participation, especially in PE. The aim of this study was to investigate the relationship between BMCs, social integration, and HRQoL in children in their first years of (pre)school.

2. Materials and Methods

The present study was a cross-sectional study based on the first measurement point for a longitudinal research project, funded by the Zurich University of Teacher Education and Health Promotion Switzerland (Gesundheitsförderung Schweiz, GFCH) and utilized convenience sampling. Although it was not a representative sample for Switzerland, we ensured that all three language regions, as well as urban and rural areas, were equally represented in the sample. In spring and summer 2021, we measured the BMCs of preschoolers

(4–6 years) and children from the first and second grades (6–8 years) in the German-, Italian-, and French-speaking parts of Switzerland. Preschool in Switzerland is part of mandatory schooling and includes a two-year entrance stage for primary school.

2.1. Participants

In total, we contacted the parents or legal guardians of 1840 preschoolers and 1163 children from the first two years of primary school in the German-, Italian-, and French-speaking parts of Switzerland. For preschoolers, 1334 parents (72.5%) gave their written consent for their children to participate in the study and sent back the questionnaire. Inclusion criteria were the presence of consent for the assessment of the BMC test and the parent questionnaire. Age ranges were formed based on the dates of entry to preschool (55–80 months) and primary school (77–105 months) in order to exclude much younger and older children from the study. We were thus able to include 1163 preschoolers (M = 5.7 years, SD = 0.57, 52% boys) from 95 classes (average class size, n = 13). In the first and second grades of primary school, 901 parents (77.5%) agreed to their children's participation in the study. We included 880 (M = 7.5 years, SD = 0.58, 51% boys) children from the first and second grades from 64 classes in the study (average class size, n = 14). We received assessments from the teachers (M = 39.7 years, SD = 10.2, 90% female teachers) and the parents (M = 38.5 years, SD = 5.9, 76% female).

2.2. Test Instruments and Data Collection

- Basic motor competencies (BMCs; children tests):

To measure BMCs, we used the MOBAK test instruments for preschool (MOBAK-KG) and the first two years of primary school (MOBAK-1-2). The MOBAK instrument is a curriculum-valid instrument that measures the level of BMC and can be used easily in PE lessons [1,32]. Moreover, it is oriented toward the elementary learning goals of PE (e.g., [5]). The BMCs in the two competence areas of self-movement and object movement (Table 1; for details, see [1,32]) are measured via four items each. A standardized task with corresponding evaluation criteria is described per item. The children performed two trials per test item (six trials for the throwing and catching items). Both attempts were rated dichotomously (0 = fail, 1 = successful). The individual results per test item were summed up to calculate the final item score (0 points = no successful attempts, 1 point = one successful attempt, 2 points = two successful attempts). The throwing and catching scores were calculated differently. In these cases, 0–2 successful attempts were scored as 0 points, 3–4 successful attempts as 1 point, and 5–6 successful attempts as 2 points. For each competency domain, a maximum sum score of eight points could be achieved (for details, see [1,32]). The data collection took 30–40 min and was carried out during a regular PE lesson of 45 min duration. The classes were split up and an examiner led three to four children through the eight test stations and gave a standardized explanation and one demonstration of each test item.

Table 1. Descriptions of the test items (see Herrmann, 2018 (p. 15) and 2020 (p. 8–9) [1,32]). Note: 0 = no attempt completed, 1 = task completed once, 2 = task completed twice.

	MOBAK-KG	MOBAK-1-2
	Object movement	
Throwing	The child throws six juggling balls at a target of 1.1 m height from a distance of 1.5 m with overhead throws.	The child throws six juggling balls at a target of 1.3 m height from a distance of 2.0 m.
Catching	The tester drops a small basketball to the ground from a height of 1.5 m so that the ball bounces back up at least 1.1 m from the ground. The child catches the ball after it has reached the highest point.	The tester drops a small ball to the ground from a height of 2.0 m so that the ball bounces back up at least 1.3 m from the ground. The child catches the ball after it has reached the highest point.

Table 1. Cont.

	MOBAK-KG	MOBAK-1-2
Bouncing	The child bounces a small volleyball with both hands and catches it again without losing the ball.	The child bounces a small basketball through a marked corridor (5.0 × 1.0 m) without losing the ball.
Dribbling	The child dribbles a futsal ball through a marked corridor (2.8 × 9.0 m) around two obstacles without stopping or losing the ball.	The child dribbles a futsal ball through a marked corridor (5.0 × 1.0 m) without losing the ball.
	Self-movement	
Balancing	The child walks across an overturned long bench without stepping off the bench.	The child walks across an overturned see-sawing long bench without stepping off the bench.
Rolling	The child performs a forward roll down an inclined mat and is able to land fluently in a standing position on his/her feet.	The child performs a forward roll on a mat and is able to land fluently in a standing position on his/her feet.
Jumping	The child jumps a distance of 3.0 m on one foot, turns around, and jumps back 3.0 m on the other foot.	The child jumps between and beneath carpet tiles fluently with one leg between the tiles and with straddled legs beneath the tiles.
Running	The child runs forward along a corridor (0.6 m × 4.0 m) to a wall, touches it with his/her hand, and then runs back backwards.	The child moves sideways from one cone to another placed at a distance of 3 m from each other.

The factorial validity of the MOBAK instruments for preschool and primary education has already been investigated and confirmed in various studies (e.g., [33,34]).

- Social integration (PIQ; teacher questionnaires):

The teachers measured the children's social integration using the subscale of the perception of inclusion (PIQ) questionnaire [15]. The teachers rated the children individually via four items (e.g., "He/she gets along very well with his/her classmates.") on a four-point scale. The teachers received the questionnaire for each child in advance along with the information on the study. We asked the teachers to complete the questionnaire and bring it with them on the day of the MOBAK test. The Cronbach's alpha of the scale was calculated for preschool (0.82) and primary school (0.83) and showed satisfactory internal consistency [35]. The factorial validity of the instrument was confirmed in a validation study by Venetz and colleagues. [15].

- General health-related quality of life (general HRQoL; parent questionnaires):

The low reading literacy of children, especially in early childhood, has led to the development of instruments that measure children's HRQoL via parental assessments [36]. General health-related quality of life (HRQoL) was measured via the KIDSCREEN-10 instrument [36,37] in a subsample of $N = 943$ preschool children and the total sample of $N = 880$ primary school children (subsample 1), with a short version used in one canton due to the construction of the questionnaire. This instrument contains ten items (e.g., "Has your child felt sad?") and provides a valid measure of a general HRQoL factor. Moreover, the parents filled out the children's date of birth and gender. The parents received the questionnaire along with the declaration of consent, both of which were collected by the teachers. The internal consistency of the KIDSCREEN-10 instrument was acceptable, with a Cronbach's alpha of 0.73 for preschool and 0.76 for primary school (overall 0.74) [35]. For the analyses, the sum score (10–50) was transformed into the t-value (mean: 50, standard deviation: 10). Higher values indicate a higher general HRQoL [36,37].

- Physical well-being (parent questionnaires):

In a subsample of $N = 348$ preschool children (subsample 2), the physical well-being subscale of the KIDSCREEN-27 instrument [36] was used exploratively. The subscale consists of five items (e.g., "Has your child felt fit and well?") and had an acceptable Cronbach's alpha of 0.71. For the analyses, the sum score (5–23) was transformed into the t-value (mean: 50, standard deviation: 10). Higher values indicate higher physical well-being [37].

2.3. Data Analysis

SPSS 28 was employed for the data editing, descriptive statistics, t-tests, and Cronbach's alpha estimations [38]. Descriptive statistics were calculated for all variables. T-tests were used to calculate differences between boys and girls in the variables of interest. In addition to the 95% confidence intervals, Cohen's d was calculated to examine the strength of the differences. Therefore, effect sizes were interpreted following Cohen (1988) as small (d = 0.10), medium (d = 0.50), and large (d = 0.80) [39]. We used Mplus 8.4 to perform multivariate analyses [40]. We calculated interclass correlations (ICCs) to test the influences of the multilevel structure (pupils from different classes) due to class associations. A high ICC value means that there are large differences between classes for the corresponding characteristics, the cause of which is to be sought at the class level (e.g., class composition). Raudenbush and Bryk (2002) recommend accounting for the multi-level structure of the data for advanced analyses with ICCs > 0.05 [41].

Model 1: In this first model, we used structural equation models to examine the relationships between the two MOBAK factors self-movement and object movement, social integration, and general HRQoL, with age as a covariate. Self-movement and object movement, as well as social integration, were included as latent factors.

Following Ravens-Sieberer and colleagues, we summed up general HRQoL, transformed it into the t-value, and included it as a manifest variable in the model [37] (Figure 1). This model was separately examined for both age groups of interest (MOBAK-KG, model 1a; MOBAK-1-2, model 1b). Since KIDSCREEN-10 was not used (in its entirety) at all study locations, model 1 was calculated for a subsample of N = 943 preschool children and N = 880 primary school children (subsample 1).

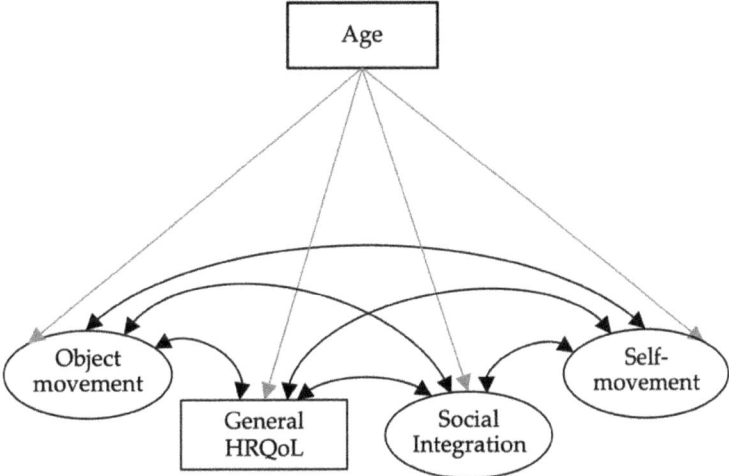

Figure 1. Model 1. Structural equation model with object movement, self-movement, general HRQoL, and social integration with the covariate age.

Model 2: Next, we re-calculated model 1 as a multigroup model to investigate the correlations between the model components separately for boys and girls. This allowed for a model test for boys and girls. All parameters were estimated freely. Only the factor structure was kept equal between boys and girls [42–44]. This served to ensure that the factor structure (numbers and types of latent factors and loadings) was the same for boys and girls. We calculated model 2 separately for both MOBAK-KG (model 2a) and MOBAK-1-2 (model 2b).

Model 3: In a subsample of N = 384 preschool children (subsample 2), we used the physical well-being subscale of the KIDSCREEN-27 instrument (5 items [36]) to assess the children's physical well-being from the parents' perspective. The sum score of the five items was t-transformed into a manifest variable. We used structural equation models to calculate the relationship between the latent factors self-movement, object movement, and social integration and the manifest variable physical well-being. Age was included as a covariate (Figure 2).

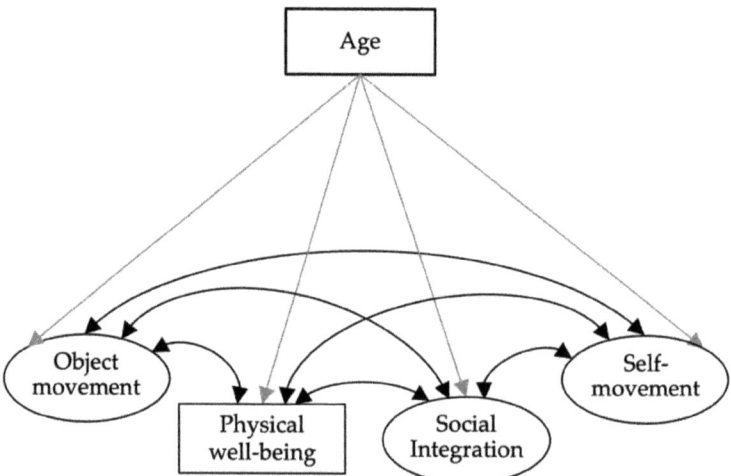

Figure 2. Model 3. Structural equation model showing object movement, self-movement, physical well-being, and social integration with the covariate age.

Model 4: We then re-calculated model 3 as a multigroup model for boys and girls. We examined the configural invariance in a multiple group model. This allowed for a model test for boys and girls simultaneously.

In all models, we treated the MOBAK test items as ordinal-scaled and the questionnaire items as interval-scaled data. Accordingly, we applied the mean- and variance-adjusted weighted least squares (WLSMV) estimator.

The "type = complex" function for nested datasets implemented in Mplus was needed to correct the standard error and ensure that dependencies within the multilevel structure ($0.01 \leq ICC \leq 0.19$; Table 2) were accounted for in all model estimations [41]. The goodness of fit of the models was assessed using fit indices proposed in the literature [45]. Effect sizes were interpreted as small ($r > 0.10$, $\beta > 0.05$), medium ($r > 0.30$, $\beta > 0.25$), and large ($r > 0.50$, $\beta > 0.45$) [39,46].

Table 2. Descriptive analyses of sum scores of the motor competency domains, social integration, general HRQoL, and physical well-being.

	Preschool						Primary School				
	Overall		Boys	Girls			Overall		Boys	Girls	
	M [95% CI]	ICC	M [95% CI]	M [95% CI]	d		M [95% CI]	ICC	M [95% CI]	M [95% CI]	d
Object movement [a]	4.0 [3.8; 4.1]	0.02	4.4 [4.2; 4.5]	3.5 [3.4; 3.7]	0.42		5.5 [5.4; 5.6]	0.12	5.9 [5.7; 6.0]	5.1 [5.0; 5.3]	0.43
Self-movement [a]	4.5 [4.4; 4.7]	0.05	4.3 [4.1; 4.5]	4.8 [4.6; 5.0]	0.21		4.9 [4.8; 5.1]	0.14	4.8 [4.6; 5.0]	5.1 [4.9; 5.3]	0.14
Social integration [a]	13.5 [13.4; 13.7]	0.19	13.4 [13.2; 13.5]	13.7 [13.6; 13.9]	0.17		13.7 [13.6; 13.8]	0.25	13.5 [13.3; 13.8]	13.9 [13.7; 14.1]	0.15
General HRQoL sum score [b]	41.5 [41.2; 41.7]	0.04	41.4 [41.1; 41.8]	41.5 [41.1; 41.8]	0.004		41.2 [40.9; 41.5]	0.03	40.8 [40.4; 41.2]	41.5 [41.2; 41.9]	0.18
General HRQoL t-value [1,b]	51.9 [51.4; 52.4]	0.02	51.8 [51.1; 52.5]	51.9 [51.2; 52.7]	0.02		51.7 [51.1; 52.2]	0.02	51.1 [50.3; 51.8]	52.3 [51.5; 53.1]	0.15

Table 2. Cont.

	Preschool					Primary School		
	Overall		Boys	Girls		Overall	Boys	Girls
Physical well-being sum score [c]	21.9 [21.7; 22.2]	0.04	22.3 [21.9; 22.6]	21.6 [21.1; 22.0]	0.27			
Physical well-being t-value [1,c]	53.2 [52.6; 53.8]	0.003	54.1 [53.3; 54.8]	52.2 [51.3; 53.1]	0.33			

Note: M = mean, 95% CI = 95% confidence interval. Point ranges: object movement (0–8), self-movement (0–8), social integration (5–20), KIDSCREEN-10 sum score (10–50), KIDSCREEN physical well-being (5–25). [1] The sum score (range: 10–50) was transformed into t-values (mean: 50, standard deviation: 10). Higher values indicate better general health-related quality of life or physical well-being [37]. [a] Complete sample (preschool: N = 1163, primary school N = 880), [b] subsample 1 (preschool: N = 943, primary school N = 880), [c] subsample 2 (preschool: N = 384).

We accounted for missing values by generating model estimates using the full information maximum likelihood (FIML) procedure. This procedure prevents bias in the sample composition by preventing a reduction in the sample size [47].

3. Results

As the descriptive analyses (Table 2) show, there were already gender-specific differences in motor performance levels. Girls were better in self-movement, while boys performed better in object movement. Girls were rated as more socially integrated by their teachers in both preschool and primary school. In preschool, there were no gender differences regarding general HRQoL, whereas boys showed higher physical well-being than girls. In primary school, general HRQoL was higher in girls than in boys. The ICC values for BMCs, general HRQoL, and physical well-being were low (ICC < 0.05). The ICC value for social integration was 0.19. This means that there were large differences between the classes due to the assessment of social integration by the teacher at the class level.

Latent Structural Equation Models

Model 1: Both model 1a (preschool) and model 1b (primary school) fit the data well (Table 3).

Table 3. Data fit of the calculated models.

Model	Analysis	Sample	n	χ^2	df	p	CFI	RMSEA
1a	MIMIC	SS 1 preschool	943	115.947	69	<0.001	0.961	0.027
1b	MIMIC	SS 1 primary school	880	92.865	69	0.029	0.967	0.020
2a	MGM	SS 1 preschool	943	201.069	160	0.015	0.971	0.023
2b	MGM	SS 1 primary school	880	180.123	160	0.132	0.977	0.017
3	MIMIC	SS 2 preschool	384	88.459	69	0.057	0.962	0.027
4	MGM	SS 2 preschool	384	175.645	160	0.188	0.971	0.023

Note: CFI = comparative fit index; RMSEA = root mean square error of approximation; MIMIC = structural equation model with covariate age; MGM = multigroup model; SS = subsample.

Table 4 shows that the associations of the latent constructs of BMC and social integration with general HRQoL differed between preschool and primary school children. A positive small to moderate association between children's BMCs and their social integration (assessed by the teachers) was found in both preschool and primary school. In preschool, no correlations were found between general HRQoL (assessed by the parents) and BMCs or between general HRQoL and social integration.

Table 4. Intercorrelations between variables in model 1 (subsample 1).

Factors	Preschool (Model 1a)				Primary School (Model 1b)			
	(1)	(2)	(3)	(4)	(1)	(2)	(3)	(4)
(1) Object movement								
(2) Self-movement	0.74 ***				0.56 ***			
(3) Social integration	0.27 ***	0.26 ***			0.22 ***	0.18 **		
(4) General HRQoL	0.01	0.04	0.04		0.003	0.14 **	0.13 ***	
(5) Age	0.59 ***	0.47 ***	0.15 ***	−0.01	0.49 ***	0.33 ***	0.10	<0.01

Note: (1) object movement, (2) self-movement, (3) social integration, (4) general HRQoL. ** $p < 0.01$, *** $p < 0.001$.

In primary school, positive significant associations were found between general HRQoL and self-movement ($r = 0.14$, $p = 0.005$), as well as general HRQoL and social integration ($r = 0.13$, $p < 0.001$), whereas no correlations were found between general HRQoL and object movement. The results show that children who were better with self-movement and children who were better socially integrated obtained higher values for general HRQoL. The correlations with age show that older children had better BMCs and seemed to be better socially integrated than younger children. No correlation with age was found for general HRQoL.

Model 2: Taking model 1 as a starting point, the correlations between the latent factors, as well as with age as a covariate, were calculated for both genders separately in a multigroup model (Table 5). This model achieved a good fit for preschool (model 2a, Table 3) and primary school (model 2b, Table 3). Deviation estimates for boys and girls appeared to be comparable in preschool (boys: $\chi^2 = 106.924$, $n = 484$; girls: $\chi^2 = 94.146$, $n = 459$) and within primary school (boys: $\chi^2 = 62.191$, $n = 450$; girls: $\chi^2 = 117.932$, $n = 430$).

Table 5. Intercorrelations between the variables in model 2 (subsample 1).

Factors	Preschool (Model 2a)					Primary School (Model 2b)				
	(1)	(2)	(3)	(4)	(5)	(1)	(2)	(3)	(4)	(5)
(1) Object movement		0.85 ***	0.34 ***	−0.01	0.53 ***		0.64 ***	0.21 **	0.11	0.44 ***
(2) Self-movement	0.84 ***		0.22 *	0.01	0.44 ***	0.68 ***		0.12	0.12	0.26 ***
(3) Social integration	0.26 ***	0.27 ***		0.07	0.15 ***	0.32 ***	0.24 **		0.16 **	0.09
(4) General HRQoL	0.06	0.05	0.01		−0.02	−0.03	0.18 **	0.10		−0.001
(5) Age	0.71 ***	0.52 ***	0.15 ***	−0.02		0.58 ***	0.44 ***	0.10	−0.001	

Note: (1) object movement, (2) self-movement, (3) social integration, (4) general HRQoL. * $p < 0.05$, ** $p < 0.01$, *** $p < 0.001$. Girls below the diagonal, boys above the diagonal

In model 2, the results were similar for boys and girls. Boys and girls with better BMCs were rated higher for their social integration by their teachers in both preschool and primary school. Regarding general HRQoL, there were no associations with BMCs or social integration for either boys or girls in preschool. For primary school, significant relationships with general HRQoL, as assessed by the parents, were only found for self-movement among girls ($r = 0.18$, $p = 0.007$) and social integration among boys ($r = 0.16$, $p = 0.004$). The finding that age was positively associated with BMCs and social integration was evident for girls and boys.

Model 3: The structural equation model with object movement, self-movement, social integration, and the subscale physical well-being (t-value of subscale sum score) achieved a good model fit (Table 3). A high correlation between object movement and self-movement was found ($r = 0.79$, $p < 0.001$). As already became clear from model 1 and model 2, older children showed higher BMCs and were assessed as being better socially integrated. Moreover social integration was significantly correlated with object movement ($r = 0.29$, $p < 0.001$) and self-movement ($r = 0.40$, $p < 0.001$). No significant correlation was found between social integration and physical well-being. The BMCs of the children were positively correlated with both object movement ($r = 0.20$, $p = 0.004$) and self-movement ($r = 0.29$, $p < 0.001$) (Table 6).

Table 6. Intercorrelations between the variables in model 3 (subsample 2).

Factors	(1)	(2)	(3)	(4)
(1) Object movement				
(2) Self-movement	0.79 ***			
(3) Social integration	0.29 ***	0.40 ***		
(4) Physical well-being	0.20 **	0.29 ***	0.07	
(5) Age	0.54 ***	0.39 ***	0.17 **	−0.04

Note: (1) object movement, (2) self-movement, (3) social integration, (4) physical well-being. ** $p < 0.01$, *** $p < 0.001$.

Model 4: Taking model 3 as a starting point, the correlations between the factors, as well as with age as a covariate, were calculated for both genders separately. This multi-group model achieved a good fit (Table 3). Separate deviation estimates were $\chi^2 = 67.209$, $n = 198$ for boys and $\chi^2 = 108.436$, $n = 186$ for girls. For both genders, the children's social integration, as assessed by their teachers, was moderately related to BMCs. Correlations with BMCs could also be found for physical well-being. Both boys and girls showed high correlations between self-movement and physical well-being ($r = 0.35/0.34$, $p < 0.001$). In the competency domain of object movement, a significant correlation was only observed for boys ($r = 0.21$, $p = 0.009$). No significant correlation was found between physical well-being and social integration (Table 7).

Table 7. Intercorrelations between the variables in model 4 (subsample 2).

Factors	Boys				Girls			
	(1)	(2)	(3)	(4)	(1)	(2)	(3)	(4)
(1) Object movement								
(2) Self-movement	0.83 ***				0.88 ***			
(3) Social integration	0.40 ***	0.26 **			0.24 **	0.48 ***		
(4) Physical well-being	0.21 **	0.35 ***	0.05		0.15	0.34 **	0.18	
(5) Age	0.45 ***	0.29 ***	0.19 ***	−0.05	0.68 ***	0.58 ***	0.20 ***	−0.04

(1) Object movement, (2) self-movement, (3) social integration, (4) physical well-being. ** $p < 0.01$, *** $p < 0.001$.

4. Discussion

The objective of the present study was to investigate the relationship between BMCs, social integration, and health-related quality of life in (pre)school children. The results of this study support earlier findings that children with poor BMCs are less integrated socially and show poorer general HRQoL in primary school and physical well-being in preschool.

Moreover, girls' general HRQoL was rated higher than boys' general HRQoL in primary school, whereas there were no gender differences in preschool. Physical well-being, on the other hand, was rated higher for boys than for girls. Differences in HRQoL between age and gender have only previously been studied from eight years onwards [48].

The findings of this study are consistent with previous studies indicating that children with lower motor competencies show lower HRQoL and are less integrated socially [16,26]. The relationship between motor competence and HRQoL has mostly been investigated in children with developmental coordination disorder, as these children are more likely to have psychological issues, which may result from poor social skills or decreased quality of life [18,24,49,50]. Moreover, children with DCD show lower scores in HRQoL than typically developing children [24]. Redondo-Tébar and colleagues (2021) studied the relationship between motor competence and HRQoL in a sample of typically developing children and found a positive association between HRQoL and motor competence [26]. In contrast to previous studies in which motor competence instruments were used in a clinical context (e.g., MABC-2 [24]), our study used curriculum-valid instruments that examine BMCs in self-movement and object movement.

Children with better BMCs seemed to be better integrated in both preschool and primary school, although this correlation was higher in preschool. This could have been due to the fact that activities other than play and sports become more important for friendships in primary school. From primary school onwards, extracurricular activities, such as musical or artistic activities, are increasingly offered, and these activities could become more important for friendships with increasing age. The increasing importance of academic achievement in school could also be a reason for the lower correlations.

Differences in the association between BMCs and general HRQoL were found between preschool and primary school. Whereas no correlations between BMCs and general HRQoL were found in preschool, primary school children with better performance in self-movement also showed higher values in general HRQoL. No connection with object movement was found. It is possible that general HRQoL in preschool is more strongly influenced by other factors, such as family factors (e.g., parents, siblings). Moreover, it could be that BMC is related to general HRQoL in more informal play settings (e.g., outside, with friends or siblings).

Due to the fact that motor competencies may be important for children's physical well-being, we additionally used the physical well-being subscale of KIDSCREEN-27 in a subsample of $N = 384$ preschool children [26,36]. Physical well-being was higher in children with better BMCs, with a stronger association for self-movement than for object movement. The results indicate a significant relationship between BMCs and physical well-being, which has already been demonstrated in other studies [26,50].

Social integration and interaction with friends and peers are important factors for children's well-being, since popularity, mutual friendships, and engagement in social play are positively associated with children's quality of life [19,28]. In the present study, primary school children who were assessed to be better integrated socially also showed higher values in general HRQoL, although the association was stronger in boys. In accordance with previous studies, it appears that children who seem to be better socially integrated show higher general HRQoL.

One strength of the study was that the investigated constructs (BMCs (motor competence test [1,32]), social integration (teacher perspective [15]), and general HRQoL or physical well-being (parent perspective [36,51])) were examined from different perspectives. Thus, we took into account the perspective of the child but also those of the parents and teachers, as home and school are important environments in children's everyday lives. Another strength was the high sample size achieved in this study. Nevertheless, a few limitations should be pointed out. While the KIDSCREEN-10 instrument is a valid measurement tool for general HRQoL and is especially useful in identifying subgroups of children who are at risk for health problems, it does not represent most of the dimensions captured in KIDSCREEN-27 [51]. This suggests that the different dimensions of the multidimensional construct of health-related quality of life should be considered in further studies. As was evident in the subsample, physical well-being is related to both BMCs and social integration. It should also be taken into account that the KIDSCREEN instrument is a validated instrument for children above eight years, and a validation study in a younger cohort has yet to be conducted [51]. Moreover, we used the teacher and parent perspective to assess social integration, general HRQoL, and physical well-being because of the young age of the children. Factors that influence HRQoL, such as socioeconomic status [52], should also be considered in future studies.

Due to the cross-sectional study design, it was not possible to identify the direction of causality. Accordingly, future longitudinal studies should examine the extent to which (basic) motor competencies influence children's social integration and HRQoL and vice versa and how (basic) motor competencies can be targeted.

The findings of the study raise the pedagogical–didactic question of how to design a careful and effective setting for PE in (pre)school. As early as preschool, there are differences between boys and girls regarding BMCs that cannot be attributed to gender alone [53,54]. Teachers should be aware of gender-specific sports socialization and try to remove gender-specific role models (boys play with the ball, girls do gymnastics) in PE. This can happen, for example, through a polysportive approach or the inclusion of different combinations of movement, balls, or equipment in PE.

As PE addresses both BMCs and interdisciplinary competencies, such as interpersonal relationship skills, it should be held in an inclusive setting that promotes not only learning outcomes but also interpersonal relationship skills. Both BMCs and interpersonal relationship skills seem to be important for children's social integration. For this purpose, PE classes should promote BMCs in social situations (e.g., open learning tasks that can be solved in a group and that do not reward the individual's performance), as well as interaction with classmates. This could involve the creation of learning tasks for children with different levels of BMCs in which children can vary the difficulty, find different ways of solving the tasks, and cooperate with other children. This could help children to integrate better and feel more comfortable in the class setting. Teachers and practitioners should be aware of the connections between BMCs, social integration, and HRQoL in children. Children with poor motor competencies in particular should be encouraged to participate in sport activities and play interaction to improve both social integration and BMCs.

5. Conclusions

This study showed a positive association between BMCs, social integration, and HRQoL. In both preschool and primary school, children with better BMCs seemed to be better integrated socially in the class. Children with better BMCs showed better general HRQoL in primary school and better physical well-being in preschool. The improvement of BMCs and social integration in the class could contribute to higher HRQoL. Furthermore, additional opportunities for movement with an integrative character and opportunities for co-determination could be implemented both in PE and in extracurricular activities. Since both BMCs and social integration are linked to better HRQoL, we recommend creating inclusive situations in physical settings in which it is possible to improve both BMCs and social integration. Consequently, BMCs should be considered to improve both social integration and HRQoL.

Author Contributions: Conceptualization, C.H., K.B., I.F., R.K., J.K. and H.S.; methodology, C.H., K.B. and H.S.; validation, C.H. and H.S.; formal analysis, K.B.; investigation, S.S., I.F., J.K. and K.B.; data curation, K.B. and H.S.; writing—original draft preparation, K.B.; writing—review and editing, K.B., H.S., I.F., R.K., J.K, S.S. and C.H.; supervision, C.H.; project administration, C.H., S.S., J.K. and K.B..; funding acquisition, K.B., H.S., I.F., R.K., J.K., S.S. and C.H. All authors have read and agreed to the published version of the manuscript.

Funding: This research was funded by Health Promotion Switzerland (Gesundheitsförderung Schweiz, GFCH) and the Zurich University of Teacher Education (PHZH).

Institutional Review Board Statement: The study was conducted in accordance with the Declaration of Helsinki and approved by the Ethics Committees of the University of Zurich (Nr. 21.2.5, 08.03.2021) and the Ticino canton (Nr. 2021-00252, Rif CE Ti 3819, 03.02.2021).

Informed Consent Statement: Informed consent was obtained from all subjects involved in the study or their parents.

Data Availability Statement: The data presented in this study are available on request from the corresponding author. The data are not publicly available due to the ethical guidelines of the Cantonal School Authorities.

Acknowledgments: The authors would like to thank all schools, teachers, pupils, and parents for participating in this study.

Conflicts of Interest: The authors declare no conflict of interest. The funders had no role in the design of the study; in the collection, analyses, or interpretation of data; in the writing of the manuscript; or in the decision to publish the results.

References

1. Herrmann, C. *MOBAK 1-4: Test Zur Erfassung Motorischer Basiskompetenzen Für Die Klassen 1-4*; Hogrefe Schultests: Göttingen, Germany, 2018.
2. Hulteen, R.M.; Morgan, P.J.; Barnett, L.M.; Stodden, D.F.; Lubans, D.R. Development of Foundational Movement Skills: A Conceptual Model for Physical Activity Across the Lifespan. *Sports Med.* **2018**, *48*, 1533–1540. [CrossRef] [PubMed]
3. Chambers, M.W.; Sudgen, D.A. *Early Years Movement Skills: Description, Diagnosis and Intervention*; Wiley Publishers Limited: West Sussex, UK, 2006.
4. Gallahue, D.L.; Ozmun, J.C. *Motor Development: A Theoretical Model. Understanding Motor Development: Infants, Children, Adolescents, Adults*, 6th ed.; McGraw-Hill: New York, NY, USA, 2006.
5. Bildungsdirektion des Kantons Zürich. *Lehrplan 21 für die Volksschule. Broschüre Bewegung und Sport*; Bildungsdirektion des Kantons Zürich: Zurich, Switzerland, 2017.
6. World Health Organization. *Life Skills Education for Children and Adolescents in Schools. Introduction and Guidelines to Facilitate the Development and Implementation of Life Skills Programmes*; World Health Organization: Geneva, Switzerland, 1994.
7. Bildungsdirektion des Kantons Zürich. *Lehrplan 21 für die Volksschule. Gesamtausgabe*; Bildungsdirektion des Kantons Zürich: Zürich, Switzerland, 2017.
8. Rubin, K.H.; Schulz Begle, A.; McDonald, K.L. Peer Relations and Social Competence in Childhood. In *Developmental Social Neuroscience and Childhood Brain Insult*; Beauchamp, M.H., Anderson, V., Eds.; Guilford Press: New York, NY, USA, 2012; ISBN 978-1-4625-0429-9.
9. Opstoel, K.; Chapelle, L.; Prins, F.J.; De Meester, A.; Haerens, L.; van Tartwijk, J.; De Martelaer, K. Personal and Social Development in Physical Education and Sports: A Review Study. *Eur. Phys. Educ. Rev.* **2020**, *26*, 797–813. [CrossRef]
10. Stanton-Chapman, T.L. Promoting Positive Peer Interactions in the Preschool Classroom: The Role and the Responsibility of the Teacher in Supporting Children's Sociodramatic Play. *Early Child. Educ. J.* **2015**, *43*, 99–107. [CrossRef]
11. Xiao, S.X.; Hanish, L.D.; Malouf, L.M.; Martin, C.L.; Lecheile, B.; Goble, P.; Fabes, R.A.; DeLay, D.; Bryce, C.I. Preschoolers' Interactions with Other-Gender Peers Promote Prosocial Behavior and Reduce Aggression: An Examination of the Buddy Up Intervention. *Early Child. Res. Q.* **2022**, *60*, 403–413. [CrossRef]
12. Siegler, R.; Eisenberg, N.; DeLoache, J.; Saffran, J. Beziehungen Zu Gleichaltrigen. In *Entwicklungspsychologie im Kindes-und Jugendalter*; Siegler, R., Eisenberg, N., DeLoache, J., Saffran, J., Eds.; Springer: Berlin/Heidelberg, Germany, 2011; pp. 483–527.
13. Martin, C.L.; Kornienko, O.; Schaefer, D.R.; Hanish, L.D.; Fabes, R.A.; Goble, P. The Role of Sex of Peers and Gender-Typed Activities in Young Children's Peer Affiliative Networks: A Longitudinal Analysis of Selection and Influence. *Child Dev.* **2013**, *84*, 921–937. [CrossRef] [PubMed]
14. Rose, A.J.; Rudolph, K.D. A Review of Sex Differences in Peer Relationship Processes: Potential Trade-Offs for the Emotional and Behavioral Development of Girls and Boys. *Psychol. Bull.* **2006**, *132*, 98–131. [CrossRef] [PubMed]
15. Venetz, M.; Zurbriggen, C.L.A.; Schwab, S. What Do Teachers Think About Their Students' Inclusion? Consistency of Students' Self-Reports and Teacher Ratings. *Front. Psychol.* **2019**, *10*, 1637. [CrossRef] [PubMed]
16. Herrmann, C.; Bretz, K.; Kühnis, J.; Seelig, H.; Keller, R.; Ferrari, I. Connection between Social Relationships and Basic Motor Competencies in Early Childhood. *Children* **2021**, *8*, 53. [CrossRef]
17. Livesey, D.; Lum Mow, M.; Toshack, T.; Zheng, Y. The Relationship between Motor Performance and Peer Relations in 9- to 12-Year-Old Children. *Child Care Health Dev.* **2011**, *37*, 581–588. [CrossRef]
18. Mancini, V.O.; Rigoli, D.; Cairney, J.; Roberts, L.D.; Piek, J.P. The Elaborated Environmental Stress Hypothesis as a Framework for Understanding the Association Between Motor Skills and Internalizing Problems: A Mini-Review. *Front. Psychol.* **2016**, *7*, 239. [CrossRef]
19. Lezhnieva, N.; Fredriksen, P.M.; Bekkhus, M. Peer Relationships and Quality of Life in 11–12-Year-Old Children: The Health Oriented Pedagogical Project (HOPP). *Scand. J. Public Health* **2018**, *46*, 74–81. [CrossRef] [PubMed]
20. The World Health Organization Quality of Life Assessment (WHOQOL): Position Paper from the World Health Organization. *Soc. Sci. Med.* **1995**, *41*, 1403–1409. [CrossRef]
21. Solans, M.; Pane, S.; Estrada, M.-D.; Serra-Sutton, V.; Berra, S.; Herdman, M.; Alonso, J.; Rajmil, L. Health-Related Quality of Life Measurement in Children and Adolescents: A Systematic Review of Generic and Disease-Specific Instruments. *Value Health* **2008**, *11*, 742–764. [CrossRef] [PubMed]
22. Ravens-Sieberer, U.; Gosch, A.; Abel, T.; Auquier, P.; Bellach, B.M.; Bruil, J.; Dür, W.; Power, M.; Rajmil, L.; European KIDSCREEN Group. Quality of Life in Children and Adolescents: A European Public Health Perspective. *Soz. Prav.* **2001**, *46*, 294–302. [CrossRef]
23. Barthel, D.; Ravens-Sieberer, U.; Nolte, S.; Thyen, U.; Klein, M.; Walter, O.; Meyrose, A.-K.; Rose, M.; Otto, C. Predictors of Health-Related Quality of Life in Chronically Ill Children and Adolescents over Time. *J. Psychosom. Res.* **2018**, *109*, 63–70. [CrossRef] [PubMed]
24. Redondo-Tébar, A.; Ruiz-Hermosa, A.; Martínez-Vizcaíno, V.; Martín-Espinosa, N.M.; Notario-Pacheco, B.; Sánchez-López, M. Health-Related Quality of Life in Developmental Coordination Disorder and Typical Developing Children. *Res. Dev. Disabil.* **2021**, *119*, 104087. [CrossRef]
25. Goswami, H. Social Relationships and Children's Subjective Well-Being. *Soc. Indic. Res.* **2012**, *107*, 575–588. [CrossRef]

26. Redondo-Tébar, A.; Fatouros, I.G.; Martinez-Vizcaino, V.; Ruíz-Hermosa, A.; Notario-Pacheco, B.; Sanchez-Lopez, M. Association between Gross Motor Competence and Health-Related Quality of Life in (Pre)Schoolchildren: The Mediating Role of Cardiorespiratory Fitness. *Phys. Educ. Sport Pedagog.* **2021**, *26*, 51–64. [CrossRef]
27. Masini, A.; Gori, D.; Marini, S.; Lanari, M.; Scrimaglia, S.; Esposito, F.; Campa, F.; Grigoletto, A.; Ceciliani, A.; Toselli, S.; et al. The Determinants of Health-Related Quality of Life in a Sample of Primary School Children: A Cross-Sectional Analysis. *Int. J. Environ. Res. Public Health* **2021**, *18*, 3251. [CrossRef]
28. Kennedy-Behr, A.; Rodger, S.; Mickan, S. Play or Hard Work: Unpacking Well-Being at Preschool. *Res. Dev. Disabil.* **2015**, *38*, 30–38. [CrossRef]
29. Cairney, J.; Rigoli, D.; Piek, J. Developmental Coordination Disorder and Internalizing Problems in Children: The Environmental Stress Hypothesis Elaborated. *Dev. Rev.* **2013**, *33*, 224–238. [CrossRef]
30. Katagiri, M.; Ito, H.; Murayama, Y.; Hamada, S.; Nakajima, S.; Takayanagi, N.; Uemiya, A.; Myogan, M.; Nakai, A.; Tsujii, M. Fine and Gross Motor Skills Predict Later Psychosocial Maladaptation and Academic Achievement. *Brain Dev.* **2021**, *43*, 605–615. [CrossRef] [PubMed]
31. Giske, R.; Ugelstad, I.; Meland, A.T.; Kaltvedt, E.; Eikeland, S.; Tonnessen, F.; Reikerås, E. Toddlers' Social Competence, Play, Movement Skills and Well-Being: An Analysis of Their Relationship Based on Authentic Assessment in Kindergarten. *Eur. Early Child. Educ. Res. J.* **2018**, *26*, 362–374. [CrossRef]
32. Herrmann, C.; Ferrari, I.; Wälti, M.; Wacker, S.; Kühnis, J. *MOBAK-KG: Motorische Basiskompetenzen Im Kindergarten: Testmanual*, 3rd ed.; Pädagogische Hochschule Zürich: Zurich, Switzerland, 2020. [CrossRef]
33. Herrmann, C.; Gerlach, E.; Seelig, H. Motorische Basiskompetenzen in der Grundschule. *Sportwissenschaft* **2016**, *46*, 60–73. [CrossRef]
34. Herrmann, C.; Heim, C.; Seelig, H. Construct and Correlates of Basic Motor Competencies in Primary School-Aged Children. *J. Sport Health Sci.* **2019**, *8*, 63–70. [CrossRef]
35. Nunnally, J.C.; Bernstein, I.H. *Psychometric Theory*, 3rd ed.; Mc-Graw-Hill: New York, NY, USA, 1994.
36. Robitail, S.; Ravens-Sieberer, U.; Simeoni, M.-C.; Rajmil, L.; Bruil, J.; Power, M.; Duer, W.; Cloetta, B.; Czemy, L.; Mazur, J.; et al. Testing the Structural and Cross-Cultural Validity of the KIDSCREEN-27 Quality of Life Questionnaire. *Qual. Life Res.* **2007**, *16*, 1335–1345. [CrossRef] [PubMed]
37. Ravens-Sieberer, U. *The Kidscreen Questionnaires: Quality of Life Questionnaires for Children and Adolescents: Handbook*, 3rd ed.; Pabst Science Publishers: Lengerich, Germany, 2016; ISBN 3-89967-334-4.
38. IBM Corp. *IBM SPSS Statistics, Version 28*; IBM Corp.: Armonk, NY, USA, 2021.
39. Cohen, J. *Statistical Power Analysis for the Behavioral Sciences*, 2nd ed.; Erlbaum: Hillsdale, NJ, USA, 1988.
40. Muthén, L.K.; Muthén, B.O. *Mplus User's Guide: Statistical Analysis with Latent Variables*, 8th ed.; Muthén & Muthén: Los Angeles, CA, USA, 2017.
41. Raudenbush, S.W.; Bryk, A.S. *Hierarchical Linear Models: Applications and Data Analysis Methods*, 2nd ed.; Sage Publications: Thousand Oaks, CA, USA, 2002; ISBN 978-0-7619-1904-9.
42. Dimitrov, D. Comparing Groups on Latent Variables: A Structural Equation Modeling Approach. *Work* **2006**, *26*, 429–436.
43. Geiser, C. *Datenanalyse Mit Mplus: Eine Anwendungsorientierte Einführung*; Springer: Wiesbaden, Germany, 2011; ISBN 978-3-531-18002-1.
44. Widaman, K.F.; Reise, S.P. Exploring the Measurement Invariance of Psychological Instruments: Applications in the Substance Use Domain. In *The science of prevention*; Bryant, K.J., Windle, M.T., West, S.G., Eds.; American Psychological Association: Washington, DC, USA, 1997; pp. 281–324. ISBN 1-55798-439-5.
45. Schreiber, J.B.; Nora, A.; Stage, F.K.; Barlow, E.A.; King, J. Reporting Structural Equation Modeling and Confirmatory Factor Analysis Results: A Review. *J. Educ. Res.* **2006**, *99*, 323–338. [CrossRef]
46. Peterson, R.A.; Brown, S.P. On the Use of Beta Coefficients in Meta-Analysis. *J. Appl. Psychol.* **2005**, *90*, 175–181. [CrossRef]
47. Urban, D.; Mayerl, J. *Strukturgleichungsmodellierung: Ein Ratgeber Für Die Praxis*; Springer: Wiesbaden, Germany, 2014; ISBN 978-3-658-01919-8.
48. Michel, G.; Bisegger, C.; Fuhr, D.C.; Abel, T. The KIDSCREEN group Age and Gender Differences in Health-Related Quality of Life of Children and Adolescents in Europe: A Multilevel Analysis. *Qual. Life Res.* **2009**, *18*, 1147. [CrossRef]
49. Wuang, Y.-P.; Wang, C.-C.; Huang, M.-H. Health-Related Quality of Life in Children with Developmental Coordination Disorder and Their Parents. *OTJR Occup. Particip. Health* **2012**, *32*, 142–150. [CrossRef]
50. Karras, H.C.; Morin, D.N.; Gill, K.; Izadi-Najafabadi, S.; Zwicker, J.G. Health-Related Quality of Life of Children with Developmental Coordination Disorder. *Res. Dev. Disabil.* **2019**, *84*, 85–95. [CrossRef] [PubMed]
51. Ravens-Sieberer, U.; Erhart, M.; Rajmil, L.; Herdman, M.; Auquier, P.; Bruil, J.; Power, M.; Duer, W.; Abel, T.; Czemy, L.; et al. Reliability, Construct and Criterion Validity of the KIDSCREEN-10 Score: A Short Measure for Children and Adolescents' Well-Being and Health-Related Quality of Life. *Qual. Life Res.* **2010**, *19*, 1487–1500. [CrossRef]
52. Rajmil, L.; Herdman, M.; Ravens-Sieberer, U.; Erhart, M.; Alonso, J.; The European KIDSCREEN Group. Socioeconomic Inequalities in Mental Health and Health-Related Quality of Life (HRQOL) in Children and Adolescents from 11 European Countries. *Int. J. Public Health* **2014**, *59*, 95–105. [CrossRef]

53. Gramespacher, E.; Herrmann, C.; Ennigkeit, F.; Heim, C.; Seelig, H. Geschlechtsspezifische Sportsozialisation Als Prädiktor Motorischer Basiskompetenzen–Ein Mediationsmodell. *Motorik* **2020**, *43*, 69–77. [CrossRef]
54. Kress, J.; Seelig, H.; Bretz, K.; Ferrari, I.; Keller, R.; Kühnis, J.; Storni, S.; Herrmann, C. Associations between Basic Motor Competencies, Club Sport Participation, and Social Relationships among Primary School Children. *CISS* **2022**. (*submitted*).

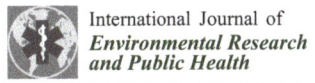

Review

Gender Differences in Fundamental Motor Skills Proficiency in Children Aged 3–6 Years: A Systematic Review and Meta-Analysis

Yunfei Zheng [1], Weibing Ye [2], Mallikarjuna Korivi [2], Yubo Liu [2,*] and Feng Hong [3,*]

1. College of Physical Education and Health Sciences, Zhejiang Normal University, Jinhua 321004, China; zyf123@zjnu.edu.cn
2. Institute of Human Movement and Sports Engineering, Zhejiang Normal University, Jinhua 321004, China; ywbls@zjnu.cn (W.Y.); mallik.k5@gmail.com (M.K.)
3. Department of Sports Operation and Management, Jinhua Polytechnic, Jinhua 321007, China
* Correspondence: liuyubo0124@outlook.com (Y.L.); fenghong0313@outlook.com (F.H.); Tel.: +86-183-2904-1023 (Y.L.)

Abstract: The age range of 3–6 years is considered as a critical period in developing and learning fundamental motor skills (FMS). To make the formulation of future FMS guidance programs more targeted, we examined gender differences in children's FMS proficiency using a meta-analysis. Structured electronic databases including PubMed, Scopus and Web of Science were systematically searched using key terms, and the Joanna Briggs Institute (JBI) was used to assess the quality of included literature. Finally, 38 articles (39 studies) met the pre-specified inclusion criteria. The results showed that boys had higher proficiency in total FMS and object control skills than girls (SMD = 0.17 (95% CI 0.03, 0.31), p = 0.02; SMD = 0.48 (95% CI 0.38, 0.58), p < 0.00001), and gender differences in locomotor skill proficiency approached significance, trending in favor of girls (SMD = −0.07 (95 % CI −0.15, 0.01), p = 0.09, I^2 = 66%). Meta-regression shows that age is associated with gender differences in object control skills (p < 0.05). In addition, through subgroup analysis, we found that boys' advantage in object control skills increased with age (3 years: SMD = 0.27 (95% CI 0.00, 0.54), p < 0.00001; 4 years: SMD = 0.58 (95% CI 0.38, 0.77), p < 0.00001; 5 years: SMD = 0.59 (95% CI 0.31, 0.88), p < 0.00001; 6 years: SMD = 0.81 (95% CI 0.61, 1.01), p < 0.00001). In this meta-analysis, we found gender differences in FMS levels in children aged 3–6 years. Notably, gender differences in skill proficiency in object control were influenced by age. We recommend focusing on and developing girls' object control skills starting at age 3.

Keywords: motor skills; child; Test of Gross Motor Development; sex differences

Citation: Zheng, Y.; Ye, W.; Korivi, M.; Liu, Y.; Hong, F. Gender Differences in Fundamental Motor Skills Proficiency in Children Aged 3–6 Years: A Systematic Review and Meta-Analysis. *Int. J. Environ. Res. Public Health* 2022, 19, 8318. https://doi.org/10.3390/ijerph19148318

Academic Editors: Clemens Drenowatz and Klaus Greier

Received: 28 May 2022
Accepted: 6 July 2022
Published: 7 July 2022

Publisher's Note: MDPI stays neutral with regard to jurisdictional claims in published maps and institutional affiliations.

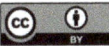

Copyright: © 2022 by the authors. Licensee MDPI, Basel, Switzerland. This article is an open access article distributed under the terms and conditions of the Creative Commons Attribution (CC BY) license (https://creativecommons.org/licenses/by/4.0/).

1. Introduction

Regular participation in physical activity (PA) has potential benefits for children to improve obesity [1,2], bone health [3], psychological health [4] and cognitive function [5,6]. However, children's physical activity levels worldwide are not positive. A study comparing physical activity behaviors of children from 15 countries found that PA behavioral indicator scores were generally low [7]. Studies have found a positive correlation between children's fundamental motor skills (FMS) and PA, and FMS have been identified as a potential mechanism for the development of PA [8–11]. FMS refer to the basic abilities and skills for children to perform a series of organized basic movements, and they includes locomotor skills (e.g., running, jumping, sliding, etc.) and object control skills (e.g., hitting, catching ball, kicking, etc.) [12]. FMS play a vital role in using more professional and complex skills in playing, games and sports [13,14]. The learning and mastery of FMS play an important role in the healthy development of children. A previous study concluded that FMS in children were significantly associated with health-related fitness (HRF) components (body composition, muscular strength, muscular endurance, cardiovascular endurance) and that the effect increases with age [15]. Despite the many benefits of FMS, a recent systematic review showed that there is still much room for improvement in FMS globally in children of all ages within the range of 3–10 years [16].

It has been well established that FMS are crucial to a child's development. When children are provided with few or no opportunities to achieve appropriate FMS levels, they are at risk of suffering from slowed motor development, thus limiting their chances for successful participation in an active and healthy sports culture [8]. Given the above, it seems crucial to improve children's FMS. A recently published study protocol presents detailed experimental designs to investigate the effects of different physical activity interventions on FMS in children [17]. However, to meet the physical developmental needs of children, exercise programs should also be tailored to their unique developmental needs, so it is important to understand gender characteristics in FMS.

However, no unified conclusion has been reached on whether there are gender differences in FMS proficiency in children. Several studies have found gender differences in FMS in children [16,18–20], with boys having higher proficiency in object control skills than girls [16,18,19,21,22], In contrast, boys and girls have been found to have similar locomotor skills proficiency [18,19,21]. Pieces of evidence suggest gender differences in locomotor skills proficiency in children, with girls showing higher proficiency [20,22]. These inconsistent results may be clarified via a meta-analysis. To the best of our knowledge, no study has investigated age variation points for gender differences in motor skills. Hence, the main aim of the present study was to systematically review and provide a meta-analysis of the gender differences in FMS, locomotor skills and object control skills in children aged 3–6 years. Secondarily, this study aims to investigate the age pattern of gender differences in motor skill proficiency by meta-regression analysis and determine the age inflection points at which gender differences emerge.

2. Materials and Methods

The systematic review was performed in accordance with the Preferred Reporting Items for Systematic Reviews and Meta-Analyses (PRISMA) guidelines [23], and the study was registered with PROSPERO (CRD42021281160).

2.1. Eligibility Criteria

Articles assessing proficiency in FMS, locomotor skills and object control skills in children aged 3 to 6 years were included in this systematic review and meta-analysis. Studies were selected if they met the following criteria: (1) children aged 3–6 years; (2) scores reported by age and gender, if the study is an intervention study, with a baseline data report required; (3) results assessed using the Test of Gross Motor Development scale (TGMD), including modified versions; and (4) outcome measures reported using raw scores.

We excluded studies that met any of the following criteria: (1) review articles, conference abstracts or books; (2) participants not being assessed simultaneously according to age and gender; (3) inclusion of special populations such as those with disabilities or diseases; and (4) studies not published in English. We calculated the pooled effect size through meta-analysis.

Inclusion and exclusion criteria were formulated and applied by two reviewers (Y.Z. and M.K.) independently, and in the case of disagreement, they were confirmed by another reviewer (W.Y.).

2.2. Search Strategy

The literature search was conducted until 10 July 2021 by two independent reviewers (Y.Z. and Y.L.) with the following electronic databases: PubMed, Scopus and Web of Science (Supplementary Materials). Search terms included "child" OR "children" OR "preschoolers" OR "boy" OR "girl" AND "fundamental movement skills" OR "motor skills" OR "motor development" OR "gross motor" AND "TGMD" OR "Test of Gross Motor Development". Specific search strategies can be found in the Supplementary Materials. In addition, we manually searched reference lists in some key previously published studies and reviews.

2.3. Data Extraction and Quality Assessment

Data were independently extracted by two reviewers (W.Y. and F.H.) and cross-checked, and controversial issues were discussed based on the original text to determine the final outcome. The extracted information included study characteristics (author name, publication time, country, study type), participant characteristics (environment, age, gender, sample), measurement information (outcome measures, outcome indicators, outcome), etc.

The two reviewers (M.K. and F.H.) independently assessed the quality of each included article using the Joanna Briggs Institute (JBI) quality appraisal checklists for cross-sectional, case–control, cohort studies, quasi-experimental and randomized control trials [24] (Supplementary Materials). If there were disagreements, we discussed these together until consensus was reached. The critical evaluation checklist for various research methods has 8 to 13 items, and positive responses were rated as "yes". We identified studies with an overall positive response between 50% and 75% as studies with moderate quality, and studies with a positive response over 75% were considered to be of high quality.

2.4. Synthesis Methods

In this study, differences in FMS proficiency among boys and girls were compared using Review Manager version 5.4.1 from the Cochrane Assistance Network. The data in this paper are continuous variables, and the comprehensive effect index is the Standard Mean Difference (SMD) and its 95% CI. SMD was interpreted as very small (<0.2), small (0.2–0.5), moderate (0.5–0.8) and large (>0.8) [25], where $p < 0.05$ indicates significant differences between the genders. The I-squared (I^2) statistic was used to test the heterogeneity between studies. When $I^2 \leq 50$, there was no heterogeneity between studies, and a fixed-effects model was used for meta-analysis; when $I^2 > 50$, there was heterogeneity between studies, and a random-effects model was used for meta-analysis [26]. The pooled results showed heterogeneity between studies, which was addressed by meta-regression analysis and subgroup analysis. In addition, we sequentially excluded literature for sensitivity analysis, evaluated the stability of the combined results of the meta-analysis and verified the existence of publication bias in the included studies using Egger's test.

When more than two subgroups needed to be merged in the research, the first two subgroups were merged first, then the third subgroup was merged, and so on. The merge formula is as follows [27]:

$$SD = \sqrt{\frac{(N_1-1)SD_1^2 + (N_2-1)SD_2^2 + \frac{N_1 N_2}{(N_1+N_2)}(M_1^2 + M_2^2 - 2M_1 M_2)}{N_1 + N_2 - 1}}$$

where SD is standard deviation; Group 1 sample size is N_1, mean is M_1, standard deviation is SD_1; and Group 2 sample size is N_2, mean is M_2, and standard deviation is SD_2.

3. Results

3.1. Search Results

A total of 2543 articles were retrieved through PubMed, Scopus and Web of Science databases, and 68 articles were obtained from reference lists of previously published studies and reviews. In the beginning, 623 duplicate records were removed from the 2543 articles. Of the remaining 1920 studies, 1688 irrelevant articles were excluded by reading the titles and abstracts, resulting in 232 items. After 15 articles that were not found were excluded, 217 articles were finally reviewed by full-text reading. From this stage, 44 articles were excluded due to age mismatch, 98 articles were removed because of insufficient information, 7 articles were excluded as they used other assessment tools, and 32 records were excluded due to other outcome measures. Ultimately, 36 articles met the inclusion criteria. In addition, 68 articles retrieved from the reference list were screened layer by layer, and 2 articles were finally included for the analysis. The detailed flow chart of the literature search, screening and selection is shown in Figure 1.

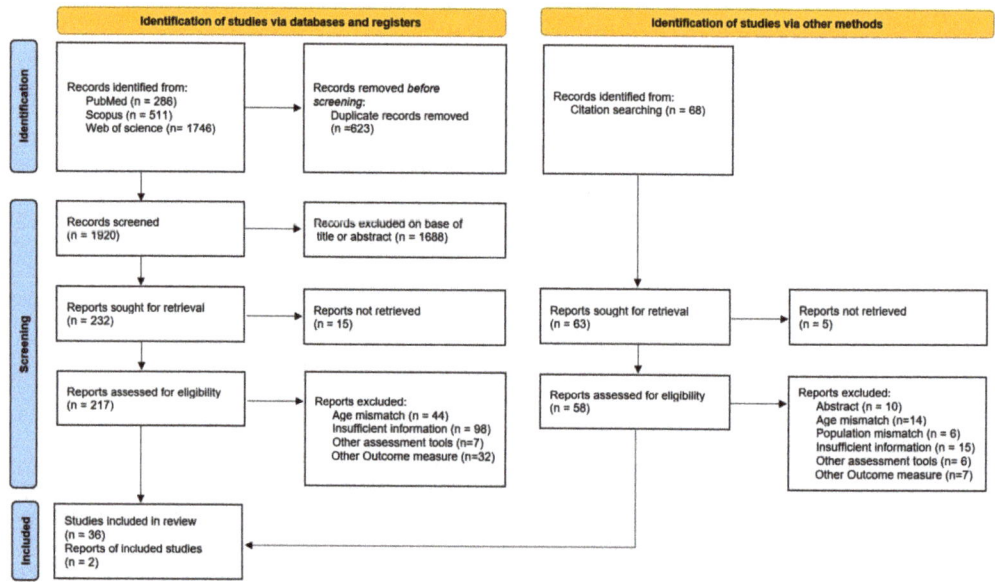

Figure 1. Flowchart of the study selection according to the Preferred Reporting Items for the Systematic Reviews and Meta-Analysis (PRISMA 2020) method.

3.2. Characteristics of Included Studies and Quality Assessment

After the inclusion and exclusion criteria had been applied, a total of 38 articles (39 studies) were included in the systematic review and meta-analysis. These studies were carried out in 19 different countries as follows: Australia [28], Belgium [29], Brazil [30–34], Britain [35–37], China [38–43], Croatia [44], Germany [45], Iran [46], Indonesia [47,48], Ireland [49,50], Japan [51], Korea [52], Myanmar [53], Poland [54,55], Portugal [56,57], Puerto Rico [58], Singapore [59], South Africa [60,61] and the USA [29,62–65]. A total of 2598 children participated in the FMS assessment, 8837 children participated in the locomotor skills assessment, and 8394 children participated in the object control skills assessment, ranging in age from 3 to 6 years old. A total of 33 studies were cross-sectional studies [28–38,40,43–45,47–63,65], one was a case–control study [39], one was a cohort study [42], two were quasi-experimental studies [46,64], and one was a randomized controlled study [41]. There were 2 studies that used TGMD-1 [44,58], 30 that used TGMD-2 [28–32,35–41,43,46,47,50–57,59–64], 1 that used the modified version of TGMD-2 [33], 5 that used TGMD-3 [42,45,48,49,65], and 1 that used the modified version of TGMD-3 [34]. Based on the JBI quality evaluation criteria, the quality scores of the included studies ranged from 60% to 100%. Most of the included articles are of high quality, a few are of medium quality, and none of them are of low quality. Test locations, test items, score reports and quality assessments are shown in Table 1.

Table 1. Characteristics of the included studies.

Author	Country	Design	Age	Sample N (Boy/Girl)	Scale	Test Items	Outcome	Assessment
Alessandro et al. 2018 [30]	Brazil	CS	5–6	158 (82/76)	TGMD-2	LM, OC, FMS	FMS: ← LM: ↔ OC: ↔	7
Aponte et al. 1990 [58]	Puerto Rico	CS	5–6	200 (102/98)	TGMD-1	FMS	FMS: ←	5
Aye et al. 2017 [53]	Myanmar	CS	5	472 (237/235)	TGMD-2	LM, OC	LM: ↔ OC: ←	7
Aye et al. 2018 [51]	Japan	CS	5	60 (34/26)	TGMD-2	LM, OC	LM: → OC: ←	7
Bakhtiar 2014 [47]	Indonesia	CS	6	67 (28/39)	TGMD-2	LM, OC	LM: ↔ OC: ↔	6
Behan et al. 2019 [49]	Ireland	CS	5–6	FMS: 357 (200/157) LM: 360 (202/158) OC: 359 (200/159)	TGMD-3	LM, OC, FMS	FMS: ↔ LM: → OC: ←	6
Bolger et al. 2017 [50]	Ireland	CS	6	102 (52/50)	TGMD-2	LM, OC	LM: → OC: ←	7
Brian et al. 2018 [29]	Belgium/USA	CS	4–5	Belgium: 170 (97/73) USA:156 (66/90)	TGMD-2	LM, OC	Belgium: LM: ↔ OC: ← USA: LM: ↔ OC: ←	6
Brian et al. 2019 [62]	USA	CS	3–6	580 (284/296)	TGMD-2	LM, OC	LM: → OC: ←	7
Capio et al. 2021 [38]	China	CS	4–6	230 (109/121)	TGMD-2	LM, OC	LM: ↔ OC: ←	6
Cheung et al. 2020 [39]	China	CC	4–6	295 (162/133)	TGMD-2	LM, OC, FMS	FMS: ↔ LM: ↔ OC: ↔	10
Cliff et al. 2009 [28]	Australia	CS	3–5	46 (25/21)	TGMD-2	LM, OC	LM: → OC: ←	6
Famelia et al. 2018 [48]	Indonesia	CS	3–6	66 (30/36)	TGMD-3	LM, OC	LM: ↔ OC: ←	7
Freitas et al. 2018 [56]	Portugal	CS	3–6	314 (155/159)	TGMD-2	LM, OC	LM: ↔ OC: ←	8
Hall et al. 2018 [35]	Britain	CS	3–5	166 (91/75)	TGMD-2	LM, OC, FMS	FMS: ↔ LM: ↔ OC: ↔	7
Hall et al. 2019 [36]	Britain	CS	4–6	38 (24/14)	TGMD-2	LM, OC, FMS	FMS: ↔ LM: ↔ OC: ←	8
Henrique et al. 2020 [31]	Brazil	CS	3–5	472 (248/224)	TGMD-2	LM, OC	LM: ↔ OC: ←	7
Jiang et al. 2018 [40]	China	CS	3–6	60 (30/30)	TGMD-2	LM, OC, FMS	FMS: ↔ LM: ↔ OC: ↔	6
Kim et al. 2016 [52]	Korean	CS	5–6	216 (102/114)	TGMD-2	LM, OC	LM: ↔ OC: ←	5
Kit et al. 2017 [63]	United States	CS	3–5	LM: 330 (167/163) OC: 338 (170/168)	TGMD-2	LM, OC	LM: → OC: ←	7
Korbecki et al. 2017 [54]	Poland	CS	6	64 (35/29)	TGMD-2	LM, OC	LM: ↔ OC: ←	5
Kordi et al. 2012 [46]	Iran	QE	4–6	147 (75/72)	TGMD-2	LM, OC	LM: ↔ OC: ↔	7
Lopes et al. 2017 [57]	Portugal	CS	5–6	57 (26/31)	TGMD-2	LM, OC	LM: ↔ OC: ←	8
Mukherjee et al. 2017 [59]	Singapore	CS	6	95 (50/45)	TGMD-2	LM, OC	LM: ↔ OC: ←	6
Nikolić et al. 2016 [44]	Croatia	CS	4–4.5	67 (34/33)	TGMD-1	LM, OC, FMS	FMS: → LM: ↔ OC: ←	5
Palmer et al. 2020 [64]	USA	QE	3.5–5	54 (27/27)	TGMD-2	LM, OC, FMS	FMS: ↔ LM: ↔ OC: ↔	8
Roscoe et al. 2019 [37]	Britain	CS	3–4	185 (97/81)	TGMD-2	LM, OC, FMS	FMS: ↔ LM: ↔ OC: ↔	6
Saczuk et al. 2021 [55]	Poland	CS	5	441 (255/186)	TGMD-2	LM, OC	LM: → OC: ↔	5
Shi et al. 2020 [41]	China	RCT	5–6	43 (22/21)	TGMD-2	LM, OC, FMS	FMS: ↔ LM: ↔ OC: ←	9
Soares et al. 2020 [32]	Brazil	CS	3–5	251 (127/124)	TGMD-2	LM, OC, FMS	FMS: ← LM: ↔ OC: ←	7
Tietjens et al. 2018 [45]	Germany	CS	3–6	27 (11/16)	TGMD-3	LM, OC	LM: ↔ OC: ←	6
Tomaz et al. 2019 (1) [60]	South African	CS	3–6	259 (130/129)	TGMD-2	LM, OC, FMS	FMS: ← LM: ↔ OC: ←	7

Table 1. *Cont.*

Author	Country	Design	Sample Age	N (Boy/Girl)	Scale	Test Items	Outcome	Assessment
Tomaz et al. 2019 (2) [61]	South African	CS	3–5	78 (39/39)	TGMD-2	LM, OC, FMS	FMS: ↔ LM: ↔ OC: ←	8
Valentini et al. 2012 [33]	Brazil	CS	3–6	LM: 786 (394/392) OC: 796 (394/402)	TGMD-2-BR	LM, OC	LM: ↔ OC: ←	6
Valentini et al. 2017 [34]	Brazil	CS	3–6	281 (135/146)	TGMD-3-BR	LM, OC	LM: ↔ OC: ←	6
Wang et al. 2020 [42]	China	Cs	3–6	268 (126/142)	TGMD-3	LM, OC, FMS	FMS: ↔ LM: ↔ OC: ↔	8
Webster et al. 2019 [65]	USA	CS	3–4	126 (58/68)	TGMD-3	LM, OC, FMS	FMS: ← LM: ↔ OC: ←	7
Wong & Cheung 2006 [43]	China	CS	3–6	797 (424/373)	TGMD-2	LM, OC	LM: ↔ OC: ←	7

CS: cross-sectional; CC: case–control; QE: quasi-experimental; Cs: cohort study RCT: randomized control trial; TGMD: test of gross motor development; FMS: fundamental movement skills; LM: locomotor skill; OC: object control skill; ←: favors boys; →: favors girls; ↔: no difference.

3.3. Gender Difference in Total FMS

Sixteen studies assessed total FMS [30,32,35–37,39–42,44,49,58,60,61,64,65], including 1351 boys and 1247 girls. Figure 2 displays the forest plots of standardized mean differences and 95% CI for the total FMS score (16 studies) based on the random effects meta-analysis results. Significant differences favor boys vs. girls (SMD = 0.17 (95% CI 0.03, 0.31), p = 0.02, I^2 = 64).

Study or Subgroup	Favours girls Mean	SD	Total	Favours boys Mean	SD	Total	Weight	Std. Mean Difference IV, Random, 95% CI
Alessandro et al. 2018	61	11.2	82	56.4	8.9	76	6.8%	0.45 [0.13, 0.77]
Aponte et al. 1990	26.57	5.89	102	24.81	6.3	98	7.4%	0.29 [0.01, 0.57]
Behan et al. 2019	72.08	15.65	200	71.84	14.34	157	8.6%	0.02 [-0.19, 0.22]
Cheung et al. 2020	67.57	8.82	162	68.56	7.48	133	8.2%	-0.12 [-0.35, 0.11]
Hall et al. 2018	45.73	13.01	91	45.88	10.75	75	7.0%	-0.01 [-0.32, 0.29]
Hall et al. 2019	61.19	8.56	24	58.01	8.56	14	3.1%	0.36 [-0.30, 1.03]
Jiang et al. 2018	54.24	11.45	30	51.29	10.88	30	4.3%	0.26 [-0.25, 0.77]
Nikolić et al. 2016	34.47	13.37	34	42.15	14.55	33	4.6%	-0.54 [-1.03, -0.06]
Palmer et al. 2020	19.8	9.8	27	16.7	9.2	27	4.1%	0.32 [-0.22, 0.86]
Roscoe et al. 2019	50.2	15.5	97	53.5	14.6	81	7.2%	-0.22 [-0.51, 0.08]
Shi et al. 2020	54.82	4.55	22	52.47	6.46	21	3.5%	0.41 [-0.19, 1.02]
Soares et al. 2020	37.59	11.07	127	34.15	10.82	124	7.9%	0.31 [0.06, 0.56]
Tomaz et al. 2019 (1)	67.9	8.9	130	63	10.5	129	8.0%	0.50 [0.25, 0.75]
Tomaz et al. 2019 (2)	76.1	5.7	39	74.1	5	39	5.0%	0.37 [-0.08, 0.82]
Wang et al. 2020	45.97	16.34	126	45.1	16.92	142	8.1%	0.05 [-0.19, 0.29]
Webster et al. 2019	40.6	12.3	58	35.2	10.7	68	6.2%	0.47 [0.11, 0.82]
Total (95% CI)			**1351**			**1247**	**100.0%**	**0.17 [0.03, 0.31]**

Heterogeneity: Tau² = 0.05; Chi² = 41.85, df = 15 (P = 0.0002); I² = 64%
Test for overall effect: Z = 2.41 (P = 0.02)

Figure 2. Forest plot of total FMS scores [30,32,35–37,39–42,44,49,58,60,61,64,65].

3.4. Gender Difference in Locomotor Skills

Thirty-seven articles (thirty-eight studies) assessed proficiency in locomotor skills [28–57,59–65], including 4290 boys and 4087 girls. Figure 3 displays the forest plots of standardized mean differences and 95% CI for the locomotor skills score (38 studies) based on the random effects meta-analysis results. Gender differences in locomotor skill proficiency approached significance, trending in favor of girls (SMD = −0.07 (95 % CI −0.15, 0.01), p = 0.09, I^2 = 66%).

3.5. Gender Difference in Object Control Skills

Thirty-seven articles (thirty-eight studies) assessed proficiency in object control skills [28–57,59–65], including 4291 boys and 4103 girls. Figure 4 displays forest plots of the standardized mean differences and 95% CI for the object control skills score (38 studies) based on the random effects meta-analysis results. Significant differences were found, favoring boys vs. girls (SMD = 0.48 (95% CI 0.38, 0.58), p < 0.00001). Meta-regression displays that age is associated with gender differences in object control skills (p < 0.05). To further explore the effect of age, we divided studies with age-specific assessments into a 3 year-old group, a 4 year-old group, a 5 year-old group and a 6 year-old group. In subgroup analyses (Figure 5), we found marginally significant results favoring boys vs. girls in children aged 3 (SMD = 0.27 (95% CI 0.00, 0.54), p = 0.05) and significant results favoring boys vs. girls aged 4, 5 and 6 years (SMD = 0.58 (95% CI 0.38, 0.77), p < 0.00001; SMD = 0.59 (95% CI 0.31, 0.88), p < 0.00001; SMD = 0.81 (95% CI 0.61, 1.01), p < 0.00001), which increased with age.

3.6. Sensitivity Analysis and Publication Bias

After excluding 39 studies one by one, it was found that there was no significant change in the magnitude or direction of differences in the proficiency of children of different genders in terms of FMS, locomotor skills or object control skills.

Egger's test was used to assess publication bias in FMS, locomotor skills and object control skills. The results showed that none of the studies included in the above review had publication bias (p > 0.05), as shown in Table 2.

Table 2. The result of publication bias estimation.

Item	Coef.	Std. Err.	t	$p > |t|$	95% Conf. Interval	
FMS	0.8661726	1.340221	0.65	0.529	−2.008316	3.740662
LM	−0.2382333	0.6962142	−0.34	0.734	−1.650221	1.173755
OC	−0.4231878	0.8376626	−0.51	0.616	−2.122046	1.275671

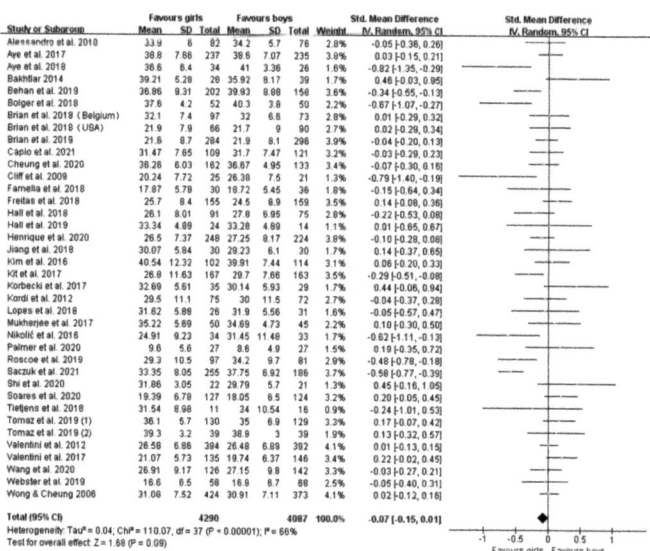

Figure 3. Forest plot of locomotor skills scores [28–57,59–65].

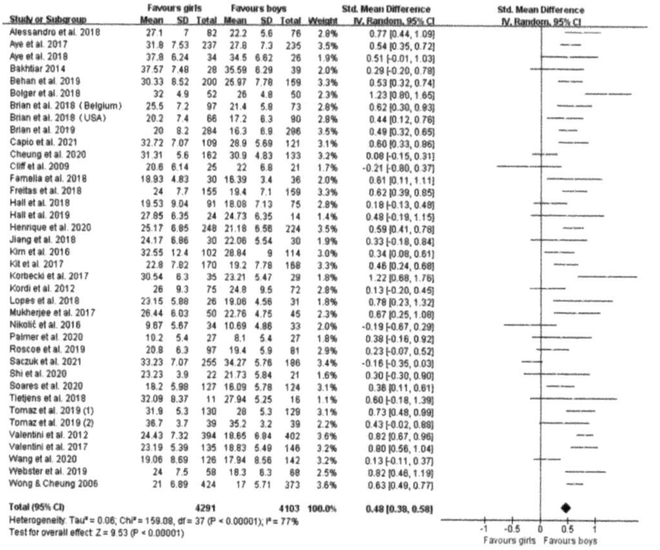

Figure 4. Forest plot of object control skills scores [28–57,59–65].

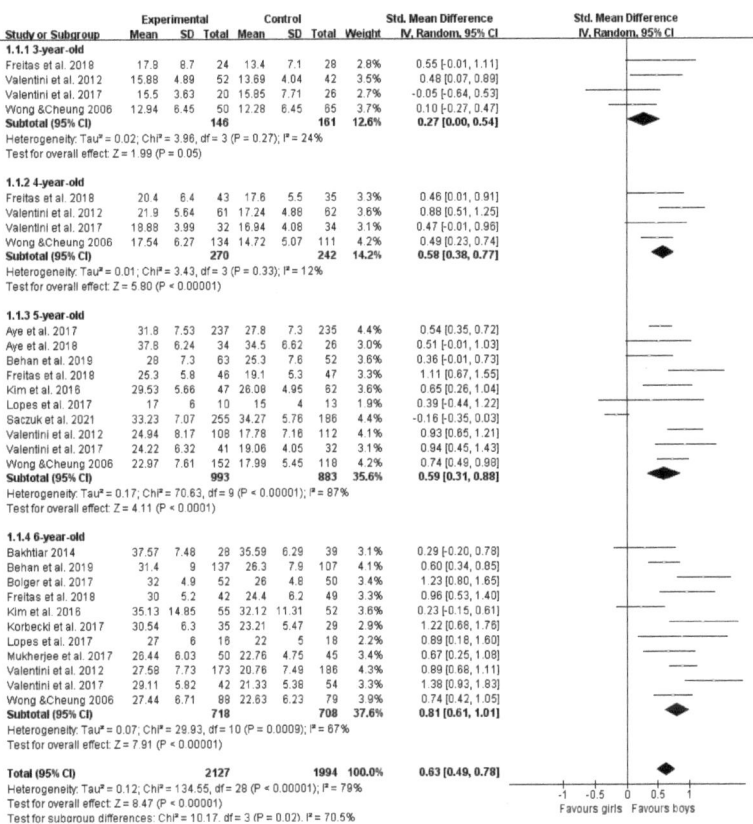

Figure 5. Forest plot of object control skills (age subgroups) [28–57,59–65].

4. Discussion

This systematic review and meta-analysis aggregated studies from Asia (China [38–43], Iran [46], Indonesia [47,48], Korean [52], Myanmar [53], Japan [51] and Singapore [59]), Africa (South Africa [60,61]), Europe (Belgium [29], Britain [35–37], Croatia [44], Germany [45], Ireland [49,50], Poland [54,55] and Portugal [56,57]), North America (the United States (US) [29,62–65] and Puerto Rico), Oceania (Australia [28]) and South America (Brazil [30–34]) and demonstrated gender differences in FMS proficiency in children aged 3–6 years. Combined results show that boys are more proficient than girls in total FMS proficiency. From the two dimensions of proficiency in locomotor skills and in object control skills, marginally significant differences were found favoring girls, and significant differences were found favoring boys in object control skills.

Differences in proficiency in object control skills between boys and girls seem to take some cues from biology. A study reported that boys are more likely to use finely segmented pelvic–torso–shoulder rotation when throwing [66]. Young explained the differences in human throwing and hitting behavior from an evolutionary perspective. Early humans made a living by throwing stones and swinging clubs. Women invested more resources into reproduction, and men were more likely to be hunters and warriors. These kinds of patterns are inherited through natural selection [67]. A previous study speculates that mature throwing is more likely an innate skill whose development is biologically determined and somewhat difficult to be influenced by nurture, and the same may be true of striking [68]. Sociological factors and behavior habits may also contribute to gender differences in proficiency in object control. Physical education programs are important for the development of FMS in preschoolers. Research shows that structured physical activity lessons can improve children's FMS [69]. A meta-analysis shows that three or more teacher-led physical activity sessions per week significantly improved FMS [11]. Furthermore, studies have shown a correlation between FMS proficiency and physical activity levels in children. A study using TGMD-2 and accelerometers measured data on FMS and physical activity in kindergartners and found a positive relationship between object control skills and moderate-intensity physical activity (MVPA) [70]. However, it has been shown that girls are significantly less likely to participate in physical activity than boys during the preschool years, especially at moderate to high intensity [71]. A systematic review including 10,316 children aged 3–6 years (5236 boys and 5080 girls) demonstrated that boys were more physically active than girls [72]. A survey in Norway showed that among children aged 3–4, only 32% of girls and 67% of boys were able to achieve the recommended 60 min of moderate to vigorous physical activity per day [73]. Therefore, different levels of physical activity may be responsible for the gender differences in object control scores. In addition, differences in exercise content may also contribute to gender differences in object control. A cross-sectional study from Japan showed that 5 year-old boys had significantly higher raw scores in terms of object control than girls of the same age (37.8 ± 6.24 vs. 34.5 ± 6.62, respectively), which is consistent with our findings, and the difference is mainly reflected in hitting, kicking and throwing [51]. A study in Australia showed that girls opted for dance and aerobic exercises far more often than boys [74]. A study found that Taiwanese girls prefer to play hopscotch, balance beam and house, while boys prefer ball games and slapstick games [75]. Previous studies have indicated that girls tend to lack opportunities to practice ball games, while boys generally spend more time participating in these games [76,77], which may also be related to parental educational attitudes [78]. In addition, an interesting study in Canada showed that 5 year-old girls' perception of physical ability was related to their proficiency in locomotor skills, but not to object control skills, which may be because girls do not value object control skills [79].

Object control skills are more important than locomotor skills in childhood and continue to affect adolescence [44]. Evidence shows that gender disparities are reduced if girls have the same opportunities for mentoring, feedback, practice and encouragement [64]. Our meta-regression analysis revealed that age was the main factor influencing differences in proficiency in object control skills between boys and girls. Using subgroup analysis to further explore the effect of age, we found that gender differences in children's proficiency in object control skill tend to be significant at age 3, and the advantage tends to favor boys. The difference is significant at the age of 4, and the advantage of boys begins to gradually increase with age, reaching a maximum at the age of 6. We recommend that parents and teachers should start paying attention to children's movements when they are 3 years old and consciously guide children's sports participation types; in particular, girls are encouraged to participate in ball games. Scholars should comprehensively consider the growth and development patterns, types of exercise and professional guidance of boys and girls when studying FMS guidance plans for children.

This meta-analysis provides evidence for gender differences in FMS proficiency in children aged 3–6 years, but some limitations should be considered. First, there are fewer articles and a smaller sample size for children aged 3 and 4 years, which requires more data to confirm. Second, our study only included children aged 3–6 years, and gender differences in FMS in children of other ages are also an important topic. Third, due to the limited number of articles, the study could not be specific to each item in the TGMD subscale (e.g., running, jumping, dribbling, etc.). Studies on specific TGMD items will therefore also be an interesting and useful topic as the number of high-quality studies increases. Finally, because TGMD is the most common tool for measuring FMS proficiency in educational, clinical and research settings, our study only included articles using TGMD or any modified version (TGMD-2 or TGMD-3), but this may have led to inconsistent results. Currently, assessments of children's FMS competencies are primarily conducted through process-oriented and product-oriented approaches. TGMD is a process-oriented assessment that examines children's motor performance on locomotor and object control tasks. We suggest that future research use product-oriented tools to further explore the gendered characteristics of FMS proficiency in young children.

5. Conclusions

Our findings demonstrated that there were gender differences in total FMS proficiency in children aged 3–6, with boys being more proficient than girls, and locomotor proficiency differences between gender approached significance, with a trend favoring girls. In the performance of proficiency in object control skills, boys were better than girls, and this difference gradually increased with age. We recommend focusing on and developing girls' object control skills starting at age 3.

Supplementary Materials: The following supporting information can be downloaded at: https://www.mdpi.com/article/10.3390/ijerph19148318/s1.

Author Contributions: Conceptualization: Y.Z. and W.Y.; methodology: Y.Z. and Y.L.; software: Y.Z. and Y.L.; validation: M.K. and F.H.; formal analysis: Y.Z., W.Y. and Y.L.; investigation: Y.Z. and M.K.; resources: W.Y.; data curation: W.Y., Y.L. and F.H.; writing—original draft preparation: Y.Z.; writing—review and editing: M.K., Y.L. and F.H.; visualization: Y.Z.; supervision: W.Y.; project administration: Y.Z. All authors have read and agreed to the published version of the manuscript.

Funding: This study was supported by the grant (KYH06Y21383) provided by Open Research Fund of College of Teacher Education, for the early development of infants and children aged 0–3 years old in China: A study on the characteristics and evaluation of physical and motor development.

Institutional Review Board Statement: Not applicable.

Informed Consent Statement: Not applicable.

Data Availability Statement: Not applicable.

Acknowledgments: The authors are thankful to the Institute of Human Movement and Sports Engineering, Zhejiang Normal University for support.

Conflicts of Interest: The authors declare no conflict of interest.

References

1. Psaltopoulou, T.; Tzanninis, S.; Ntanasis-Stathopoulos, I.; Panotopoulos, G.; Kostopoulou, M.; Tzanninis, I.G.; Tsagianni, A.; Sergentanis, T.N. Prevention and treatment of childhood and adolescent obesity: A systematic review of meta-analyses. *World J. Pediatr.* **2019**, *15*, 350–381. [CrossRef] [PubMed]
2. Arhab, A.; Messerli-Bürgy, N.; Kakebeeke, T.H.; Stülb, K.; Zysset, A.; Leeger-Aschmann, C.S.; Schmutz, E.A.; Meyer, A.H.; Munsch, S.; Kriemler, S.; et al. Association of physical activity with adiposity in preschoolers using different clinical adiposity measures: A cross-sectional study. *BMC Pediatr.* **2019**, *19*, 397. [CrossRef] [PubMed]
3. Loprinzi, P.D.; Cardinal, B.J.; Loprinzi, K.L.; Lee, H. Benefits and environmental determinants of physical activity in children and adolescents. *Obes. Facts* **2012**, *5*, 597–610. [CrossRef]
4. Eime, R.M.; Young, J.A.; Harvey, J.T.; Charity, M.J.; Payne, W.R. A systematic review of the psychological and social benefits of participation in sport for children and adolescents: Informing development of a conceptual model of health through sport. *Int. J. Behav. Nutr. Phys. Act.* **2013**, *10*, 98. [CrossRef]
5. Martin, A.; Booth, J.N.; Laird, Y.; Sproule, J.; Reilly, J.J.; Saunders, D.H. Physical activity, diet and other behavioural interventions for improving cognition and school achievement in children and adolescents with obesity or overweight. *Cochrane Database Syst. Rev.* **2018**. [CrossRef] [PubMed]
6. Donnelly, J.E.; Hillman, C.H.; Castelli, D.; Etnier, J.L.; Lee, S.; Tomporowski, P.; Lambourne, K.; Szabo-Reed, A.N. Physical activity, fitness, cognitive function, and academic achievement in children: A systematic review. *Med. Sci. Sports Exerc.* **2016**, *48*, 1197. [CrossRef]
7. Tremblay, M.S.; Gray, C.E.; Akinroye, K.; Harrington, D.M.; Katzmarzyk, P.T.; Lambert, E.V.; Prista, A. Physical activity of children: A global matrix of grades comparing 15 countries. *J. Phys. Act. Health* **2014**, *11*, S113–S125. [CrossRef]
8. Stodden, D.F.; Goodway, J.D.; Langendorfer, S.J.; Roberton, M.A.; Rudisill, M.E.; Garcia, C.; Garcia, L.E. A developmental perspective on the role of motor skill competence in physical activity: An emergent relationship. *Quest* **2008**, *60*, 290–306. [CrossRef]
9. Lubans, D.R.; Morgan, P.J.; Cliff, D.P.; Barnett, L.M.; Okely, A.D. Fundamental movement skills in children and adolescents. *Sports Med.* **2010**, *40*, 1019–1035. [CrossRef]

10. Williams, H.G.; Pfeiffer, K.A.; O'neill, J.R.; Dowda, M.; McIver, K.L.; Brown, W.H.; Pate, R.R. Motor skill performance and physical activity in preschool children. *Obesity* **2008**, *16*, 1421–1426. [CrossRef]
11. Engel, A.C.; Broderick, C.R.; van Doorn, N.; Hardy, L.L.; Parmenter, B.J. Exploring the relationship between fundamental motor skill interventions and physical activity levels in children: A systematic review and meta-analysis. *Sports Med.* **2018**, *48*, 1845–1857. [CrossRef] [PubMed]
12. Wick, K.; Leeger-Aschmann, C.S.; Monn, N.D.; Radtke, T.; Ott, L.V.; Rebholz, C.E.; Cruz, S.; Gerber, N.; Schmutz, E.A.; Puder, J.J. Interventions to promote fundamental movement skills in childcare and kindergarten: A systematic review and meta-analysis. *Sports Med.* **2017**, *47*, 2045–2068. [CrossRef] [PubMed]
13. Logan, S.W.; Ross, S.M.; Chee, K.; Stodden, D.F.; Robinson, L.E. Fundamental motor skills: A systematic review of terminology. *J. Sports Sci.* **2018**, *36*, 781–796. [CrossRef]
14. Zhang, L.; Cheung, P. Making a difference in PE lessons: Using a low organized games approach to teach fundamental motor skills in China. *Int. J. Environ. Res. Public Health* **2019**, *16*, 4618. [CrossRef]
15. Behan, S.; Belton, S.; Peers, C.; O'connor, N.E.; Issartel, J. Exploring the relationships between fundamental movement skills and health related fitness components in children. *Eur. J. Sport Sci.* **2022**, *22*, 171–181. [CrossRef]
16. Bolger, L.E.; Bolger, L.A.; O'Neill, C.; Coughlan, E.; O'Brien, W.; Lacey, S.; Burns, C.; Bardid, F. Global levels of fundamental motor skills in children: A systematic review. *J. Sports Sci.* **2021**, *39*, 717–753. [CrossRef] [PubMed]
17. Wang, G.; Zi, Y.; Li, B.; Su, S.; Sun, L.; Wang, F.; Ren, C.; Liu, Y. The Effect of Physical Exercise on Fundamental Movement Skills and Physical Fitness among Preschool Children: Study Protocol for a Cluster-Randomized Controlled Trial. *Int. J. Environ. Res. Public Health* **2022**, *19*, 6331. [CrossRef]
18. Robinson, L.E. The relationship between perceived physical competence and fundamental motor skills in preschool children. *Child Care Health Dev.* **2011**, *37*, 589–596. [CrossRef]
19. Robinson, L.E.; Wadsworth, D.D.; Peoples, C.M. Correlates of school-day physical activity in preschool students. *Res. Q. Exerc. Sport* **2012**, *83*, 20–26. [CrossRef]
20. Niemistö, D.; Finni, T.; Cantell, M.; Korhonen, E.; Sääkslahti, A. Individual, family, and environmental correlates of motor competence in young children: Regression model analysis of data obtained from two motor tests. *Int. J. Environ. Res. Public Health* **2020**, *17*, 2548. [CrossRef]
21. Barnett, L.M.; Van Beurden, E.; Morgan, P.J.; Brooks, L.O.; Beard, J.R. Gender differences in motor skill proficiency from childhood to adolescence: A longitudinal study. *Res. Q. Exerc. Sport* **2010**, *81*, 162–170. [CrossRef]
22. Temple, V.A.; Crane, J.R.; Brown, A.; Williams, B.-L.; Bell, R.I. Recreational activities and motor skills of children in kindergarten. *Phys. Educ. Sport Pedagog.* **2016**, *21*, 268–280. [CrossRef]
23. Page, M.J.; McKenzie, J.E.; Bossuyt, P.M.; Boutron, I.; Hoffmann, T.C.; Mulrow, C.D.; Shamseer, L.; Tetzlaff, J.M.; Akl, E.A.; Brennan, S.E.; et al. The PRISMA 2020 statement: An updated guideline for reporting systematic reviews. *Syst. Rev.* **2021**, *10*, 89. [CrossRef]
24. Moola, S.; Munn, Z.; Tufanaru, C.; Aromataris, E.; Mu, P.F. Chapter 7: Systematic Reviews of Etiology and Risk. In *JBI Manual for Evidence Synthesis*; Aromataris, E., Munn, Z., Eds.; JBI: Adelaide, Australia, 2020.
25. Cohen, J. *Statistical Power Analysis for the Behavioral Sciences*; Academic Press: Cambridge, MA, USA, 1988.
26. Higgins, J.P.; Thompson, S.G.; Deeks, J.J.; Altman, D.G. Measuring inconsistency in meta-analyses. *BMJ* **2003**, *327*, 557–560. [CrossRef]
27. Higgins, J.P.; Deeks, J.; Higgins, J.; Green, S. Chapter 7: Selecting studies and collecting data. In *Cochrane Handbook of Systematic Reviews of Interventions*; Version 5.1.0; Updated March 2011; Cochrane Collaboration: London, UK, 2011.
28. Cliff, D.P.; Okely, A.D.; Smith, L.M.; McKeen, K. Relationships between fundamental movement skills and objectively measured physical activity in preschool children. *Pediatric Exerc. Sci.* **2009**, *21*, 436–449. [CrossRef] [PubMed]
29. Brian, A.; Bardid, F.; Barnett, L.M.; Deconinck, F.J.; Lenoir, M.; Goodway, J.D. Actual and perceived motor competence levels of Belgian and United States preschool children. *J. Mot. Learn. Dev.* **2018**, *6*, S320–S336. [CrossRef]
30. Ré, A.H.; Logan, S.W.; Cattuzzo, M.T.; Henrique, R.S.; Tudela, M.C.; Stodden, D.F. Comparison of motor competence levels on two assessments across childhood. *J. Sports Sci.* **2018**, *36*, 1–6. [CrossRef] [PubMed]
31. Henrique, R.S.; Stodden, D.F.; Fransen, J.; Feitoza, A.H.; Ré, A.H.; Martins, C.M.; Dos Prazeres, T.M.; Cattuzzo, M.T. Is motor competence associated with the risk of central obesity in preschoolers? *Am. J. Hum. Biol.* **2020**, *32*, e23460. [CrossRef]
32. Soares, Í.A.A.; Martins, C.M.d.L.; Nobre, G.C.; Cattuzzo, M.T. Evidences of construct validity, criteria and validation of the motor competence assessment batery of tests in preschoolers. *J. Phys. Educ.* **2020**, *31*. [CrossRef]
33. Valentini, N.C. Validity and reliability of the TGMD-2 for Brazilian children. *J. Mot. Behav.* **2012**, *44*, 275–280. [CrossRef]
34. Valentini, N.C.; Zanella, L.W.; Webster, E.K. Test of Gross Motor Development—Third edition: Establishing content and construct validity for Brazilian children. *J. Mot. Learn. Dev.* **2017**, *5*, 15–28. [CrossRef]
35. Hall, C.J.; Eyre, E.L.; Oxford, S.W.; Duncan, M.J. Relationships between motor competence, physical activity, and obesity in British preschool aged children. *J. Funct. Morphol. Kinesiol.* **2018**, *3*, 57. [CrossRef] [PubMed]
36. Hall, C.J.; Eyre, E.L.; Oxford, S.W.; Duncan, M.J. Does perception of motor competence mediate associations between motor competence and physical activity in early years children? *Sports* **2019**, *7*, 77. [CrossRef] [PubMed]
37. Roscoe, C.M.; James, R.S.; Duncan, M.J. Accelerometer-based physical activity levels, fundamental movement skills and weight status in British preschool children from a deprived area. *Eur. J. Pediatrics* **2019**, *178*, 1043–1052. [CrossRef]

38. Capio, C.M.; Eguia, K.F. Movement skills, perception, and physical activity of young children: A mediation analysis. *Pediatrics Int.* **2021**, *63*, 442–447. [CrossRef]
39. Cheung, P.; Zhang, L. Environment for Preschool Children to Learn Fundamental Motor Skills: The Role of Teaching Venue and Class Size. *Sustainability* **2020**, *12*, 9774. [CrossRef]
40. Jiang, G.-P.; Jiao, X.-B.; Wu, S.-K.; Ji, Z.-Q.; Liu, W.-T.; Chen, X.; Wang, H.-H. Balance, proprioception, and gross motor development of chinese children aged 3 to 6 years. *J. Mot. Behav.* **2018**, *50*, 343–352. [CrossRef]
41. Shi, K.; Sun, X.; Wang, Y.; Zha, P. Effects of gymnastics intervention on gross motor development in children aged 5 to 6 years: A randomized, controlled trial. *Med. Dello Sport* **2020**, *73*, 327–336. [CrossRef]
42. Wang, H.; Chen, Y.; Liu, J.; Sun, H.; Gao, W. A follow-up study of motor skill development and its determinants in preschool children from middle-income family. *BioMed Res. Int.* **2020**, *2020*, 6639341. [CrossRef]
43. Wong, A.K.Y.; Cheung, S.Y. Gross Motor Skills Performance of Hong Kong Chinese Children. *Asian J. Phys. Educ. Recreat.* **2006**, *12*, 23–29. [CrossRef]
44. Nikolić, I.; Mraković, S.; Kunješić, M. Gender differences of preschool children in fundamental movement skills. *Croat. J. Educ.* **2016**, *18*, 123–131. [CrossRef]
45. Tietjens, M.; Dreiskaemper, D.; Utesch, T.; Schott, N.; Barnett, L.M.; Hinkley, T. Pictorial scale of physical self-concept for younger children (P-PSC-C): A feasibility study. *J. Mot. Learn. Dev.* **2018**, *6*, S391–S402. [CrossRef]
46. Kordi, R.; Nourian, R.; Ghayour, M.; Kordi, M.; Younesian, A. Development and evaluation of a basic physical and sports activity program for preschool children in nursery schools in Iran: An interventional study. *Iran. J. Pediatrics* **2012**, *22*, 357. [CrossRef]
47. Bakhtiar, S. Fundamental motor skill among 6-year-old children in Padang, West Sumatera, Indonesia. *Asian Soc. Sci.* **2014**, *10*, 155–158. [CrossRef]
48. Famelia, R.; Tsuda, E.; Bakhtiar, S.; Goodway, J.D. Relationships among perceived and actual motor skill competence and physical activity in Indonesian preschoolers. *J. Mot. Learn. Dev.* **2018**, *6*, S403–S423. [CrossRef]
49. Behan, S.; Belton, S.; Peers, C.; O'Connor, N.E.; Issartel, J. Moving Well-Being Well: Investigating the maturation of fundamental movement skill proficiency across sex in Irish children aged five to twelve. *J. Sports Sci.* **2019**, *37*, 2604–2612. [CrossRef]
50. Bolger, L.E.; Bolger, L.A.; O'Neill, C.; Coughlan, E.; O'Brien, W.; Lacey, S.; Burns, C. Age and sex differences in fundamental movement skills among a cohort of Irish school children. *J. Mot. Learn. Dev.* **2018**, *6*, 81–100. [CrossRef]
51. Aye, T.; Kuramoto-Ahuja, T.; Sato, T.; Sadakiyo, K.; Watanabe, M.; Maruyama, H. Gross motor skill development of kindergarten children in Japan. *J. Phys. Ther. Sci.* **2018**, *30*, 711–715. [CrossRef]
52. Kim, C.-I.; Lee, K.-Y. The relationship between fundamental movement skills and body mass index in Korean preschool children. *Eur. Early Child. Educ. Res. J.* **2016**, *24*, 928–935. [CrossRef]
53. Aye, T.; Oo, K.S.; Khin, M.T.; Kuramoto-Ahuja, T.; Maruyama, H. Gross motor skill development of 5-year-old Kindergarten children in Myanmar. *J. Phys. Ther. Sci.* **2017**, *29*, 1772–1778. [CrossRef]
54. Korbecki, M.; Wawrzyniak, S.; Rokita, A. Fundamental movement skills of six-to seven-year-old children in the first grade of elementary school: A pilot study. *Balt. J. Health Phys. Act.* **2017**, *9*, 2. [CrossRef]
55. Saczuk, J.; Wasiluk, A. Assesment of the relationship between fitness abilities and motor skills of 5-year-olds by taking into account dimorphic differences. *J. Phys. Educ. Sport* **2021**, *21*, 115–121. [CrossRef]
56. Freitas, D.; Lausen, B.; Maia, J.; Gouveia, É.; Antunes, A.; Thomis, M.; Lefevre, J.; Malina, R. Skeletal maturation, fundamental motor skills, and motor performance in preschool children. *Scand. J. Med. Sci. Sports* **2018**, *28*, 2358–2368. [CrossRef] [PubMed]
57. Lopes, V.P.; Saraiva, L.; Rodrigues, L.P. Reliability and construct validity of the test of gross motor development-2 in Portuguese children. *Int. J. Sport Exerc. Psychol.* **2018**, *16*, 250–260. [CrossRef]
58. Aponte, R.; French, R.; Sherrill, C. Motor development of Puerto Rican children: Cross-cultural perspectives. *Percept. Mot. Ski.* **1990**, *71*, 1200–1202. [CrossRef]
59. Mukherjee, S.; Ting Jamie, L.C.; Fong, L.H. Fundamental motor skill proficiency of 6-to 9-year-old Singaporean children. *Percept. Mot. Ski.* **2017**, *124*, 584–600. [CrossRef]
60. Tomaz, S.; Jones, R.A.; Hinkley, T.; Bernstein, S.; Twine, R.; Kahn, K.; Norris, S.A.; Draper, C.E. Gross motor skills of South African preschool-aged children across different income settings. *J. Sci. Med. Sport* **2019**, *22*, 689–694. [CrossRef]
61. Tomaz, S.A.; Prioreschi, A.; Watson, E.D.; McVeigh, J.A.; Rae, D.E.; Jones, R.A.; Draper, C.E. Body mass index, physical activity, sedentary behavior, sleep, and gross motor skill proficiency in preschool children from a low-to middle-income urban setting. *J. Phys. Act. Health* **2019**, *16*, 525–532. [CrossRef]
62. Brian, A.; Pennell, A.; Taunton, S.; Starrett, A.; Howard-Shaughnessy, C.; Goodway, J.D.; Wadsworth, D.; Rudisill, M.; Stodden, D. Motor competence levels and developmental delay in early childhood: A multicenter cross-sectional study conducted in the USA. *Sports Med.* **2019**, *49*, 1609–1618. [CrossRef]
63. Kit, B.K.; Akinbami, L.J.; Isfahani, N.S.; Ulrich, D.A. Gross motor development in children aged 3–5 years, United States 2012. *Matern. Child Health J.* **2017**, *21*, 1573–1580. [CrossRef]
64. Palmer, K.K.; Harkavy, D.; Rock, S.M.; Robinson, L.E. Boys and girls have similar gains in fundamental motor skills across a preschool motor skill intervention. *J. Mot. Learn. Dev.* **2020**, *8*, 569–579. [CrossRef]
65. Webster, E.K.; Martin, C.K.; Staiano, A.E. Fundamental motor skills, screen-time, and physical activity in preschoolers. *J. Sport Health Sci.* **2019**, *8*, 114–121. [CrossRef] [PubMed]

66. Butterfield, S.A.; Angell, R.M.; Mason, C.A. Age and sex differences in object control skills by children ages 5 to 14. *Percept. Mot. Ski.* **2012**, *114*, 261–274. [CrossRef]
67. Young, R.W. The ontogeny of throwing and striking. *Hum. Ontog. Int. J. Interdiscip. Dev. Res.* **2009**, *3*, 19–31. [CrossRef]
68. Angell, R.M.; Butterfield, S.A.; Tu, S.; Loovis, E.M.; Mason, C.A.; Nightingale, C.J. Children's throwing and striking: A longitudinal study. *J. Mot. Learn. Dev.* **2018**, *6*, 315–332. [CrossRef]
69. Jones, R.A.; Okely, A.D.; Hinkley, T.; Batterham, M.; Burke, C. Promoting gross motor skills and physical activity in childcare: A translational randomized controlled trial. *J. Sci. Med. Sport* **2016**, *19*, 744–749. [CrossRef] [PubMed]
70. Crane, J.R.; Naylor, P.J.; Cook, R.; Temple, V.A. Do Perceptions of Competence Mediate The Relationship Between Fundamental Motor Skill Proficiency and Physical Activity Levels of Children in Kindergarten? *J. Phys. Act. Health* **2015**, *12*, 954–961. [CrossRef]
71. Pate, R.R.; Pfeiffer, K.A.; Trost, S.G.; Ziegler, P.; Dowda, M. Physical activity among children attending preschools. *Pediatrics* **2004**, *114*, 1258–1263. [CrossRef]
72. Tucker, P. The physical activity levels of preschool-aged children: A systematic review. *Early Child. Res. Q.* **2008**, *23*, 547–558. [CrossRef]
73. Andersen, E.; Borch-Jenssen, J.; Øvreås, S.; Ellingsen, H.; Jørgensen, K.A.; Moser, T. Objectively measured physical activity level and sedentary behavior in Norwegian children during a week in preschool. *Prev. Med. Rep.* **2017**, *7*, 130–135. [CrossRef]
74. Dudley, D.A.; Cotton, W.G.; Peralta, L.R.; Winslade, M. Playground activities and gender variation in objectively measured physical activity intensity in Australian primary school children: A repeated measures study. *BMC Public Health* **2018**, *18*, 1101. [CrossRef] [PubMed]
75. Tsai, C.; Yang, S. Study on the appearance of childhood games. *J. Educ. Stud.* **2012**, *46*, 1–19.
76. Ogden, C.L.; Flegal, K.M.; Carroll, M.D.; Johnson, C.L. Prevalence and trends in overweight among US children and adolescents, 1999–2000. *JAMA* **2002**, *288*, 1728–1732. [CrossRef] [PubMed]
77. Thornton, M. *Life Span Motor Development*, 4th ed.; Physiotherapy Canada: Ottawa, ON, Canada, 2006; Volume 58, p. 240. [CrossRef]
78. Fagot, B.I.; Leinbach, M.D. The young child's gender schema: Environmental input, internal organization. *Child Dev.* **1989**, *60*, 663–672. [CrossRef] [PubMed]
79. LeGear, M.; Greyling, L.; Sloan, E.; Bell, R.I.; Williams, B.L.; Naylor, P.J.; Temple, V.A. A window of opportunity? Motor skills and perceptions of competence of children in kindergarten. *Int. J. Behav. Nutr. Phys. Act.* **2012**, *9*, 29. [CrossRef]

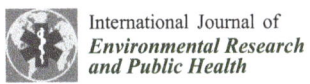

Article

Association of Body Weight and Physical Fitness during the Elementary School Years

Clemens Drenowatz [1,*], Si-Tong Chen [2], Armando Cocca [3], Gerson Ferrari [4], Gerhard Ruedl [3] and Klaus Greier [3,5]

1. Division of Sport, Physical Activity and Health, University of Education Upper Austria, 4020 Linz, Austria
2. Institute for Health and Sport, Victoria University, Melbourne 8001, Australia; sitong.chen@live.vu.edu.au
3. Department of Sport Science, University of Innsbruck, 6020 Innbruck, Austria; armando.cocca@uibk.ac.at (A.C.); gerhard.ruedl@uibk.ac.at (G.R.); nikolaus.greier@kph-es.at (K.G.)
4. Escuela de Ciencias de la Actividad Física, El Deporte y la Salud, Universidad de Santiago de Chile (USACH), Santiago 7500618, Chile; gersonferrari08@yahoo.com.br
5. Division of Physical Education and Sports, University of Education Stams—KPH-ES, 6422 Stams, Austria
* Correspondence: clemens.drenowatz@ph-ooe.at; Tel.: +43-732-7470-7426

Abstract: Physical fitness and body weight are key correlates of health. Nevertheless, an increasing number of children display poor physical fitness and high body weight. The aim of this study was to examine the prospective association of physical fitness with body weight throughout the elementary school years with a special emphasis on children with high body weight or poor physical fitness at baseline. A total of 303 Austrian children (55.1% male) completed the German motor test up to eight times over a 4-year time span (between the ages 6 and 10 years). Physical fitness did not differ across quartiles of body weight at baseline. A more pronounced weight gain, however, was associated with an impaired development of physical fitness and this association was more pronounced in children with higher baseline body weight. In addition, the detrimental effects of an impaired development of physical fitness on subsequent body weight were more pronounced in children with higher baseline body weight. No differences in the longitudinal association between body weight and physical fitness, on the other hand, were observed across quartiles of baseline fitness. These results emphasize the importance of the promotion of physical fitness, particularly in children with increased body weight, to ensure future health.

Keywords: overweight; obesity; youth; cardiorespiratory fitness; muscular strength; BMI percentile; motor competence

1. Introduction

Excess body weight is one of the major health risks in modern society due to the association with various non-communicable diseases [1,2]. Overweight/obesity during childhood is associated with cardiovascular dysfunction and asthma [3–5], in addition to psychological problems including lower self-esteem, underachievement in school, and overall quality of life [6]. Children with excess body weight are also at increased risk to become overweight/obese adults [7] and, even in the absence of overweight/obesity during adulthood, children with excess body weight have an increased risk for cardiovascular disease later in life [8].

Physical fitness, which consists of cardiorespiratory endurance, muscular strength, and endurance, in addition to flexibility and body composition, is also a critical marker of health [9]. Various components of physical fitness have been associated with beneficial effects on cardiovascular and metabolic disease risk, bone health, and psychological and cognitive outcomes, which contribute to an enhanced quality of life [9–13]. As physical fitness is defined as a person's ability to perform daily tasks without undue fatigue and adequate energy to enjoy leisure-time pursuits [14], it should also be considered a critical aspect in the promotion of an active lifestyle. The beneficial associations of physical fitness with various health parameters, however, are independent of physical activity [15], and children with a better physical fitness have a lower risk for metabolic and cardiovascular disease in adulthood independent of confounding factors [9,16]. Given these long-term effects, both physical fitness and body weight have been recognized as predictors of morbidity and mortality [9,10,17,18].

There is also extensive evidence on an inverse association between physical fitness and body weight [19–22], in addition to the independent association of these entities with several health outcomes. Longitudinal studies further showed that current body weight affects the development of physical fitness [23–25] and that poor physical fitness increases the risk for excess weight gain [23,26]. Despite considerable efforts to control excess weight gain and promote physical fitness in youth, overweight/obesity rates in children remain high and physical fitness levels have declined over the last several decades [27–29]. These trends are further associated with low motor competence in children, which is critical for the promotion of physical activity that, in turn, enhances physical fitness and facilitates weight management [30]. Given the long-term health implications, such a development not only affects the individual but also puts a substantial burden on the health care system [31–33]. Accordingly, additional actions are required to prevent the potential adverse health outcomes associated with poor physical fitness and high body weight. Recent efforts addressing low physical fitness and high body weight in children, however, have achieved limited success and it appears that a more targeted approach is warranted. This also requires a better understanding of the reciprocal association between physical fitness and body weight. The present study, therefore, examined potential differences in the cross-sectional and longitudinal association between these two entities across different levels of physical fitness and body weight in Austrian elementary school children. Given the potentially greater deficiencies in functional capacity and future health risks, a special focus was given to participants with low initial fitness and those with high body weight.

2. Materials and Methods

The study was conducted in the largest county of the federal state of Tyrol, Austria. Of the total 71 elementary schools in the county, 15 schools were selected via a random number generator and received information about the study. One school declined to participate due to organizational problems. The final sample, therefore, consisted of 14 schools that participated in data collection throughout the 4-year observation period. In order to track participants throughout their entire elementary school time, only students who were in first grade at baseline were eligible for participation. In addition, participants needed to be able to complete a physical fitness test battery, and children with mental, neurological, or physical diagnoses were excluded from the study. This resulted in a sample size of 392 children (55.4% male; age: 6.9 ± 0.5 years). The study protocol was approved by the Institutional Review Board of the University of Innsbruck (certificate of good standing, 16/2014), the school authorities of the federal state of Tyrol, and the school board of each participating school. Written parental consent was obtained prior to baseline data collection and children provided oral assent at the time of data collection. All study procedures were in accordance with the ethical standards of the Declaration of Helsinki (as amended in 2013).

Participants completed anthropometric measurements and physical fitness tests during each fall and spring semester over their four years in elementary school, which resulted in up to eight measurements throughout the entire observation period. Baseline data collection occurred during the school entry evaluation in October 2014 and the final follow-up measurements were completed in June 2018 when children were in their final grade (fourth grade) of elementary school. In order to be included in the analysis, participants needed to provide valid and complete data for at least five measurements, including at baseline and the last follow-up assessment.

Data collection occurred in the participating school's gymnasium during regular class time in a single session. Anthropometric measurements and fitness tests were administered by exercise science graduate students, who were well trained in conducting these measurements in a pediatric population during the course of a research seminar prior to data collection. A total of 14 students were involved in the measurements throughout the 4-year study period, with 6 to 7 students present during each measurement session in the schools. An overview of the procedures for each testing session is provided in Figure 1.

Anthropometry	Warm Up	Physical Fitness (German Motor Test)		Time
Body Height (cm) Body Weight (kg)	Standardized Exercise (5 min)	20m Sprint (sec)	Sit Ups (#/40 sec) Push Ups (#/40 sec) Longjump (cm) Side Jumps (#/15 sec) Back Balance (steps) Stand & Reach (cm) [Random Order]	6-Minute Run (m)

Figure 1. Data collection procedure at each measurement time.

Body height (cm) was measured with a portable stadiometer (SECA® 217, Hamburg, Germany) and weight (kg) was measured with a calibrated digital scale (SECA® 803, Hamburg, Germany) to the nearest 0.1 cm and 0.1 kg, respectively, with children wearing gym clothes and barefoot. Body mass index (BMI) was calculated (kg/m^2) and converted to BMI percentiles (BMIPCT) using German reference values [34]. Children with a BMIPCT above the 90th percentile were classified as overweight/obese. For the statistical analyses, quartiles of baseline BMI percentiles were established (Quartile 1: BMIPCT < 29.0; Quartile 2: $29 \leq$ BMIPCT < 50.2; Quartile 3: $50.2 \leq$ BMIPCT < 76; Quartile 4: BMIPCT > 76.0).

Upon the completion of anthropometric measurements, participants completed the German Motor Test (DMT6-18) [35], which has been shown to provide valid and reliable information on physical fitness in children and adolescents [35,36]. The DMT6-18 consists of eight test items that assess cardiorespiratory endurance, muscular endurance, muscular strength, power, speed and agility, and balance and flexibility. Specifically, participants performed a 6 min run, sit ups, push ups, a standing long jump, a 20 m sprint, 20 s sideways jumping, backwards balancing, and a stand and reach test, with practice trials and measured attempts as specified in the test manual. Fitness tests were administered in random order after a standardized 5 min warm up, except for the 20 m sprint, which was completed at the beginning, and the 6 min run, which was completed at the end of the test session. In addition to raw performance values, the DMT6-18 provides sex- and age-standardized scores. The average of these scores is used as an indicator for overall physical fitness, with a value of 100 indicating average physical fitness for the respective age and sex; higher scores indicate above average physical fitness and lower scores indicate below average physical fitness [35]. As shown for baseline BMIPCT, quartiles for baseline physical fitness were established based on overall physical fitness scores (Quartile 1: overall physical fitness < 100; Quartile 2: $100 \leq$ overall physical fitness < 105; Quartile 3: $105 \leq$ overall physical fitness < 108; Quartile 4: overall physical fitness ≥ 108).

Statistical Analysis. Normal distribution of the data was confirmed prior to statistical analyses. Cross-sectional associations between BMIPCT and components of physical fitness were examined via Pearson correlation analysis. Linear mixed models (LMMs) were used to determine change in BMIPCT and overall physical fitness throughout the observation period in order to account for different time intervals between measurement periods. Subsequently, ANOVA was used to examine differences in the development of BMIPCT and physical fitness across quartiles of baseline BMIPCT and baseline physical fitness, respectively. Additionally, quantile regression analyses were performed to determine the effect of change in physical fitness and BMIPCT on physical fitness and BMIPCT at follow-up, respectively, across baseline quartiles of BMIPCT and baseline quartiles of physical fitness. In addition to change in BMIPCT or physical fitness (based on LMM), baseline

BMIPCT and physical fitness were included in the regression models. Secondary analyses included sex as a co-variate to examine potential sex-specific associations. All statistical tests were performed in SPSS V26.0 software (SPSS Inc., IBM Corp., Armonk, NY, USA) with the significance level set at $\alpha < 0.05$.

3. Results

Of the 392 eligible participants 303 children between 6 and 8 years of age at baseline (55.1% male; 9.3% overweight/obese) provided valid measurements for at least five time points, including baseline and the last follow-up measurement. There were no differences in sex distribution and anthropometric characteristics at baseline between children included in the analyses and those excluded due to missing follow-up data. Children with sufficient follow-up measurements, however, displayed better overall physical fitness at baseline compared to those excluded (104.2 ± 5.9 vs. 100.9 ± 6.5, $p < 0.01$).

Descriptive characteristics of participants included in the analyses are shown in Table 1. Boys were taller and heavier compared to girls but there was no difference in BMIPCT. Accordingly, there was also no difference in weight status and sex distribution did not differ across quartiles of BMIPCT. There was also no sex difference in overall physical fitness and sex distribution across quartiles of physical fitness. Absolute performance for the 6 min run, sit ups, standing long jump and 20 m sprint, however, was better in boys, whereas balance and flexibility was better in girls ($p < 0.05$).

Table 1. Descriptive characteristics at baseline for the total sample and separately for boys and girls. Values are Mean ± SD.

	Total Sample (n = 303)	Girls (n = 135)	Boys (n = 166)
Age (years)	6.9 ± 0.5	6.9 ± 0.5	6.9 ± 0.5
Height (cm) **	122.4 ± 5.7	121.2 ± 5.3	123.4 ± 5.9
Weight (kg) *	24.3 ± 4.4	23.6 ± 4.2	24.8 ± 4.5
BMI percentile	51.8 ± 27.3	50.2 ± 26.4	53.0 ± 28.1
6 min run (m) **	854 ± 140	823 ± 130	879 ± 143
Sit ups (# in 40 s) **	15.1 ± 5.6	14.0 + 6.0	16.0 ± 5.2
Push ups (# in 40 s)	11.6 ± 3.7	11.5 ± 3.7	11.7 ± 3.6
Long jump (cm) **	113.5 ± 17.9	106.2 ± 15.8	119.4 ± 17.3
20 m sprint (s) **	4.8 ± 0.5	5.0 ± 0.6	4.6 ± 0.4
Side jumps (# in 15 s)	23.0 ± 5.8	22.3 ± 5.6	23.5 ± 5.9
Balance (steps) *	26.7 ± 9.8	28.0 ± 10.2	25.7 ± 9.5
Stand and reach (cm) [1],**	0.8 ± 5.6	1.9 ± 5.2	−0.1 ± 5.7
Overall fitness score (Z)	104.2 ± 5.9	103.5 ± 6.2	104.7 ± 5.6

[1] positive values indicate reaching beyond the toes, while negative values indicate not reaching toes. * sig. sex difference ($p < 0.05$); ** sig. sex difference ($p < 0.01$).

Pearson correlation analyses did not show significant cross-sectional correlations between BMIPCT and components of physical fitness at baseline, except for a low inverse association between BMIPCT and 6 min run performance (Table 2). Nevertheless, the prevalence of overweight/obesity differed significantly across fitness quartiles (Q1: 4.0%, Q2: 3.0%, Q3: 1.7%, Q4: 0.7%; $p = 0.02$). However, during the last follow-up assessment, when children were 10.4 ± 0.5 years of age, significant cross-sectional associations were observed between BMIPCT and all components of physical fitness, except for flexibility. Accordingly, overall physical fitness was negatively associated with BMIPCT (r= −0.43, $p < 0.01$) when participants were in fourth grade, whereas there was no significant correlation between overall physical fitness and BMIPCT in children when they were in first grade. In addition, low significant negative correlations between weight change and change in various components of physical fitness were observed, which also resulted in a negative association of weight change with change in overall physical fitness during the elementary school years (r = −0.25, $p < 0.01$).

Table 2. Association between body weight and physical fitness at baseline and last follow-up, and between change in body weight and change in physical fitness. Values are Pearson correlation coefficients.

		6 Min Run (m)	Sit Ups (Reps)	Push Ups (Reps)	Long-Jump (cm)	20 m Sprint (sec)	Side Jumps (Reps)	Balance (Steps)	Stand and Reach (cm)
Baseline Age: 6.9 years	BMI PCT	−0.21 **	0.02	−0.02	−0.02	−0.06	0.03	−0.06	0.12
Follow-Up Age: 10.4 years	BMI PCT	−0.36 **	−0.24 **	−0.27 **	−0.32 **	0.30 **	−0.22 **	−0.29 **	−0.01
Change (Δ 4 years)	BMI PCT	−0.15 **	−0.16 **	−0.11	−0.17 **	0.17 **	−0.13 *	−0.13 *	−0.11

* $p < 0.05$; ** $p < 0.01$; BMIPCT—BMI (body mass index) percentile; reps—repetitions in 40 s for sit ups and push ups, and repetitions in 15 s for sideways jumping.

Longitudinal analyses showed a significant increase in the prevalence of overweight/obesity from 9.3% in first grade to 17.5% in the fourth grade. Across the entire sample, participants with a higher baseline BMIPCT displayed a lower improvement in all components of physical fitness (p for trend < 0.05), except for balance and flexibility (Figure 2). Change in BMIPCT, however, did not differ across quartiles of baseline BMIPCT and baseline fitness. Accordingly, the increase in the prevalence of overweight/obesity did not differ across quartiles of physical fitness (Figure 3). There were also no differences in changes in various components of physical fitness across quartiles of baseline fitness, except for the 20 m sprint (p for trend < 0.01), where a more pronounced improvement was detected in participants with lower baseline performance.

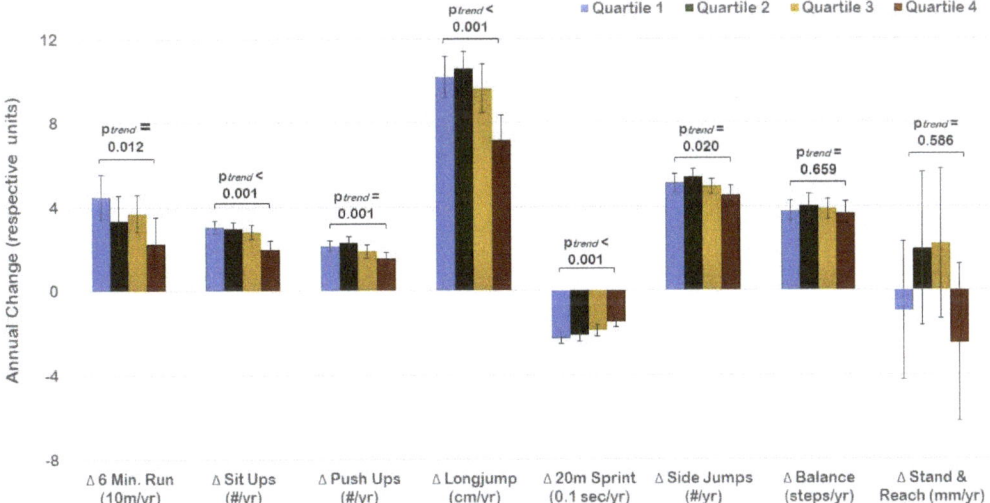

Figure 2. Change in physical fitness across quartiles of baseline BMI percentile (Quartile 1 indicates lowest BMI percentiles). Values are Mean with 95% CI.

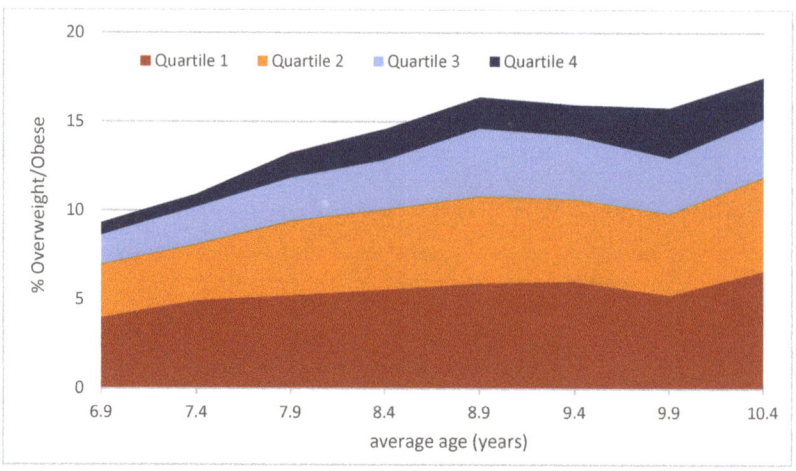

Figure 3. Cumulative prevalence of overweight/obesity throughout the observation period across quartiles of baseline physical fitness (Q1 indicates low physical fitness).

Linear regression analyses further showed a significant negative association between change in BMIPCT and subsequent fitness (Table 3). The detrimental effect of higher weight gain on fitness development was particularly pronounced in participants with higher BMIPCT at baseline. No clear pattern of this association was observed across baseline fitness quartiles. The association between baseline fitness and fitness at the last follow-up, however, was stronger in participants with lower baseline fitness. These results remained essentially unchanged after including sex as covariate.

Table 3. Regression coefficients based on linear regression analysis for overall physical fitness at last measurement.

	BL Fitness (β)	BL BMIPCT (β)	Δ BMIPCT (β)	R^2
Total Sample	0.525 **	−0.309 **	−0.252 **	0.456
Low BMIPCT	0.490 **	−0.015	−0.008	0.241
<avg. BMIPCT	0.596 **	0.042	−0.238 *	0.416
>avg. BMIPCT	0.516 **	−0.126	−0.427 **	0.530
High BMIPCT	0.560 **	−0.054	−0.427 **	0.523
Low BL Fitness	0.444 **	−0.502 **	−0.211 *	0.508
Avg. BL Fitness	0.222 *	−0.287 **	−0.359 **	0.268
Above avg. BL Fitness	0.198	−0.302 **	−0.150	0.179
High BL Fitness	−0.006	0.244 *	−0.485 **	0.269

BL—baseline; BMIPCT—BMI percentile; Δ—annual change based on linear mixed model. * $p < 0.05$, ** $p < 0.01$. Low BMIPCT—BMIPCT < 29; below average BMIPCT—29 ≤ BMIPCT < 50.2; above average BMIPCT—50.2 ≤ BMIPCT < 76; high BMIPCT—BMIPCT ≥ 76. Low fitness—overall fitness < 100; average fitness—100 ≤ overall fitness < 105; above average Fitness—105 ≤ overall fitness < 108; high fitness—overall fitness ≥ 108.

Change in physical fitness was negatively associated with subsequent BMIPCT as well (Table 4). This association was also more pronounced in participants with higher baseline BMIPCT, whereas no clear pattern was observed across baseline fitness quartiles. Further, the association between baseline BMIPCT and BMIPCT at follow-up was less pronounced in participants with below-average baseline BMIPCT compared to those with higher baseline BMIPCT. The inclusion of sex as additional independent variable in the regression models did not have a significant impact on the previously reported results.

Table 4. Regression coefficients based on linear regression analysis for overall BMI percentile at last measurement.

	BL Fitness (β)	BL BMIPCT (β)	Δ Fitness (β)	R^2
Total Sample	−0.102 **	0.742 **	−0.203 **	0.686
Low BMIPCT	−0.144	0.235 *	−0.006	0.075
<avg. BMIPCT	−0.068	0.227 *	−0.326 **	0.155
>avg. BMIPCT	−0.289 **	0.342 **	−0.541 **	0.495
High BMIPCT	−0.104	0.372 **	−0.387 **	0.291
Low BL Fitness	0.020	0.644 **	−0.239 **	0.631
Avg. BL Fitness	−0.110	0.761 **	−0.238 **	0.740
Above avg. BL Fitness	−0.044	0.813 **	−0.101	0.733
High BL Fitness	−0.105	0.746 **	−0.261 **	0.671

BL—baseline; BMIPCT—BMI percentile; Δ—annual change based on linear mixed model. * $p < 0.05$, ** $p < 0.01$. Low BMIPCT—BMIPCT < 29; below average BMIPCT—29 ≤ BMIPCT < 50.2; above average BMIPCT—50.2 ≤ BMIPCT < 76; high BMIPCT—BMIPCT ≥ 76. Low fitness—overall fitness < 100; average fitness—100 ≤ overall fitness < 105; above average Fitness—105 ≤ overall fitness < 108; high fitness—overall fitness ≥ 108.

4. Discussion

The results of the present study show an inverse association between body weight and physical fitness in older children, whereas the association was limited in younger children. Increased body weight and low physical fitness at younger ages, however, were associated with an attenuated development of physical fitness and increased weight gain throughout the elementary school years, respectively. In addition, this study showed that the inverse reciprocal longitudinal association between body weight and physical fitness was more pronounced in children with high body weight at young ages, whereas no differences in the prospective association between body weight and physical fitness were observed across quartiles of baseline physical fitness.

These results are consistent with previous studies that showed an inverse association between body weight and physical fitness in children [20,26,37]. Musálek et al. further showed that even children who have increased body fat despite being considered normal weight displayed poorer performances on endurance and strength tests [38]. A reduction in body fat, on the other hand, was associated with an improvement in physical fitness [39]. Thus, body weight has been shown to account for a substantial portion of the variability in physical fitness during childhood [40,41] and the increase in population body weight has been associated with declines in physical fitness. Accordingly, today's youth display lower physical fitness than those of previous generations [27,42]. The detrimental effect of increased body weight is particularly pronounced in weight-bearing activities, whereas associations between body weight and muscular strength have been less consistent [37,39,41,43,44]. This may be attributed to the fact that excess body weight may be a morphological constraint, particularly when the body needs to be moved against gravity, which potentially results in less efficient movement patterns and lower exercise tolerance, increasing the risk for withdrawal from various forms of physical activity [45,46]. Increased body weight is also associated with lower motor competence [30], which provides the foundation for engagement in various forms of physical activity [47]. The resulting lower engagement in various forms of physical activity also reduces the opportunities for the development of physical fitness [48], which results in a vicious cycle of increased body weight, poor physical fitness, and low physical activity [49]. High motor competence, on the other hand, enables children to engage in more physical activity over time, which enhances physical fitness and facilitates the maintenance of a healthy body weight. Accordingly, a recent review showed significantly higher fitness levels and lower body weight, and particularly body fat, in active compared to inactive adolescents [50]. The fact that low physical activity tracks from childhood into adolescence and adulthood [51], and increases the risk for various health problems later in life [52], further emphasizes the need for early intervention strategies.

The inverse association between body weight and physical fitness, however, appears to be limited at younger ages but strengthens with age [20,53,54]. Accordingly, change in body weight was negatively associated with the development of various aspects of physical fitness throughout the elementary school years. This, however, also implies that overweight/obese children who changed their weight status to normal weight can achieve similar fitness levels as those who were always normal weight [55]. Strategies targeting excessive fat accumulation in children, therefore, have been recommended to ensure functional capacity later in life [39]. In particular, middle childhood is considered a critical period, where positive trajectories of high physical fitness and healthy body weight or negative trajectories of poor physical fitness and increased body weight start to diverge [56]. The lack of differences in the development of body weight and physical fitness across quartiles of baseline fitness at the beginning of elementary school also indicates the high potential for the promotion of physical fitness at young ages as all children can benefit from the promotion of physical fitness, independent of their current fitness level. In particular, exercise programs of higher intensity have been shown to improve physical fitness [9,57]. Physical education in elementary school and movement programs in pre-schools, and youth sports, therefore, should be considered important intervention settings for ensuring sufficient physical fitness early in life [58]. The importance of early interventions is further emphasized by the fact that low fitness levels are sustained during adolescence, which can have major effects at the individual level and for society due to the associated health risks [39]. The results of the present study additionally highlight the importance of focusing on children with increased body weight as these have a higher risk for entering a vicious cycle of excess weight gain and poor physical fitness, which is most likely accompanied by lower physical activity levels and associated health problems.

Given the importance of physical fitness for future health among children and youth, independent of physical activity [59,60], monitoring physical fitness levels in children and adolescents has shifted from a performance-related focus to the assessment of health-related fitness [12]. At least partially due to low physical activity levels in youth, there has been a resurgence of research on health outcomes related to physical fitness in recent years [12]. Such research may be even more important in light of the observed recent declines in physical fitness due to movement restrictions in response to the COVID-19 pandemic [61]. The collection of fitness data at national and school levels, therefore, should be considered a public health priority [12]. Nevertheless, only a few countries have implemented national surveillance systems for physical fitness. One example in Europe is Slovenia, which can also be used to highlight the benefits of such efforts. Slovenia has collected physical fitness data for all children and adolescents for more than three decades via the "SLOfit" initiative [62]. In response to the observed decline in physical fitness that started in the 1990s, Slovenia implemented a national health-promotion program in 2010 that included two additional hours of physical education per week [63]. As a result, physical fitness levels have notably improved, and Slovenia was the only European country to receive an "A–" grade for physical fitness and overall physical activity in the recent Global Physical Activity Report Card [64]. In addition to highlighting poor physical fitness in European youth, it was shown that only 9 of the 20 European countries participating in the Global Physical Activity Report Card provided adequate data to determine a grade for physical fitness in youth. This aspect further emphasizes the need for the implementation of national fitness testing initiatives that can guide the implementation of policies targeting physical fitness in youth [15].

Despite the important insights provided by the present study, there are some limitations that need to be considered when interpreting the results. There was no information on physical activity and, therefore, it was not possible to examine the association of changes in physical activity with alterations in body weight and physical fitness. The small sample size along with higher fitness levels of children that were included in the analyses compared to those excluded due to missing data may also limit generalizability of the findings. Furthermore, even though BMI is a well-accepted proxy measure for the assessment of weight status, it does not directly measure body fatness and fat distribution [65]. A higher BMI could also be associated with higher lean body mass, rather than fat mass, which has a stronger association with health compared to body weight [66]. Nevertheless, BMI is commonly used in epidemiological studies and has been shown to correlate well with body fat percentage in youth [67]. The utilization of a validated test battery that assesses various components of physical fitness, which was administered by trained personnel, on the other hand, should be considered a strength of the present study. Additionally, a total of eight measurements were administered over four years throughout the entire elementary school period, which allows for an investigation of the dynamic, prospective relationship of physical fitness and body weight. Causality, however, cannot be established due to the observational nature of this study. The insights gained, nevertheless, enhance the understanding of the complex interaction between body weight and physical fitness and, therefore, support evidence-based practice. In order to examine causal relationships, randomized controlled trials that explore effects of different exercise programs on physical fitness in youth are needed. Such longitudinal studies should also include other critical correlates of leisure time physical activity, such as self-efficacy and socio-environmental aspects, along with the assessment of health markers in order to provide further evidence on the impact of physical fitness on future health and well-being. With an increased public awareness on the influence of physical fitness and body weight on future health, there may also be a stronger commitment to emphasize the promotion of physical fitness in children as a critical contributor to public health.

5. Conclusions

In conclusion, the results of the present study show an inverse reciprocal relationship between body weight and physical fitness in elementary school children. The fact that this association starts to emerge during the elementary school years emphasizes the importance of early intervention strategies that minimize excess fat accumulation to ensure adequate physical fitness later in life. Additionally, it was shown that the inverse association between body weight and physical fitness was more pronounced in heavier children, whereas no differences in the progression of physical fitness were observed across different levels of baseline fitness. This highlights the potential of promoting physical fitness for each child, independent of their current fitness level. Intervention efforts, nevertheless, should pay particular attention to children with non-optimal weight status as they are at an increased risk for entering a vicious cycle of excess body weight, poor physical fitness, and low physical activity, which has a significant impact on general development and health later in life.

Author Contributions: Conceptualization, K.G.; methodology, K.G.; formal analysis, C.D. resources, G.R.; data curation, K.G.; writing—original draft preparation, C.D.; writing—review and editing, S.-T.C., A.C., G.F., G.R. and K.G.; project administration, K.G. All authors have read and agreed to the published version of the manuscript.

Funding: This research received no external funding.

Institutional Review Board Statement: The study was conducted in accordance with the Declaration of Helsinki, and approved by the Institutional Review Board of the University of Innsbruck (certificate of good standing 16/2014).

Informed Consent Statement: Informed consent was obtained from all subjects involved in the study.

Data Availability Statement: The data presented in this study are available on request from the corresponding author.

Conflicts of Interest: The authors declare no conflict of interest.

References

1. Pi-Sunyer, F.X. The obesity epidemic: Pathophysiology and consequences of obesity. *Obes. Res.* **2002**, *10* (Suppl. 2), 97S–104S. [CrossRef] [PubMed]
2. Poirier, P.; Giles, T.D.; Bray, G.A.; Hong, Y.; Stern, J.S.; Pi-Sunyer, F.X.; Eckel, R.H. Obesity and cardiovascular disease: Pathophysiology, evaluation, and effect of weight loss: An update of the 1997 American Heart Association Scientific Statement on Obesity and Heart Disease from the Obesity Committee of the Council on Nutrition, Physical Activity, and Metabolism. *Circulation* **2006**, *113*, 898–918. [PubMed]
3. Cote, A.T.; Harris, K.C.; Panagiotopoulos, C.; Sandor, G.G.; Devlin, A.M. Childhood obesity and cardiovascular dysfunction. *J. Am. Coll. Cardiol.* **2013**, *62*, 1309–1319. [CrossRef] [PubMed]
4. Ayer, J.; Charakida, M.; Deanfield, J.E.; Celermajer, D.S. Lifetime risk: Childhood obesity and cardiovascular risk. *Eur. Heart J.* **2015**, *36*, 1371–1376. [CrossRef]
5. Lang, J.E.; Bunnell, H.T.; Hossain, M.J.; Wysocki, T.; Lima, J.J.; Finkel, T.H.; Bacharier, L.; Dempsey, A.; Sarzynski, L.; Test, M.; et al. Being Overweight or Obese and the Development of Asthma. *Pediatrics* **2018**, *142*, e20182119. [CrossRef]
6. Lobstein, T.; Jackson-Leach, R.; Moodie, M.L.; Hall, K.D.; Gortmaker, S.L.; Swinburn, B.A.; James, W.P.T.; Wang, Y.; McPherson, K. Child and adolescent obesity: Part of a bigger picture. *Lancet* **2015**, *385*, 2510–2520. [CrossRef]
7. Simmonds, M.; Llewellyn, A.; Owen, C.G.; Woolacott, N. Predicting adult obesity from childhood obesity: A systematic review and meta-analysis. *Obes. Rev.* **2016**, *17*, 95–107. [CrossRef]
8. Umer, A.; Kelley, G.A.; Cottrell, L.E.; Giacobbi, P.; Innes, K.E.; Lilly, C.L. Childhood obesity and adult cardiovascular disease risk factors: A systematic review with meta-analysis. *BMC Public Health* **2017**, *17*, 683. [CrossRef]
9. Ortega, F.B.; Ruiz, J.R.; Castillo, M.J.; Sjöström, M. Physical fitness in childhood and adolescence: A powerful marker of health. *Int. J. Obes.* **2008**, *32*, 1–11. [CrossRef]
10. Ruiz, J.R.; Castro-Piñero, J.; Artero, E.G.; Ortega, F.B.; Sjöström, M.; Suni, J.; Castillo, M.J. Predictive validity of health-related fitness in youth: A systematic review. *Br. J. Sports Med.* **2009**, *43*, 909–923. [CrossRef]
11. Zaqout, M.; Michels, N.; Bammann, K.; Ahrens, W.; Sprengeler, O.; Molnar, D.; Hadjigeorgiou, C.; Eiben, G.; Konstabel, K.; Russo, P.; et al. Influence of physical fitness on cardio-metabolic risk factors in European children. The IDEFICS study. *Int. J. Obes.* **2016**, *40*, 1119–1125. [CrossRef] [PubMed]
12. Sacheck, J.; Hall, M. Current evidence for the impact of physical fitness on health outcomes in youth. *Am. J. Lifestyle Med.* **2015**, *9*, 388–397. [CrossRef]
13. Smith, J.J.; Eather, N.; Morgan, P.J.; Plotnikoff, R.C.; Faigenbaum, A.D.; Lubans, D.R. The health benefits of muscular fitness for children and adolescents: A systematic review and meta-analysis. *Sports Med.* **2014**, *44*, 1209–1223. [CrossRef] [PubMed]
14. Caspersen, C.J.; Powell, K.E.; Christenson, G.M. Physical activity, exercise, and physical fitness: Definitions and distinctions for health-related research. *Public Health Rep.* **1985**, *100*, 126–131. [PubMed]
15. Lang, J.J.; Tomkinson, G.R.; Janssen, I.; Ruiz, J.R.; Ortega, F.B.; Léger, L.; Tremblay, M.S. Making a Case for Cardiorespiratory Fitness Surveillance Among Children and Youth. *Exerc. Sport Sci. Rev.* **2018**, *46*, 66–75. [CrossRef] [PubMed]
16. Grøntved, A.; Ried-Larsen, M.; Møller, N.C.; Kristensen, P.L.; Froberg, K.; Brage, S.; Andersen, L.B. Muscle strength in youth and cardiovascular risk in young adulthood (the European Youth Heart Study). *Br. J. Sports Med.* **2015**, *49*, 90–94. [CrossRef] [PubMed]
17. García-Hermoso, A.; Ramírez-Campillo, R.; Izquierdo, M. Is Muscular Fitness Associated with Future Health Benefits in Children and Adolescents? A Systematic Review and Meta-Analysis of Longitudinal Studies. *Sports Med.* **2019**, *49*, 1079–1094. [CrossRef]
18. Ajala, O.; Mold, F.; Boughton, C.; Cooke, D.; Whyte, M. Childhood predictors of cardiovascular disease in adulthood. A systematic review and meta-analysis. *Obes. Rev.* **2017**, *18*, 1061–1070. [CrossRef]
19. Janssen, I.; Leblanc, A.G. Systematic review of the health benefits of physical activity and fitness in school-aged children and youth. *Int. J. Behav. Nutr. Phys. Act.* **2010**, *7*, 40. [CrossRef]
20. Fiori, F.; Bravo, G.; Parpinel, M.; Messina, G.; Malavolta, R.; Lazzer, S. Relationship between body mass index and physical fitness in Italian prepubertal schoolchildren. *PLoS ONE* **2020**, *15*, e0233362.
21. Barnett, L.M.; Lai, S.K.; Veldman, S.L.; Hardy, L.L.; Cliff, D.P.; Morgan, P.J.; Zask, A.; Lubans, D.R.; Shultz, S.P.; Ridgers, N.D.; et al. Correlates of Gross Motor Competence in Children and Adolescents: A Systematic Review and Meta-Analysis. *Sports Med.* **2016**, *46*, 1663–1688. [CrossRef] [PubMed]
22. Tsiros, M.D.; Coates, A.M.; Howe, P.R.; Walkley, J.; Hills, A.P.; Wood, R.E.; Buckley, J.D. Adiposity is related to decrements in cardiorespiratory fitness in obese and normal-weight children. *Pediatr. Obes.* **2016**, *11*, 144–150. [CrossRef]
23. Greier, K.; Drenowatz, C. Bidirectional association between weight status and motor skills in adolescents: A 4-year longitudinal study. *Wien. Klin. Wochenschr.* **2018**, *130*, 314–320. [CrossRef] [PubMed]
24. Ruedl, G.; Franz, D.; Frühauf, A.; Kopp, M.; Niedermeier, M.; Drenowatz, C.; Greier, K. Development of physical fitness in Austrian primary school children: A longitudinal study among overweight and non-overweight children over 2.5 years. *Wien. Klin. Wochenschr.* **2018**, *130*, 321–327. [CrossRef]
25. Albrecht, C.; Hanssen-Doose, A.; Oriwol, D.; Bös, K.; Worth, A. Beeinflusst ein Veränderung des BMI die Entwicklung der motorischen Leistungsfähigkeit im Kindes- und Jugendalter? Ergebnisse der Motorik-Modul Studie (MoMo). *Beweg. und Gesundh.* **2016**, *32*, 168–172.

26. Lopes, V.; Maia, J.; Rodrigues, L.; Malina, R. Motor coordination, physical activity and fitness as predictors of longitudinal change in adiposity during childhood. *Eur. J. Sport Sci.* **2012**, *12*, 384–391. [CrossRef]
27. Tomkinson, G.R.; Lang, J.J.; Tremblay, M.S. Temporal trends in the cardiorespiratory fitness of children and adolescents representing 19 high-income and upper middle-income countries between 1981 and 2014. *Br. J. Sports Med.* **2019**, *53*, 478–486. [CrossRef]
28. NCD Risk Factor Collaboration (NCD-RisC). Worldwide trends in body-mass index, underweight, overweight, and obesity from 1975 to 2016: A pooled analysis of 2416 population-based measurement studies in 128·9 million children, adolescents, and adults. *Lancet* **2017**, *390*, 2627–2642. [CrossRef]
29. Brunner, F.; Kornexl, E.; Kastner, H.; Drenowatz, C.; Greier, K. Fitness trend analysis in male Austrian middle and high school students from 1975 to 2010. *Curr. Issues Sport Sci.* **2021**, *6*, 007. [CrossRef]
30. Bolger, L.E.; Bolger, L.A.; O'Neill, C.; Coughlan, E.; O'Brien, W.; Lacey, S.; Burns, C.; Bardidd, F. Global levels of fundamental motor skills in children: A systematic review. *J. Sports Sci.* **2021**, *39*, 717–753. [CrossRef]
31. Drozdz, D.; Alvarez-Pitti, J.; Wójcik, M.; Borghi, C.; Gabbianelli, R.; Mazur, A.; Herceg-Čavrak, V.; Lopez-Valcarcel, B.G.; Brzeziński, M.; Lurbe, E.; et al. Obesity and Cardiometabolic Risk Factors: From Childhood to Adulthood. *Nutrients* **2021**, *13*, 4176. [CrossRef] [PubMed]
32. Muka, T.; Imo, D.; Jaspers, L.; Colpani, V.; Chaker, L.; van der Lee, S.J.; Mendis, S.; Chowdhury, R.; Bramer, W.M.; Falla, A.; et al. The global impact of non-communicable diseases on healthcare spending and national income: A systematic review. *Eur. J. Epidemiol.* **2015**, *30*, 251–277. [CrossRef] [PubMed]
33. Spieker, E.A.; Pyzocha, N. Economic Impact of Obesity. *Prim. Care* **2016**, *43*, 83–95. [CrossRef] [PubMed]
34. Kromeyer-Hauschild, K.; Wabitsch, M.; Kunze, D.; Geller, F.; Geiß, H.; Hesse, V.; von Hippel, A.; Jaeger, U.; Johnsen, D.; Korte, W.; et al. Perzentile für den Body-mass-Index für das Kindes- und Jugendalter unter Heranziehung verschiedener deutscher Stichproben. *Mon. Kinderheilkd.* **2001**, *149*, 807–818. [CrossRef]
35. Bös, K.; Schlenker, L.; Büsch, D.; Lämmle, L.; Müller, H.; Oberger, J.; Seidel, I.; Tittelbach, S. *Deutscher Motorik-Test 6-18 (DMT6-18) [German Motor Abilities Test 6-18 (DMT6-18)]*; Czwalina: Hamburg, Germany, 2009.
36. Abdelkarim, O.; Fritsch, J.; Jekauc, D.; Bös, K. Examination of Construct Validity and Criterion-Related Validity of the German Motor Test in Egyptian Schoolchildren. *Int. J. Environ. Res. Public Health* **2021**, *18*, 8341. [CrossRef]
37. Ceschia, A.; Giacomini, S.; Santarossa, S.; Rugo, M.; Salvadego, D.; Da Ponte, A.; Driussi, C.; Mihaleje, M.; Poser, S.; Lazzer, S. Deleterious effects of obesity on physical fitness in pre-pubertal children. *Eur. J. Sport Sci.* **2016**, *16*, 271–278. [CrossRef]
38. Musálek, M.; Clark, C.C.T.; Kokštejn, J.; Vokounova, Š.; Hnízdil, J.; Mess, F. Impaired Cardiorespiratory Fitness and Muscle Strength in Children with Normal-Weight Obesity. *Int. J. Environ. Res. Public Health* **2020**, *17*, 9198. [CrossRef]
39. Joensuu, L.; Kujala, U.M.; Kankaanpää, A.; Syväoja, H.J.; Kulmala, J.; Hakonen, H.; Oksanen, H.; Kallio, J.; Tammelin, T.H. Physical fitness development in relation to changes in body composition and physical activity in adolescence. *Scand. J. Med. Sci. Sports* **2021**, *31*, 456–464. [CrossRef]
40. Brunet, M.; Chaput, J.-P.; Tremblay, A. The association between low physical fitness and high body mass index or waist circumference is increasing with age in children: The 'Québec en Forme' Project. *Int. J. Obes.* **2007**, *31*, 637–643. [CrossRef]
41. Sacchetti, R.; Ceciliani, A.; Garulli, A.; Masotti, A.; Poletti, G.; Beltrami, P.; Leoni, E. Physical fitness of primary school children in relation to overweight prevalence and physical activity habits. *J. Sports Sci.* **2012**, *30*, 633–640. [CrossRef]
42. Santtila, M.; Pihlainen, K.; Koski, H.; Vasankari, T.; Kyröläinen, H. Physical Fitness in Young Men between 1975 and 2015 with a Focus on the Years 2005–2015. *Med. Sci. Sports Exerc.* **2018**, *50*, 292–298. [CrossRef]
43. Armstrong, M.E.G.; Lambert, M.I.; Lambert, E.V. Relationships between different nutritional anthropometric statuses and health-related fitness of South African primary school children. *Ann. Hum. Biol.* **2017**, *44*, 208–213. [CrossRef]
44. Gulías-González, R.; Sánchez-López, M.; Olivas-Bravo, Á.; Solera-Martínez, M.; Martínez-Vizcaíno, V. Physical fitness in Spanish schoolchildren aged 6–12 years: Reference values of the battery EUROFIT and associated cardiovascular risk. *J. Sch. Health* **2014**, *84*, 625–635. [CrossRef]
45. Kakebeeke, T.H.; Lanzi, S.; Zysset, A.E.; Arhab, A.; Messerli-Bürgy, N.; Stuelb, K.; Leeger-Aschmann, C.S.; Schmutz, E.A.; Meyer, A.H.; Kriemler, S.; et al. Association between Body Composition and Motor Performance in Preschool Children. *Obes. Facts* **2017**, *10*, 420–431. [CrossRef]
46. de Andrade Gonçalves, E.C.; Augusto Santos Silva, D.; Gimenes Nunes, H.E. Prevalence and Factors Associated with Low Aerobic Performance Levels in Adolescents: A Systematic Review. *Curr. Pediatr. Rev.* **2015**, *11*, 56–70. [CrossRef]
47. Gallahue, D.; Ozmun, J.; Goodway, J. *Understanding Motor Development. Infants, Children, Adolescents, Adults*, 7th ed.; McGraw-Hill: Boston, MA, USA, 2012.
48. Lima, R.A.; Bugge, A.; Ersbøll, A.K.; Stodden, D.F.; Andersen, L.B. The longitudinal relationship between motor competence and measures of fatness and fitness from childhood into adolescence. *J. Pediatr.* **2019**, *95*, 482–488. [CrossRef]
49. Stodden, D.; Goodway, J.; Langendorfer, S.; Roberton, M.; Rudisill, M.; Garcia, C.; Garcia, L.E. A developmental perspective on the role of motor skill competence in physical activity: An emergent relationshihp. *Quest* **2008**, *60*, 290–306. [CrossRef]
50. Mateo-Orcajada, A.; González-Gálvez, N.; Abenza-Cano, L.; Vaquero-Cristóbal, R. Differences in Physical Fitness and Body Composition Between Active and Sedentary Adolescents: A Systematic Review and Meta-Analysis. *J. Youth Adolesc.* **2022**. Epub ahead of print. [CrossRef]

51. Telama, R.; Yang, X.; Leskinen, E.; Kankaanpää, A.; Hirvensalo, M.; Tammelin, T.; Raitakari, O.T. Tracking of physical activity from early childhood through youth into adulthood. *Med. Sci. Sports Exerc.* **2014**, *46*, 955–962. [CrossRef]
52. Li, J.; Siegrist, J. Physical activity and risk of cardiovascular disease-a meta-analysis of prospective cohort studies. *Int. J. Environ. Res. Public Health* **2012**, *9*, 391–407. [CrossRef]
53. Battaglia, G.; Giustino, V.; Tabacchi, G.; Lanza, M.; Schena, F.; Biino, V.; Giuriato, M.; Gallotta, M.C.; Guidetti, L.; Baldari, C.; et al. Interrelationship Between Age, Gender, and Weight Status on Motor Coordination in Italian Children and Early Adolescents Aged 6–13 Years Old. *Front. Pediatr.* **2021**, *9*, 738294. [CrossRef]
54. Battaglia, G.; Giustino, V.; Tabacchi, G.; Alesi, M.; Galassi, C.; Modica, C.; Palma, A.; Bellafiore, M. Effectiveness of a Physical Education Program on the Motor and Pre-literacy Skills of Preschoolers From the Training-To-Health Project: A Focus on Weight Status. *Front. Sports Act. Living* **2020**, *2*, 579421. [CrossRef] [PubMed]
55. Lima, R.A.; Soares, F.C.; Queiroz, D.R.; Aguilar, J.A.; Bezerra, J.; Barros, M.V.G. The importance of body weight status on motor competence development: From preschool to middle childhood. *Scand. J. Med. Sci. Sports* **2021**, *31* (Suppl. 1), 15–22. [CrossRef] [PubMed]
56. Robinson, L.E.; Stodden, D.F.; Barnett, L.M.; Lopes, V.P.; Logan, S.W.; Rodrigues, L.P.; D'Hondt, E. Motor Competence and its Effect on Positive Developmental Trajectories of Health. *Sports Med.* **2015**, *45*, 1273–1284. [CrossRef] [PubMed]
57. Beltran-Valls, M.R.; Adelantado-Renau, M.; Moliner-Urdiales, D. Reallocating time spent in physical activity intensities: Longitudinal associations with physical fitness (DADOS study). *J. Sci. Med. Sport* **2020**, *23*, 968–972. [CrossRef] [PubMed]
58. Cocca, A.; Carbajal Baca, J.E.; Hernández Cruz, G.; Cocca, M. Does A Multiple-Sport Intervention Based on the TGfU Pedagogical Model for Physical Education Increase Physical Fitness in Primary School Children? *Int. J. Environ. Res. Public Health* **2020**, *17*, 5532. [CrossRef]
59. Kelly, A.S.; Wetzsteon, R.J.; Kaiser, D.R.; Steinberger, J.; Bank, A.J.; Dengel, D.R. Inflammation, insulin, and endothelial function in overweight children and adolescents: The role of exercise. *J. Pediatr.* **2004**, *145*, 731–736. [CrossRef]
60. Janz, K.F.; Dawson, J.D.; Mahoney, L.T. Increases in physical fitness during childhood improve cardiovascular health during adolescence: The Muscatine Study. *Int. J. Sports Med.* **2002**, *23* (Suppl. 1), S15–S21. [CrossRef]
61. Jarnig, G.; Jaunig, J.; van Poppel, M.N.M. Association of COVID-19 Mitigation Measures with Changes in Cardiorespiratory Fitness and Body Mass Index Among Children Aged 7 to 10 Years in Austria. *JAMA Netw. Open* **2021**, *4*, e2121675. [CrossRef]
62. Jurak, G.; Kovač, M.; Sember, V.; Starc, G. 30 years of SLOfit: Its legacy and perspective. *Turk. J. Sports Med.* **2019**, *54*, 23–27. [CrossRef]
63. Strel, J. *Analysis of the Program Healthy Lifestyle for the Years 2010/11 and 2011/12*; Institute for Sport Planica: Ljubljana, Slovenia, 2013.
64. Coppinger, T.; Milton, K.; Murtagh, E.; Harrington, D.; Johansen, D.; Seghers, J.; Skovgaard, T.; HEPA Europe Children & Youth Working Group; Chalkley, A. Global Matrix 3.0 physical activity report card for children and youth: A comparison across Europe. *Public Health* **2020**, *187*, 150–156. [CrossRef]
65. Freedman, D.S.; Katzmarzyk, P.T.; Dietz, W.H.; Srinivasan, S.R.; Berenson, G.S. Relation of body mass index and skinfold thicknesses to cardiovascular disease risk factors in children: The Bogalusa Heart Study. *Am. J. Clin. Nutr.* **2009**, *90*, 210–216. [CrossRef] [PubMed]
66. Lo, K.; Wong, M.; Khalechelvam, P.; Tam, W. Waist-to-height ratio, body mass index and waist circumference for screening paediatric cardio-metabolic risk factors: A meta-analysis. *Obes. Rev.* **2016**, *17*, 1258–1275. [CrossRef] [PubMed]
67. Mei, Z.; Grummer-Strawn, L.M.; Pietrobelli, A.; Goulding, A.; Goran, M.I.; Dietz, W.H. Validity of body mass index compared with other body-composition screening indexes for the assessment of body fatness in children and adolescents. *Am. J. Clin. Nutr.* **2002**, *75*, 978–985. [CrossRef] [PubMed]

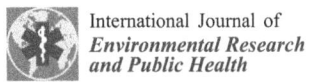

International Journal of
Environmental Research and Public Health

Article

A Study on the Subjectivity of Parents Regarding "0th-Period Physical Education Class" of Middle Schools in Korea Using Q-Methodology

Wonseok Choi [1] and Wonjae Jeon [2,*]

[1] Department of Physical Education, Keimyung University, Daegu 42601, Korea; wschoi@kmu.ac.kr
[2] Department of Physical Education, Korea National University of Education, Cheongju-si 28173, Korea
* Correspondence: wonjaejeon1228@knu.ac.kr; Tel.: +82-10-8455-4774

Abstract: The current study examined parents' subjective perception types and characteristics regarding the 0th-Period Physical Education Class of Middle School in Korea. The Q-methodology was applied, and the final 25 Q-Samples were selected through the composition of the 42 Q-population. Among Korean parents, 20 students who participated in "Physical Education Activities in Class 0" for more than one year were selected as P-Sample. Q-sorting was performed by the P-Sample. Data collected by Q-sorting were analyzed using the PQ method program version 2.35, with centroid factor analysis and varimax rotation. The finding pointed to four types, with a total explanatory variance of 63%. Type 1 (N = 7), and was named "urgent legal and institutional settlement of 0th-period physical education". Type 2 (N = 4) has the theme of "beach-head for a vibrant school life". Type 3 (N = 4) was named "enhancement of academic capability". Type 4 (N = 4) was described as "strengthening physical and mental health". Moreover, the consensus statements between each type were investigated in Q1 and Q2. These findings highlight the importance of the "0th-period physical education class" so the program could be expanded and institutionalized in Korea.

Keywords: 0th-period physical education class; adolescent; parents; Q-methodology; subjectivity

Citation: Choi, W.; Jeon, W. A Study on the Subjectivity of Parents Regarding "0th-Period Physical Education Class" of Middle Schools in Korea Using Q-Methodology. *Int. J. Environ. Res. Public Health* **2022**, *19*, 7760. https://doi.org/10.3390/ijerph19137760

Academic Editors: Paul B. Tchounwou, Clemens Drenowatz and Klaus Greier

Received: 27 May 2022
Accepted: 21 June 2022
Published: 24 June 2022

Publisher's Note: MDPI stays neutral with regard to jurisdictional claims in published maps and institutional affiliations.

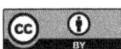

Copyright: © 2022 by the authors. Licensee MDPI, Basel, Switzerland. This article is an open access article distributed under the terms and conditions of the Creative Commons Attribution (CC BY) license (https://creativecommons.org/licenses/by/4.0/).

1. Introduction

Different cardiovascular exercises that can be practiced in everyday life, such as swimming, walking, running, cycling, and mountain climbing, improve oxygen transfer to each body cell [1]. In addition, it positively affects neurological and cognitive function in all ages, from children to the elderly [2]. Since regular exercise has been steadily reported to improve brain function in various age groups, adolescence, the most active period for nerve production and cell connection, is a critical moment to enhance cognitive function by participating in the exercise [3].

Physical activity during adolescence positively affects the brain's readiness to accept new information, improving learning memory [4] and optimizing the mental environment to increase alertness and concentration [5]. Marsh and Kleitman [6] noted that healthy children generally have better learning skills than their counterparts. Furthermore, children who practiced regular exercise also had higher memory skills and academic achievement [7]. Hence, it is well documented that adolescent exercise improves the brain's structure by supplying blood to the brain and further improves academic ability while functioning to make the brain's state optimal [8].

One interesting topic among the various studies of adolescent exercise participation is related to morning exercise. For example, a recent study revealed that routine morning exercise improved the health and weight management of the overweight population [9]. Moreover, McGowan et al. [10] suggested that completion of a morning swimming session with resistance exercise can substantially enhance sprint-swimming performance completed later the same day. In this respect, morning exercise can draw academic significance in studies targeting adolescents. For instance, consistent morning exercise participation, such as swimming in adolescents, positively affects the sleep–wake cycle [11]. In addition, Babadi et al. [12] observed that adolescents who engaged in morning exercise at school had a lower prevalence of hypertension. At the same time, the other group who spent more time on sedentary activities were at higher risk for hypertension.

A project attempted to prove the effectiveness of such early morning exercise related to academic achievement. The study showed that early morning exercise with moderate to vigorous intensity optimizes students' brain function, attentional control skills, and learning attitude [13]. In 2010, the project leader, Dr. John Lately, was invited as a guest lecturer in Korea to introduce his findings and emphasize early morning exercise in the school system. Since then, the early morning exercise program has been implemented at the public schools in the country and was named "0th-period physical activity" or "0th-period physical education class" [14]. Recently, the term "0th-period physical education class (0th-period PE class)" has been generally accepted for autonomous physical activity sessions (i.e., 7:30~8:30 a.m.) before the official class begins [15].

Various studies on "0th-period PE class" have been conducted in Korea, and Jeon et al. [15] found that the participation of middle school students had a statistically significant effect on perceived enjoyment and learning attitudes. Furthermore, an intervention study at the elementary school also concluded that the early morning exercise program significantly improves social skills, autonomy, and stability [16]. Finally, for the high school case, a 3-year long-term morning exercise program positively influenced participants' fitness test scores, physical self-concept, and academic achievement [17].

Although many studies showed positive results of adolescent morning exercise programs, parents' involvement and perception are not well documented yet. In general, parental involvement in a child's education is consistently found to be positively associated with a child's academic performance [18]. However, Lim et al. [19] pointed out that excessive parental obsession with their children's academic achievement might harm the expansion of "0th-period PE class". Furthermore, Jeon et al. [20] stressed that parents' perceptions should also be further investigated, noting that there will be great differences between middle school students' perceptions and parents' perceptions in participation in "0th-period PE class". In this respect, the Q methodology could be used as one of the prominent ways to reveal other social perspectives that exist on issues or topics related to physical activity [21]. Therefore, considering the parental influence on adolescents, investigating and analyzing parents' perceptions and demands is of great importance for successfully settling the "0th-period PE class". The results of this study will contribute to grasping parents' perspectives in exploring improvements in morning exercise programs and presenting policy directions for future program expansion.

Consequently, the current study examined the parental perception of a morning exercise program for adolescents to provide ideas and agendas for successfully implementing "0th-period PE class" in the country. Two research questions guided the methodology and data analysis. First, using the Q-methodology, how are parents' perceptions of the "0th-period PE class" categorized? Second, what are the characteristics of each type, and what are the differences, commonalities, and implications?

2. Methods

The Q-methodology was developed by William Stephenson in 1953 [22]. It is a suitable technique to recognize the "subjectivity" perceived by humans. Particularly, it is suitable for questions about personal experiences, preferences, values, and beliefs about the research topic [23]. In addition, unlike the R-methodology, the Q-methodology is an operant methodology that represents perceptions in the study subjects' own thoughts and languages, not in the researcher's operational definition [24]. For this reason, it is used in different academic fields such as psychology, nursing, and pedagogy [25]. The advantage of the Q method over other forms of discourse analysis is that since everyone responds to the same set of Q statements, researchers can directly compare participants' responses in a consistent manner. This is usually distinct from other types of qualitative discourse analysis. Hence, it could be an appropriate way to explore how Korean parents perceive their children's physical activities during the 0th period in South Korea.

2.1. Q–Population (Concourse of Statements) and Q-Sample

Q-population, called concourse, is the raw material of the Q-Sample. The Q-population can be constructed using a variety of methods, including focus group interviews, individual in-depth interviews, and literature reviews [26]. Therefore, in this study, Q-population was created through two aspects. First, a focus group interview (FGI) was conducted for a group that included parents with a lot of information about their children's "0th-period PE class", physical education (PE) teachers with experience in the class, and professors majoring in sports pedagogy [27]. Second, various documents that can indirectly understand parents' perceptions of the "0th-period PE class" were analyzed [28]. Through the above method process, 42 Q-populations were finally secured. Next, 42 statements (the "concourse") were reinterpreted and reclassified.

In the Q-methodology, the more Q-Samples, the less reliable they tend to be, and if a complex thinking process on the research topic is needed, it is necessary to adopt fewer than 30 [29]. Finally, 25 Q-Samples were confirmed. In addition, Q-sorting was conducted twice for 5 research participants. The test results were found to be r = 0.72, and reliability was secured [30]. The final Q-Sample is presented in Table 1.

Table 1. Q-Sample.

Q Number	Q Statements
1	Morning exercise can create a sense of goal and impellent.
2	Through participation in morning exercise, it has changed or is becoming a bright personality.
3	Through participation in morning exercise, the relationship with teachers is expanding and improving.
4	Through participation in morning exercise, the relationship with school friends is expanding and improving.
5	Morning exercise helps improve adaptability to overall school life.
6	Morning exercise helps develop social skills such as cooperation and thoughtfulness.
7	Participation in morning exercise is helpful in psychological stability and stress relief.
8	Muscle strength (muscle endurance) and body flexibility improved through morning exercise.
9	Participation in morning exercise helps improve exercise functions such as agility and power.
10	Morning exercise makes physical attractiveness (body, physique, etc.) even better.
11	Participation in morning exercise increases attention and interest in other sports.
12	Morning exercise has increased interest in participating in physical education(PE) class.
13	Morning exercise has given rise to awareness of the importance of future exercise (lifetime PE).
14	Morning exercise increases concentration on various tasks.
15	Through participation in morning exercise, children's grades improved.
16	Participation in morning exercise reduced the fatigue of children.
17	Participation in morning exercise can develop regular lifestyle habits.
18	Morning exercise induces active and confident daily life.
19	Morning exercise allows youths to develop regular eating habits.
20	It is necessary to change the teacher's positive perception of "0th-period PE class".
21	It is necessary to develop infrastructure (facilities, programs) for the operation of the "0th-period PE class".
22	There is a need for an incentive system for teachers who operate "0th-period PE class".
23	Research on the effectiveness of "0th-period PE class" is needed.
24	Legal and institutional settlement of "0th-period PE class" is necessary.
25	It is necessary to strengthen the publicity of "0th-period PE class" for parents.

2.2. P-Sample

The Q-methodology is a method of measuring subjective opinions within an individual. Most importantly, there is no limit to the number of P-Samples because "inter-individual difference in significance" is the core of the study rather than the "inter-individual difference" of the study respondents. This is because the characteristics of the population are not inferred from the characteristics of the P-Sample [31]. The number of P-Samples should be fewer than the number of items in the Q-Sample for statistical reasons [32]. B-middle School in a metropolitan city, South Korea, was selected as a research environment. B-middle School has been running "0th-period PE class" for more than 10 years since 2012. Among them, parents who could provide sufficient data on the "0th-period PE class" were recommended by the teacher in charge of the class. Prior to the start of the study, consent for participation in the study was received from the principal of B school and the physical education teacher. Lastly, 20 parents of students who participated in the "0th-period PE class" for more than one year were selected as P-Samples [22]. The detailed characteristics of P-Samples are as follows in Table 2.

Table 2. Summary of characteristics for P-Sample and factor weight.

Factor (Type)	P-Sample	Age	Child's Age	Gender	Participation Period (Semester)	Factor Weight
Type 1. (N = 7)	1	55	16	Male	6	0.69
	2	54	15	Male	5	0.74
	8	43	15	Female	5	0.78
	9	52	14	Male	4	0.87
	15	41	15	Female	6	0.88
	17	55	15	Male	6	0.61
	18	45	16	Female	6	0.68
Type 2. (N = 4)	3	44	15	Female	5	0.70
	10	50	16	Male	5	0.73
	16	45	16	Female	5	0.90
	19	51	16	Male	6	0.81
Type 3. (N = 4)	4	49	15	Male	5	0.92
	5	44	16	Female	6	0.70
	11	46	15	Female	5	0.69
	20	44	15	Male	5	0.81
Type 4. (N = 4)	6	56	16	Male	6	0.84
	12	49	14	Female	3	0.89
	13	50	16	Female	5	0.58
	14	58	15	Male	5	0.59
Non-significant sample	7	55	16	Male	6	0.32

2.3. Q-Sorting and Factor Analysis

Q-Sorting is the task of placing Q-Samples in a Q-sorting response table for P-Samples. To this end, a forced sorting method was applied in which 20 P-Samples were classified one by one according to the degree to which they positively or negatively agree with the concept and thoughts of the "0th-period PE class" [33]. The specific Q-Sorting process is as follows. From 1 December 2021 to 31 December 2022, Q-Sorting was conducted for P-Sample. Specifically, due to the recent COVID-19 pandemic, it was conducted through non-face-to-face video conferencing (ZOOM). The Q-Sorting method was sufficiently described to each respondent. In addition, after P-Sample read Q-Sample, the most positive (+4) to most negative (−4) questions were placed at both extremes one by one. Next, the positive, negative, and neutral questions were divided into three groups and placed in the positive (+) to negative (−3). Finally, the contents of the reasons for placing them in the questions of both extremes were written, and interviews were conducted in the background [29]. Regarding this procedure, consent to participate in the study was received before the study began. The distribution frame and score composition of the Q population are shown in Figure 1.

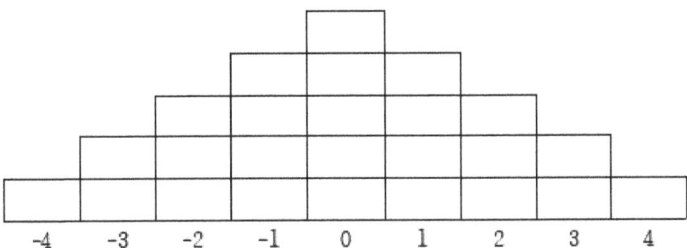

Figure 1. Q sorting response table.

The processing of the collected data was analyzed using the PQ method (VERSION 2.35) program [34]. Factor analysis was conducted through the centroid method, and factor rotation was analyzed through the Varimax rotation method [35]. To determine the ideal number of factors, only factors with an eigenvalue of 1.0 or more were extracted, and the optimal number of types was calculated by entering the number of factors from 7 to 2 [35,36].

3. Results

As a result of the parent's subjectivity in the "0th-period PE class", a total of 4 types were extracted. The eigenvalue, explanatory variance ratio, and correlation results for each type are as follows. Next, four types of parents' perceptions of "0th-period PE class" were presented.

3.1. Eigenvalues (EVs), Variance and Correlations between Factor (Type)

The EVs for each type appeared as 6.19, 3.42, 3.15, and 3.17, respectively. Furthermore, the explanatory variance was derived as 0.20, 0.15, 0.14, and 0.14, respectively. The total variance was 0.63, resulting in 69% explanatory power for all four factors. All factors met the Kaiser–Guttman criterion [36,37]. Table 3 yields the results.

Table 3. Eigenvalue (EVs) and variance between types.

	Type 1	Type 2	Type 3	Type 4
Eigenvalue (EVs)	6.19	3.42	3.15	3.17
% of explanatory variance	0.20	0.15	0.14	0.14
Total variance	0.20	0.35	0.49	0.63

Table 4 demonstrates the correlation between the four factors. Looking more closely, the correlation between Types 1 and 2 was the highest. On the other hand, Types 2 and 4 had the lowest figures. As most of the overall correlation values were derived low, explanatory power and independence for each type were secured, and it can be seen that all types were clearly distinguished [31].

Table 4. Correlations between types.

	Type 1	Type 2	Type 3	Type 4
Type 1	1.000			
Type 2	0.16	1.000		
Type 3	0.08	0.40	1.000	
Type 4	0.12	0.05	0.13	1.000

3.2. Type 1 (Factor 1): Urgent Legal and Institutional Settlement of "0th-Period PE Class": Strengthening Facilities, Programs, Instructors, and Publicity

The results of statements recognized positively or negatively by participants belonging to Type 1 are shown in Table 5. Each Z-score is also presented in Table 5. In this type, the statements that participants positively agreed with are in the following order: Q24, Q23, Q22, and Q21, with Z-scores of 1.80, 1.61, 1.40, and 1.21, respectively. The participants also had the most negative viewpoints on the Q8 statement, with a Z-score of −2.01.

Table 5. Statements with a Z score of ±1.00 or higher for each type and Z score results.

		Q Statement	Z Score
Type 1	Positive	Q 24	1.80
		Q 23	1.61
		Q 22	1.40
		Q 21	1.21
	Negative	Q 8	−2.01
		Q 9	−1.69
		Q 11	−1.35
Type 2	Positive	Q 4	1.82
		Q 6	1.52
		Q 5	1.20
	Negative	Q 9	−1.89
		Q 8	−1.41
		Q 3	−1.20
Type 3	Positive	Q 14	1.92
		Q 15	1.65
		Q 12	1.23
	Negative	Q 3	−1.92
		Q 4	−1.50
		Q 6	−1.19
Type 4	Positive	Q 10	1.82
		Q 8	1.41
		Q 12	1.17
	Negative	Q 15	−1.84
		Q 14	−1.30

A total of seven participants belonged to Type 1 and showed the largest number of respondents. The P-Sample number and the factor weight were P1 (0.69), P2 (0.74), P8 (0.78), P9 (0.87), P15 (0.88), P17 (0.61), and P18 (0.68). Respondent P15 displayed the highest factor weight, which well represents the point of view of Type 1.

3.3. Type 2 (Factor 2): Beachhead for a Vibrant School Life: Improving Interpersonal Relationships, Social Skills, and Adaptability

As shown in Table 5, The statement most agreed upon by the participants in Type 2 is Q4, followed by Q6 and Q5, with a Z-score of 1.82, 1.52, and 1.20, respectively. In addition, the most negative statements is Q9 (Z-score = −1.89), followed by Q8 (Z-score = −1.41) and Q3 (Z-score = −1.20).

Four participants belonged to Type 2. Respondents P3, P10, P16, and P 19 belonged to this type, with factor weights of 0.70, 0.73, 0.90, and 0.81, respectively. The factor weight of P 16 was the highest, indicating well with regard for this type of perspective.

3.4. Type 3 (Factor 3): Enhancement of Academic Capability: Increased Concentration, Positive Learning Attitude, and Increased Academic Performance

Table 5 illustrates the positive and negative statements for Type 3 and each Z-score. In Type 3, the most positive Q statement by participants are Q14 (Z-score = 1.92), followed by Q15 (Z-score = 1.65) and Q12 (Z-score = 1.23), whereas the most negative statement is Q3 (Z-score = −1.92).

There are four participants in this type. Participants P4, P5, P11, and P20 belonged to Type 3, and the factor weight was 0.92, 0.70, 0.69, and 0.81, respectively.

3.5. Type 4 (Factor 4): Strengthening Physical and Mental Health: Improving Exercise Function, Increasing Interest in PE Classes, and Leading a Healthy Daily Life

The statements (positive and negative) of Type 4 and each Z score are shown in Table 5. The most positively agreed-upon statement is Q10 (Z-score = 2.05), whereas the most negatively agreed statement was Q15 (Z-score = −1.84).

In the last type, Type 4, four respondents were identified. As we have seen from Table 5, participants P6, P12, P13, and P14 were included in this type, and the factor weight was 0.84, 0.89, 0.58 and 0.59, respectively.

3.6. Consensus Statements by All Types

Table 6 indicates the commonly agreed-upon statements for all types, namely Q1 and Q2, with Z-scores of 0.78 and 0.60, respectively.

Table 6. Consensus statements.

Q Statement	Z Score
Q 1. Morning exercise can create a sense of goal and impellent.	0.78
Q 2. Through participation in morning exercise, it has changed or is becoming a bright personality.	0.60

4. Discussion

The researchers have discussed the EVs, variance, and correlation between the five types and reviewed the classification results for P-Sample and Q-Sample involved in each type with Z-scores. We have also checked the consensus statements.

In terms of correlation findings regarding each type, since the correlation between all types was low, each type's independence and explanatory power were secured. A strong correlation between Type 2 and Type 4 was observed, which means that the classification intensity of respondents belonging to Type 2 and Type 4 is the highest. In other words, perceptions between the two types of respondents are different prominently. For example, in the case of Type 2, children's participation in the early morning exercise program was recognized by the participants belonging to Type 2 as having a positive effect on revitalizing school life. On the other hand, however, they had negative thoughts about physical and mental reinforcement. In the case of Type 4, they were aware of the advantages of improving their children's exercise skills and increasing interest in PE classes. However, they were not aware of the impact on school life. The discussion based on the results of this study is as follows.

Most of all, respondents from Type 1 showed great awareness of the inclusion of "0-period PE class" into a regular curriculum, not a temporal activity. That is, there is a need for a multifaceted infrastructure in which the "0th-period PE class" can be operated as a regular class. Therefore, expanding facilities, diversifying programs, and placing expert instructors should be considered first to improve the quality of early morning exercise programs. In addition, the respondents were convinced that the "0th-period PE class" helped students develop in various aspects which legitimate promotion expansion of early morning exercise. As a result, this type was titled "urgent legal and institutional settlement of "0th-period PE class": Strengthening facilities, programs, instructors, and publicity".

As mentioned earlier, the early morning exercise program has been activated in Korea since 2010. However, lack of attention from the teachers, low incentives for participating teachers and students, and recognition as an extra-curricular activity are regarded as decisive reasons for the institutional failure to settle down. Lee [21] pointed out several issues each school undergoes in the operation of the early morning exercise program. As a result, the researcher suggested optimizing the program for each school environment, strengthening the role of operating teachers, and improving program facilities. Meanwhile, cooperation between PE teachers, general teachers, and students was emphasized as the most crucial factor for the program's success [19]. For example, Jeon et al. [38] emphasized the theoretical basis for implementing the "0th-period PE class" for middle schools and applied practical measures to encourage the participation of teachers and students. Furthermore, this will be possible through stable administrative and financial support from government and local agencies [21]. Hence, the result that the most significant number of respondents were distributed in Type 1 means the possibility of legal and institutional settlement of the "0th-period PE class".

Secondly, the Type 2 participants strongly believed that early morning exercise plays a significant role in leading to successful school life. Notably, respondents recognized that the program was helpful in social development, such as cooperation with others, interpersonal skills, and leadership building [39]. Moreover, unlike in regular classes, interaction with friends and teachers frequently occurs, leading to students' social development and expansion of social networks. These results mean that "0th-period PE class" helps students adapt to overall school life. Lee et al. [40] suggested that the program not only manages stress but also prevents deviations from school for students. Jeon et al. [20] explored Korean middle school students' subjective perception types and characteristics regarding participation in the "0th-period PE class". He concluded that the program was recognized as the driving force for students to maintain a stable school and could be an advantage of the morning exercise program from a parent's point of view.

Based on the discussion above, Type 2 was named "Beachhead for a vibrant school life: Implying interpersonal relationships, social skills, and adaptability". Meanwhile, participants in Type 2 recognized that "0th-period PE class" had a positive effect on school life but showed a negative perception of improving motor skills and physical fitness such as agility, muscular strength, and endurance.

Thirdly, Type 3 was named "Enhancement of academic capability: Increased concentration, positive learning attitude, and increased academic performance". In this type, positive perceptions of academic achievement were mainly derived. Interestingly, participants in Type 3 showed a negative perception about the development of social skills through the early morning exercise program.

Recently, scholars in kinesiology have shown scientific evidence of an association between physical activity and academic achievement. Research studies on a positive relationship between physical activity and academic achievement have been discussed [41–43], especially for those adolescent populations [4,6]. For example, Hobart [8] demonstrated that the morning exercise program improves the brain's structure and condition, improving academic performance. Furthermore, there is scientific evidence that physical activity can contribute to developing and activating the hippocampus, which has a significant role in learning and memory in the limbic system [44,45].

Studies conducted in Korea related to these topics produced similar results. For example, participation in the "0th-period PE class" improved high school students' academic performance than a control group that did not receive the morning exercise program [46]. However, the results also showed that students in the control group had more stress and mental issues. Park and Moon [16] mentioned that the morning exercise program could improve academic performance through increased concentration. Thus, the logical and theoretical connection between morning exercise and academic achievement supports the response of Type 3 participants.

Lastly, Type 4 is titled "Strengthening physical and mental health: Improving exercise function, increasing interest in PE classes, and leading a healthy daily life". Participants in this category were highly aware of the direct physical effects of participation in sports and exercise. Furthermore, experiencing the morning exercise program contributed to motivation and active participation in PE classes. Based on these results, the healthy daily life of student agency was logically derived. However, respondents of Type 4 showed a negative perception of the impact on academic performance through the early morning exercise program.

The benefits of early morning exercise have been substantially proven by scientific evidence in physiology and medical science [47]. For example, regular morning exercise program participation positively improved adolescents' motor skills, cardiorespiratory endurance, and muscle strength [16,48]. Furthermore, the sports club activities in the "0th-period PE class" significantly affected elementary school students' physical self-concept [49]. For this reason, the researchers draw attention to the fact that maintaining healthy daily life is possible by participating in "0th-period PE class" in terms of physical and mental benefits for adolescents [50,51]. Based on the above academic perspective, various perceptions of parents in the results of this study were discussed. A variety of previous studies have already published the effects of early morning exercise. However, this study has the ultimate goal of institutionalizing the "0th-period PE class" based on early morning exercise. Particularly, the positive perception of parents was derived in a different aspect from the students participating [20] in the "0th-period PE class". As remarked in the introduction, the role of parents is important in the institutional development of public education in South Korea. Thus, this study's findings can be an academic driving force for "0th-period PE class" to be operated as a regular class in the near future.

5. Conclusions

The current study attempted to establish a systematic settlement of the "0th-period PE class" in Korea. The researchers mainly explored the subjective perspectives of parents regarding the morning exercise program of middle schools in Korea using the Q-methodology. The composition of the 42 Q-population resulted in selecting the final 25 Q-Samples. Among the participants, 20 students who participated in "0th-period PE class" for more than one year were selected as P-Sample. The Q-sorting process was performed by the P-Sample. Data collected by Q-sorting were analyzed using the P-Q method program (version 2.35) with centroid factor analysis and varimax rotation. The data analysis categorized the results into four types with a total explanatory variance of 63%. The four types are as follows: urgent legal and institutional settlement of the "0th-period PE class" (Type 1, $n = 7$); beachhead for a vibrant school life (Type 2, $n = 4$); enhancement of academic capability (Type 3, $n = 4$); and strengthening physical and mental health (Type 4, $n = 4$). Moreover, the consensus statements between each type were investigated in Q1 and Q2.

Based on published papers, the morning exercise program is more prevalent and widely spread in the United States, UK, and Japan. Moreover, a legitimate legal basis supports program implementation in some countries, which guarantees adolescents the right to education and a healthy lifestyle [52]. However, the Korean education community has yet to implement legal and institutional procedures to settle the "0th-period PE class". For this reason, continuous attention of the academic community should be followed [20]. The results of this study produced academic intellectual assets that could be systematically implemented in a "0th-period PE class" in Korea. Future directions include further studies to advance the "0th-period PE class", as well as better understand the roles and relationships among diverse stakeholders (policymakers, administrators, teachers, students, and parents).

Author Contributions: Conceptualization, W.J. and W.C.; methodology, W.J.; investigation, W.C.; data analysis, W.J. and W.C.; writing—original draft preparation, W.J.; writing—review and editing, W.C.; supervision, W.J. and W.C. All authors have read and agreed to the published version of the manuscript.

Funding: This research received no external funding.

Institutional Review Board Statement: The study was conducted according to the guidelines of the Declaration of Helsinki. Ethical review and approval were waived because necessary permissions were obtained from the schools (to which this study participants belonged) affiliated with this study.

Informed Consent Statement: Informed consent was obtained from all subjects involved in the study.

Data Availability Statement: The data presented in this study are available upon request from the corresponding authors.

Conflicts of Interest: The authors declare no conflict of interest.

References

1. Herting, M.M.; Chu, X. Exercise, cognition, and the adolescent brain. *Birth Defects Res.* **2017**, *109*, 1672–1679. [CrossRef] [PubMed]
2. Chaddock, L.; Pontifex, M.B.; Hillman, C.H.; Kramer, A.F. A review of the relation of aerobic fitness and physical activity to brain structure and function in children. *J. Int. Neuropsychol. Soc.* **2011**, *17*, 975–985. [CrossRef] [PubMed]
3. O'Connor, P.J.; Tomporowski, P.D.; Dishman, R.K. Age moderates the association of aerobic exercise with initial learning of an online task requiring cognitive control. *J. Int. Neuropsychol. Soc.* **2015**, *21*, 802–815. [CrossRef]
4. Blakemore, C.L. Movement is essential to learning. *J. Phys. Educ. Recreat. Danc.* **2003**, *74*, 22–41. [CrossRef]
5. Basch, C.E. Healthier students are better learners: A missing link in school reforms to close the achievement gap. *J. School Health* **2011**, *81*, 593–598. [CrossRef]
6. Marsh, H.W.; Kleitman, S. School Athletic Participation Mostly Gain with Little pain. *J. Sport Exerc. Psychol.* **2003**, *25*, 205–228. [CrossRef]
7. Donnelly, J.E.; Hillman, C.H.; Castelli, D.; Etnier, J.L.; Lee, S.; Tomporowski, P.; Lambourne, K.; SzaboReed, A.N. Physical activity, fitness, cognitive function, and academic achievement in children: A systematic review. *Med. Sci. Sports Exerc.* **2016**, *48*, 197–222. [CrossRef]
8. Hobart, M. Spark: The revolutionary new science of exercise and the brain. *Psychiatr. Serv.* **2008**, *59*, 939. [CrossRef]
9. Schumacher, L.M.; Thomas, J.G.; Raynor, H.A.; Rhodes, R.E.; Bond, D.S. Consistent morning exercise may be beneficial for individuals with obesity. *Exerc. Sport Sci. Rev.* **2020**, *48*, 201. [CrossRef]
10. McGowan, C.J.; Pyne, D.B.; Thompson, K.G.; Raglin, J.S.; Rattray, B. Morning exercise: Enhancement of afternoon sprint-swimming performance. *Int. J. Sports Physiol. Perform.* **2017**, *12*, 605–611. [CrossRef]
11. Maia, A.P.L.; Sousa, I.C.D.; Azevedo, C.V.M.D. Effect of morning exercise in sunlight on the sleep-wake cycle in adolescents. *Psychol. Neurosci.* **2011**, *4*, 323–331. [CrossRef]
12. Babadi, M.E.; Mansouri, A.; Nouri, F.; Mohammadifard, N.; Gharipour, M.; Jozan, M.; Rabiei, K.; Azarm, T.; Khosravi, A. Morning Exercise at School and Sedentary Activities are Important Determinants for Hypertension in Adolescents. *Int. J. Prev. Med.* **2021**, *12*, 131. [PubMed]
13. Ratey, J.J. *Spark: The Revolutionary New Science of Exercise and the Brain*; Little, Brown Spark: Hachette, UK, 2008.
14. Lim, S.W.; Lee, K.M.; Kim, I.H.; Lee, H.G. The Operation System and Implications of "The 0 period Physical Education Class": The Case Study about "Blue" Elementary School. *Korean J. Phys. Educ.* **2014**, *53*, 51–61.
15. Jeon, W.; Ahn, C.; Gwon, H. Causal Model of Participation, Perceived Enjoyment, and Learning Attitudes in "the 0th Period Physical Education Class" of Middle Schools in South Korea. *Int. J. Environ. Res. Public Health.* **2021**, *18*, 7668. [CrossRef]
16. Park, Y.; Moon, J. Effects of early morning physical activity on elementary school students' physical fitness and sociality: Focusing on the comprehensive school physical activity program. *Int. Electron. J. Elem. Educ.* **2018**, *10*, 441–447.
17. Park, I.S. A Case Study on Morning Exercises Conducted for Three Years in Science High School. *Korean J. Phys. Educ.* **2013**, *52*, 193–204.
18. Topor, D.R.; Keane, S.P.; Shelton, T.L.; Calkins, S.D. Parent involvement and student academic performance: A multiple mediational analysis. *J. Prev. Interv. Community* **2010**, *38*, 183–197. [CrossRef]
19. Lim, S.W.; Lee, K.M.; Kim, I.H.; Lee, H.G. Ways to activate "0 period physical education" through Delphi technique and analytic hierarchy process. *Korean J. Sociol. Sport* **2015**, *28*, 1–21.
20. Jeon, W.; Kwon, G.; Joung, K. Subjective Perceptions and Their Characteristics of Middle School Students Regarding the Effectiveness of the "0th Period Physical Education Class" in South Korea: The Q Methodology Application. *Sustainability* **2021**, *13*, 12081. [CrossRef]
21. Lee, I. Study on zero hour physical education experience of high school students. *Korean Soc. Study Phys. Educ.* **2014**, *19*, 31–47.
22. Stephenson, W. *The Study of Behavior: Q-Technique and Its Methodology*; University of Chicago Press: Chicago, IL, USA, 1953.
23. Baker, R.M. Economic rationality and health and lifestyle choices for people with diabetes. *Soc. Sci. Med.* **2006**, *63*, 2341–2353. [CrossRef] [PubMed]
24. Jeon, W.; Jang, S.; Joung, K. Subjective Perceptions of South Korean Parents Regarding the Effectiveness of Taekwondo Education for Adolescents and Its Characteristics: The Q Methodology Application. *Int. J. Environ. Res. Public Health* **2021**, *18*, 9687. [CrossRef] [PubMed]
25. Brown, S.R. Q methodology and qualitative research. *Qual. Health Res.* **1996**, *6*, 561–567. [CrossRef]
26. Akhtar-Danesh, N.; Baumann, A.; Cordingley, L. Q-methodology in nursing research: A promising method for the study of subjectivity. *West. J. Nurs. Res.* **2008**, *30*, 759–773. [CrossRef] [PubMed]
27. Alderson, S.; Foy, R.; Bryant, L.; Ahmed, S.; House, A. Using Q-methodology to guide the implementation of new healthcare policies. *BMJ Qual. Saf.* **2018**, *27*, 737–742. [CrossRef]
28. Raadgever, G.T.; Mostert, E.; Van De Giesen, N.C. Identification of stakeholder perspectives on future flood management in the Rhine basin using Q methodology. *Hydrol. Earth Syst. Sci.* **2008**, *12*, 1097–1109. [CrossRef]
29. Kerlinger, F.N. *Foundation of Behavioral Research*, 2nd ed.; Holt, Rinehart and Winston: New York, NY, USA, 1973.
30. Kim, H.Q.Q. *Methodology: Philosophy, Theories: Analysis, and Application*; Communication Books: Seoul, Korea, 2008.
31. Brown, S. *Political Subjectivity*; Yale University: New Haven, CT, USA, 1980.
32. Watts, S. Develop a Q methodological study. *Educ. Prim. Care* **2015**, *26*, 435–437. [CrossRef]
33. Brown, S.R. On the use of variance designs in Q methodology. *Psychol. Rec.* **1970**, *20*, 179–189. [CrossRef]

34. Schmolck, P. PQ Method Manual. 2014. Available online: http://schmolck.org/qmethod/pqmanual.htm (accessed on 30 January 2022).
35. Watts, S.; Stenner, P. *Doing Q Methodological Research: Theory, Method and Interpretation*; SAGE: Los Angeles, CA, USA, 2012.
36. Guttman, L. Some necessary conditions for common-factor analysis. *Psychometrika* **1954**, *19*, 149–161. [CrossRef]
37. Kaiser, H.F. The application of electronic computers to factor analysis. *Educ. Psychol. Meas.* **1960**, *20*, 141–151. [CrossRef]
38. Jeon, W.J.; Nam, Y.H. A study on the subjectivity of middle school teachers regarding 0th Period Physical Education Class. *J. Learn. Cent. Curric. Instr.* **2021**, *21*, 639–651. [CrossRef]
39. Park, S.B. The effects of 0 hour class Physical education of Middle School Students on Sociality and School Life Adaptation. *Korea J. Sports Sci.* **2013**, *22*, 97–110.
40. Lee, K.M.; Lim, S.W.; Kim, I.H.; Lee, H.G. The relationship among stress, emotion regulation strategies and school resilience of the middle school students participating in zero hour class physical activity. *Korean J. Sociol. Sport* **2014**, *27*, 133–153.
41. Ratey, J.; Loehr, J.E. The positive impact of physical activity on cognition during adulthood: A review of underlying mechanisms, evidence, and recommendations. *Rev. Neurosci.* **2001**, *22*, 171–185. [CrossRef]
42. Cotman, C.W.; Berchtold, N.C. Exercise a behavioral intervention to enhance brain health and plasticity. *Trends Neurosci.* **2002**, *25*, 295–301. [CrossRef]
43. Sibley, B.A.; Etnier, J.L. The relationship between physical activity and cognition in children: A meta-analysis. *Pediatric Exerc. Sci.* **2003**, *15*, 243–256. [CrossRef]
44. Greenwood, B.N.; Strong, P.V.; Foley, T.E.; Fleshner, M. A behavioral analysis of the impact of voluntary physical activity on hippocampus-dependent contextual conditioning. *Hippocampus* **2009**, *19*, 988–1001. [CrossRef]
45. Bolijn, S.; Lucassen, P.J. How the body talks to the brain; peripheral mediators of physical activity-induced proliferation in the adult hippocampus. *Brain Plast.* **2015**, *1*, 5–27. [CrossRef]
46. Beak, J.S. Recognition of science high school students on the 0 h class physical activity. *Korean Soc. Study Phys. Educ.* **2015**, *19*, 59–78. [CrossRef]
47. Valipour Dehnouhnou, V.; Abbasi Moghadam, M.; Soleymani Farsani, M. Effects of early morning exercise on serum brain-derived neurotrophic factor level and its relation with blood cholesterol and glucose levels in the elderly men. *Iran. J. Ageing* **2018**, *13*, 324–333. [CrossRef]
48. Lee, K.M.; Lim, S.W.; Lee, H.G.; Kim, I.H. Improvement Direction of Exercise in the Morning by IPA. *Korean J. Phys. Educ.* **2016**, *55*, 35–46.
49. Kim, Y.S.; Kim, D.K.; Chae, C.M. Effect of Early Morning Sport club Physical Activity on Academic Achievement and Learning Attitude, Physical Self-Concept of Elementary School Students. *Korean J. Phys. Educ.* **2014**, *53*, 223–233.
50. Jung, H.Y.; Lee, M.H.; Beak, S.S. Effects of 10-week physical education program in the morning on physical activity and cognitive function in the middle school students. *Korean J. Phys. Educ.* **2015**, *54*, 521–529.
51. Lee, I. Aspect of Operation and Finding Out Improvement Direction on Physical Education during Before Class in High Schools. *Korean Soc. Study Phys. Educ.* **2015**, *20*, 31–46. [CrossRef]
52. Noh, Y.K.; Kim, S.J. Case Studies for Analyzing Before School of Physical Activities in the Inside and Outside of the Country: Managerial Implications in Club Sports. *Educ. Res.* **2021**, *81*, 97–117.

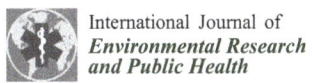

Article

Self-Rated Health Status of Upper Secondary School Pupils and Its Associations with Multiple Health-Related Factors

Armando Cocca [1,*], Martin Niedermeier [1], Vera Prünster [1], Katharina Wirnitzer [1,2,3], Clemens Drenowatz [4], Klaus Greier [1,5], Karin Labek [6] and Gerhard Ruedl [1]

1. Department of Sport Science, University of Innsbruck, 6020 Innsbruck, Austria; martin.niedermeier@uibk.ac.at (M.N.); vera.pruenster@student.uibk.ac.at (V.P.); katharina.wirnitzer@ph-tirol.ac.at (K.W.); nikolaus.greier@uibk.ac.at (K.G.); gerhard.ruedl@uibk.ac.at (G.R.)
2. Department of Research and Development in Teacher Education, University College of Teacher Education Tyrol, 6010 Innsbruck, Austria
3. Research Center Medical Humanities, Leopold-Franzens University of Innsbruck, 6020 Innsbruck, Austria
4. Division of Sport, Physical Activity and Health, University of Education Upper Austria, 4020 Linz, Austria; clemens.drenowatz@ph-ooe.at
5. Divison of Physical Education, Private Educational College (KPH-ES), 6422 Stams, Austria
6. Institute of Psychology, University of Innsbruck, 6020 Innsbruck, Austria; karin.labek@uibk.ac.at
* Correspondence: armando.cocca@uibk.ac.at

Abstract: Health is an essential part of any individual, and gains particular importance in youth, as a good health at this age is more likely to reduce health risks both in the short and long term. The aim of this study was to assess the impact of physical and contextual parameters on youths' perceived health. A total of 919 adolescents completed questionnaires on self-rated health status, electronic media use, leisure time and club physical activity, alcohol and tobacco consumption, and back pain, as well as performed the German Motor Performance Test. Participants with very good health had significantly higher physical fitness, leisure time exercise, and participated in sports clubs more often than those with poorer health. Electronic media use was significantly higher for those with poor/very poor health. Future intervention programs to improve youth health status should not only focus on active lifestyle but might also consider the impact of socioenvironmental factors, such as daily media use.

Keywords: youth; perceived health; physical fitness; structured sport activities; screen time

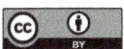

1. Introduction

Being healthy is an essential part of any adolescent life. In fact, youths with a positive health status have higher chances to grow into healthy adults, as several serious diseases (e.g., cardiorespiratory fitness, mental disorders) that generally occur in adulthood originate from health issues during adolescence [1]. Although several approaches exist to study people's health status, individual self-perception has grown as one of the most interesting methods due to several advantages. Compared to medical records, self-perception tools are easier to apply, allow for encompassing broader strata of the population at lower costs, and have been shown to be a valid assessment strategy [2]. Although there exist some differences due to sociodemographic factors compared to the objective assessment of health, these two methods are deemed to obtain comparable findings [2].

Perceived health status is influenced by several socioenvironmental and personal factors. Studies found a positive association between physical fitness and perceived health in youth, especially in terms of cardiorespiratory and muscular fitness [3,4]. Participation in organized sports activities may also be an essential contributor to perceived health as there exists a positive relationship between sports participation and perceived health regardless of the sociocultural environment [5,6]. In addition, children with healthier body mass index

(BMI) display enhanced perceived health status or higher perception of health-related self-efficacy [7,8]. Furthermore, BMI and weight status may indirectly affect perceived health through associations with active habits and nutritional and lifestyle choices [9].

On the other hand, unhealthy behaviors, such as tobacco and alcohol consumption, excessive screen time and electronic media use, and back pain, can be mentioned as prominent sources of reduced health perception in youth [9–11]. Tebar et al. [12] showed a worse health perception in youth with a higher number of sedentary activities, regardless of their physical activity habits. Prolonged sitting and excess screen time are also related to back pain at early ages [13,14], which has a detrimental effect on perceived health as well [11,15].

Although previous studies have investigated the separate effect of the factors mentioned earlier on perceived health, to date, there are only a few studies addressing their intertwined action. Perceived health, however, is the result of the combination of physical, social, environmental, and demographic agents, and its alteration cannot be fully understood without considering this wide spectrum of variables. The aims of this study, therefore, are to evaluate the current perceived health of upper secondary school pupils and its associations with multiple health-related factors; to compare physical, social, and environmental variables by health status; and to analyze the explanatory power of such variables on perceived health status.

2. Materials and Methods

2.1. Participants

Using a cross-sectional design, adolescents between grades 9 and 12 from six randomly selected public secondary schools participated in the study. Data collection occurred during spring 2018. The study protocol received formal ethical approval. Parents provided written informed consent, and participants provided assent at the time of data collection. All study procedures were in accordance with the ethical standards of the Declaration of Helsinki.

2.2. Anthropometric Measurements

In line with previous studies on Austrian adolescents [16,17], students' height and weight were measured in sport clothing and barefoot during regular physical education lessons in the school gym. Body height was measured with a mobile stadiometer "Seca 217" (Seca, Hamburg, Germany) with an accuracy of 0.1 cm, and body weight was measured with a calibrated scale "Grundig PS 2010" (Grundig AG, Neu-Isenburg, Germany) with an accuracy of 0.1 kg. BMI (kg/m^2) was calculated, and students were classified according to the BMI reference system by Kromeyer-Hauschild et al. [18] into three groups: underweight vs. normal weight vs. overweight/obese.

2.3. Questionnaire

Regarding the perceived health status of adolescents, self-rated health represents a meaningful subjective indicator for general health [19]. According to the Health Behavior in School-Aged Children (HBSC) study [20], self-rated health was measured by a single item with the question "Would you say your health in general is ... ". For answering this question, we used a five-point Likert scale (very good, good, moderate, poor, very poor). Participants were subsequently divided into four health categories (very good, good, moderate, poor/very poor), which are comparable to the four HBSC categories of self-rated health (excellent, good, fair, poor) [20]. Participants also reported their average daily time (hours/day) of electronic media use (smartphone, tablet, computer, TV, etc.) outside of school as well as the presence of a TV in their bedroom [16]. Sports club participation was determined via self-report (yes/no). In addition, participants reported mean duration (hours per week) of practicing sports in a club setting as well as during leisure time. Weekly hours of sports club participation and weekly hours of physical activity in leisure time were then summed up to obtain a total amount of weekly leisure time sports activity. Finally, smoking and alcohol consumption, as well as current back pain during the previous 7 days, were reported using a dichotomous variable (yes/no), respectively.

2.4. Physical Fitness

For testing the physical fitness, participants completed the German Motor Performance Test (GMT) 6-18 [21]. The GMT is a standardized test battery consisting of eight items that assesses various subdomains of physical fitness: 20 m sprint (sprint velocity), balancing backwards on three 3 m long beams with different width (coordination in a task requiring precision), jumping sidewards over a middle line for 15 s (coordination under time pressure), stand-and-reach (flexibility), push-ups in a period of 40 s (strength endurance), sit-ups in a period of 40 s (strength endurance), standing long jump (power), and 6 min run (endurance). With regard to the performance criteria of GMT 6-18, the inter-rater reliability (0.95) and test–retest reliability (0.82) of the test battery were good, and the battery has been validated for assessing speed, coordination, flexibility, strength, and endurance [21]. According to the exact instruction of the test manual by Bös [21], tests were carried out by trained physical education students in the gymnasiums of the participating schools. All tests were completed during a single session, lasting about 90 min in random order, except for the 20 m sprint, which was completed at the beginning, and the 6 min run, which was completed at the end of the testing session. Values of the eight test items were standardized according to age and sex-reference values resulting in so-called Z-values, with a value of 100 representing average performance in the tests. According to Bös [21], the formula for the standardization is

$$Z = (x_i - M)/SD \times 10 + 100 \qquad (1)$$

where x_i is the raw value of the test item, M is the mean, and SD the standard deviation of the age- and sex-specific norm sample. Values above 100 indicate above-average performance and values below 100 indicate below-average performance. The average of all scores was used as an indicator for overall physical fitness [21].

2.5. Statistics

Data are presented as means ± standard deviations and relative (absolute) frequencies, respectively. All statistical analyses were conducted using SPSS Statistics version 26 (IBM, New York, NY, USA). The first step of the analysis consisted of tests on differences in potentially associated factors between the four health groups group with very good perceived health (VH), good perceived health (GH), moderate perceived health (MH), and poor/very poor perceived health (PH). Since the group sizes were unequal (n = 34 for the smallest and n = 482 for the largest group), Kruskal–Wallis H-tests were calculated for continuous factors (age, BMI, mean daily electronic media use, mean weekly leisure time sports activity, and mean physical fitness). For categorical factors (sex, weight status, electronic media in bedroom, sports club participation, and prevalence of smoking and drinking alcohol, as well as of suffering from back pain), Pearson's chi-square tests were used to evaluate differences between the four health groups. In the case of a significant result, additional post hoc tests with Bonferroni correction were performed.

The second analysis step consisted of a multiple multinominal logistic regression analysis with health status as the dependent variable. A multinominal logistic regression model was chosen since proportional odds between categories of health status were not assumed. The reference level was set to the group with very good perceived health (VH). All variables with significant differences between categories were included as predictor variables to the multiple model, except for weight status to avoid redundancy with BMI. Although not significant in the simple analysis, age was included in the multiple model to account for age differences in the predictor variables (e.g., percentage of smokers, percentage of alcohol consumers, BMI). Odds ratios (OR), including 95% confidence intervals (95% CI), were calculated for all predictor variables.

All *p*-values were two-tailed, and values less than 0.05 were considered to indicate statistical significance.

3. Results

A total of 919 adolescents (55.6% girls) with a mean age of 15.5 ± 1.3 years and a mean BMI of 22.0 ± 3.9 kg/m^2 participated. With regard to the additional classification into three weight groups, 5.3% (n = 49) of students were in the underweight group, 75.3% (n = 692) in the normal weight group, and 19.4% (n = 178) in the overweight/obese group, respectively.

Regarding self-rated health status, 21.8% of adolescents stated very good health, 52.6% good, 21.9% moderate, and 3.7% poor/very poor health.

In total, 68% stated to have a TV or computer in the bedroom, and 42% participated in sports clubs. Additionally, 8.7% reported smoking, 59.8% consumed alcohol, and 42.2% reported suffering from back pain.

Mean reported daily electronic media use was 2.7 ± 1.7 h, mean reported weekly leisure time sports activity was 9.8 ± 4.9 h, and mean physical fitness (Z-value) of the cohort was 105.6 ± 6.2.

In Table 1, results of the univariate comparison of the four different health groups are presented. Significant differences between groups were found with regard to sex, BMI, weight status, electronic media in the bedroom, daily electronic media use, sports club participation, weekly leisure time sports activity, physical fitness, smoking, and prevalence of back pain.

Table 1. Group differences in factors between adolescents with a very good, good, moderate, and poor/very poor perceived health. Values are means with SD or prevalence (%).

Factors	Very Good Health (n = 200)	Good Health (n = 482)	Moderate Health (n = 201)	Poor/Very Poor Health (n = 34)	*p*-Value	Post Hoc [c]
Age [years]	15.6 ± 1.3	15.5 ± 1.3	15.5 ± 1.3	15.4 ± 1.6	0.691 [a]	none
Sex [%], girls	44.5	57.9	61.7	50.0	0.002 [b]	VH:GH, VH:MH,
BMI [kg/m^2]	21.3 ± 2.7	21.6 ± 3.4	22.8 ± 4.5	25.9 ± 7.1	<0.001 [a]	VH:MH, VH:PH, GH:MH, GH:PH
Weight status [%]					<0.001 [b]	VH:MH, GH:MH
Underweight	3.5	5.8	7.0	0		
Normal weight	87.0	77.2	63.2	52.9		
Overweight/adipose	9.5	17.0	29.9	47.1		
Electronic media in bedroom [%], yes	72.5	63.1	74.1	76.5	0.008 [b]	GH:MH
Daily electronic media use [h]	2.4 ± 1.3	2.6 ± 1.7	2.9 ± 1.7	3.8 ± 2.7	<0.001 [a]	VH:MH, VH:PH
Sports club participation [%], yes	59.0	43.4	25.4	23.5	<0.001 [b]	VH:GH, VH:MH, VH:PH, GH:MH
Weekly leisure time sports activity [h]	8.0 ± 5.4	6.2 ± 5.0	3.9 ± 3.7	3.1 ± 4.1	<0.001 [a]	VH:GH, VH:MH, VH:PH, GH:MH, GH:PH
Physical fitness [Z-value]	108.4 ± 5.4	106.0 ± 5.8	102.9 ± 5.6	99.7 ± 9.1	<0.001 [a]	VH:GH, VH:MH, VH:PH, GH:MH, GH:PH
Smoking [%], yes	4.0	8.5	13.9	5.9	0.005 [b]	VH:MH
Alcohol consumption [%], yes	56.5	61.2	61.2	52.9	0.546 [b]	none
Back pain [%], yes	35.0	41.3	47.8	61.8	0.006 [b]	VH:PH

Notes: Data are displayed as means ± standard deviations or relative frequencies, as appropriate. [a]: Kruskal–Wallis H-test, [b]: chi-square-test, [c]: significant differences specified according to Bonferroni-corrected pairwise comparisons. BMI: body mass index, VH: group with very good perceived health, GH: group with good perceived health, MH: group with moderate perceived health, PH: group with poor/very poor perceived health. Bold values indicate significant differences.

In Table 2, results of the multiple multinomial regression model are presented. Compared to the group with very good perceived health (reference group), being female (OR = 1.57) significantly increased the odds for being in the group with good perceived health. Conversely, being older (OR = 0.84), having electronic media in the bedroom (OR = 0.57), showing higher physical fitness (OR = 0.93), and not reporting back pain (OR = 0.66) significantly decreased the odds for being in the group with good perceived health compared to the group with very good perceived health.

Table 2. Results of the multiple multinomial regression analysis with the dependent variable perceived health status.

Variable	B	SE B	OR	OR 95% CI lb	OR 95% CI ub	p
GH vs. VH						
Intercept	11.52	(2.54)				<0.001
Age [years]	−0.17	(0.07)	0.84	0.74	0.97	0.015
Sex, female	0.45	(0.19)	1.57	1.09	2.27	0.016
Body mass index [kg/m^2]	0.04	(0.03)	1.04	0.98	1.11	0.170
Electronic media in bedroom, yes	−0.56	(0.20)	0.57	0.39	0.84	0.004
Daily electronic media use [h]	0.10	(0.06)	1.10	0.97	1.25	0.129
Sports club participation, yes	−0.61	(0.32)	0.54	0.29	1.02	0.057
Weekly leisure time sports activity [h]	−0.03	(0.02)	0.97	0.94	1.01	0.166
Physical fitness [Z-value]	−0.08	(0.02)	0.93	0.90	0.96	<0.001
Smoking, yes	0.73	(0.41)	2.08	0.94	4.63	0.072
Back pain, no	−0.42	(0.19)	0.66	0.46	0.95	0.024
MH vs. VH						
Intercept	15.79	(3.12)				<0.001
Age [years]	−0.21	(0.08)	0.81	0.69	0.96	0.014
Sex, female	0.42	(0.24)	1.52	0.96	2.42	0.074
Body mass index [kg/m^2]	0.10	(0.03)	1.11	1.03	1.18	0.003
Electronic media in bedroom, yes	−0.24	(0.25)	0.79	0.48	1.30	0.351
Daily electronic media use [h]	0.11	(0.07)	1.12	0.97	1.30	0.124
Sports club participation, yes	−0.89	(0.36)	0.41	0.20	0.83	0.012
Weekly leisure time sports activity [h]	−0.12	(0.03)	0.89	0.84	0.94	<0.001
Physical fitness [Z-value]	−0.13	(0.02)	0.88	0.84	0.92	<0.001
Smoking, yes	1.16	(0.44)	3.17	1.33	7.55	0.009
Back pain, no	−0.83	(0.23)	0.44	0.28	0.68	<0.001
PH vs. VH						
Intercept	17.48	(5.49)				0.001
Age [years]	−0.36	(0.16)	0.70	0.51	0.95	0.022
Sex, female	−0.06	(0.44)	0.94	0.40	2.21	0.883
Body mass index [kg/m^2]	0.20	(0.05)	1.22	1.11	1.34	<0.001
Electronic media in bedroom, yes	−0.59	(0.49)	0.55	0.21	1.46	0.233
Daily electronic media use [h]	0.26	(0.10)	1.30	1.06	1.59	0.013
Sports club participation, yes	−1.48	(0.56)	0.23	0.08	0.68	0.008
Weekly leisure time sports activity [h]	−0.13	(0.07)	0.88	0.77	1.00	0.047
Physical fitness [Z-value]	−0.15	(0.04)	0.86	0.80	0.93	<0.001
Smoking, yes	0.19	(0.86)	1.20	0.22	6.49	0.829
Back pain, no	−1.61	(0.43)	0.20	0.09	0.46	<0.001

Notes: R^2 (Nagelkerke) = 0.26, model chi-square (21) = 243.45, $p < 0.001$, B: unstandardized regression coefficient, SE: standard error, OR: odds ratio, 95% CI: 95% confidence interval, lb: lower bound, ub: upper bound. Bold values indicate $p < 0.05$. VH: group with very good perceived health (reference group), GH: group with good perceived health, MH: group with moderate perceived health, PH: group with poor/very poor perceived health.

Compared to the group with very good perceived health (reference group), the likelihood for being in the group with moderate perceived health significantly increased with higher BMI (OR = 1.11) and smoking (OR = 3.17). Conversely, being older (OR = 0.81), participating in a sports club (OR = 0.41), higher weekly leisure time sports activity (OR = 0.89), higher physical fitness (OR = 0.88), and not reporting back pain (OR = 0.44) was associated with a decreased likelihood to be in the group with moderate perceived health.

Similarly, the odds for being in the poor/very poor health group was significantly larger in adolescents with higher BMI (OR = 1.22) compared to the group with very good perceived health. Age (OR = 0.70), sports club participation (OR = 0.23), higher weekly leisure time sports activity (OR = 0.88), higher physical fitness (OR = 0.86), and not reporting back pain (OR = 0.20), on the other hand, was associated with decreased odds for being in the group with poor/very poor health perceived health compared to the group with very good perceived health. Additionally, the chance for an increased daily electronic media use was significantly higher in the poor/very poor health group (OR = 1.30).

4. Discussion

The aims of this study were to evaluate the current perceived health of upper secondary school students and its associations with multiple health-related factors; to compare physical, social, and environmental variables by health status; and to analyze the explanatory power of such variables on perceived health status.

Our findings show that almost three quarters of the studied population (74.4%) perceive their health as at least good. In accordance, the latest Austrian Health Interview Survey [22] reported that the vast majority of adolescents reported being satisfied with their health status, with less than 10% considering their health as poor or very poor.

A more detailed analysis of the results indicates that a high perception of health (very good, good) is very similar in male and female participants (44.5% and 57.9% of girls, respectively); however, two thirds of the "moderate health" group is represented by girls. This seems to be partially in line with previous studies suggesting that women tend to show a poorer perception of their health [23,24] or similar perception to men, despite the latter reporting higher incidence of health issues [25].

When analyzing the factors associated with perceived health in youth, the positive association between physical fitness and perceived health is clear. In fact, physical fitness seems to have a significant influence at all levels of health, as indicated by various studies [3,4]. In line with our findings, Liu et al. [26] proposed a significant association between overall physical fitness and general health, which, together, may predict adolescents' lifestyle choices and their willingness to engage in and promote healthy habits. The prominent role of physical fitness is also emphasized in studies focusing on different areas of youth's individual health, such as mental health [27], physical and metabolic health [28], social health [29], and overall quality of life [4]. Physical fitness, therefore, should be promoted in different settings, including the school environment, physical education, and leisure time.

Accordingly, leisure time physical activity appears to be an important determinant for perceived health, particularly discriminating between positive and low or negative perception of health [30]. Gomes et al. [31] report that leisure time exercise may positively influence mental health both directly and indirectly by reducing the time spent by youth in sedentary activities. These types of activities are also bidirectionally associated with health literacy, which may not only improve adolescents' health status, but also their knowledge and understanding of the indicators of health and, as a consequence, influence their lifestyle choices [32].

Our sample reported significantly better health for those engaging in sports club activities compared to those who did not. Participation in sports clubs, in fact, may be important not only for individual health but also as an opportunity for youth to reduce social and environmental inequities [33].

Similar to our findings on leisure time and organized physical activity, in our study, worse BMI scores were only associated with lower to poor perception of health, with no significant differences between those participants who reported being in very good or good health. This is in line with previous studies showing the impact of BMI and weight status on perceived health [7,9]. Additionally, BMI is considered a mediator of the relation between participation in physical activity and perceived health [9].

It may have been surprising that having electronic media in the bedroom did not affect the perception of health in our sample. Although some studies suggest a relation between media availability in the bedroom and certain factors associated with general health, such as sleep time and quality [34], increased screen time [35], or even depression symptoms [36], the availability of electronic media in the bedroom does not necessarily lead to their usage or over-usage. In our sample, the fact that most of the participants stated to have media available in their bedroom regardless of the health group they belonged to might simply indicate that they do not make excessive use of them. However, when we combine these results with those on the daily usage of media, the difference between adolescents in the "very good health" group and those in the "moderate" and "poor health" ones becomes significant. It is also evident from our data that only the "very good health" group members (and partially the "good health" group ones) are close to the recommendations on maximum daily screen time (2 h/day) [37], whereas those who perceived lower or poor health spent an average of 3 h and 4 h on screen, respectively. Excessive screen time, therefore, should be considered as correlation of the perception of one's own health, as already stated elsewhere [10,12].

In addition, reported back pain is significantly lower in the "very good health" group compared to all the other groups. This is in line with previous studies on the impact of this issue on perceived health [11,15]. As the authors emphasize, back pain is logically strictly related to people's consideration of their own health as positive or negative. In fact, differently than physical fitness, physical activity, and body composition, which may be perceived very differently based on cultural aspects [38], and screen time, which some individuals may at times perceive as positive for their mental health [39], back pain is embedded in one's health condition, and may be even considered as a component of it. Therefore, it is reasonable to assume that those who did not report any back pain consider their health better compared to those who experienced such a problem. Finally, it is important to keep in mind that our results on back pain may not be sufficiently accurate, as the onset and duration of this issue (for instance, chronic vs. acute), as well as its intensity and source (mechanical, neurological, etc.), were not considered in the present study.

Limitations

This study presents some limitations. Although perceived health status evaluated with a single item is considered a valid measurement method, using self-rating tools may encompass risks, such as invalid responses, social desirability biases, or general response biases [40]. Additionally, health status has been evaluated with a single item. Given the complex structure of such a variable, a single item might not reflect such condition in full. However, we decided not to burden the participants with an excessively long series of items, in accordance with previous literature on the topic [41,42], and based it on single-item assessment that has been validated [43]. Additionally, our analysis of potential agents of perceived health could not include several other variables that are also known to be associated with it, such as personality traits [44], dietary patterns [45], or family situation and social support networks [46].

In the future, this type of study could also expand to explore potential differences in such network of variables based on school location (for instance, type of neighborhood, urban vs. rural) or school type (public or private). Another interesting addition to this research could be represented by a deeper analysis of participants' sports habits both within sports clubs and during leisure time, since the type of exercise is known to potentially affect health-related parameters [47].

5. Conclusions

Perceived health status may be influenced by many factors, both environmental and personal. Among them, the overall level of physical fitness, which includes cardiorespiratory endurance, muscular strength, and flexibility, among others, seem to be central determinants for the perception of adolescents' health. Accordingly, sports club participation and overall leisure time physical activities appear to be critical correlates of perceived health. In addition, screen time needs to be considered in strategies targeting health in adolescents. Therefore, future investigations/approaches should be multifocal and include robust physical fitness developmental plans through physical education curricula in school while also emphasizing participation in organized sport club activities and replacing sedentary leisure time, such as screen time, with more active tasks. All these attempts/interventions may enhance youth health literacy as well, which could reduce other detrimental health behaviors such as smoking and alcohol consumption. Any intervention should also include parental counseling and a coordinated effort of families, teachers, and administrators in order to pursue appropriate strategies targeting the diverse contributors of adolescents' health.

Author Contributions: Conceptualization, G.R. and K.G.; methodology, G.R. and V.P.; software, M.N. and A.C.; validation, A.C. and C.D.; formal analysis, M.N. and C.D.; investigation, V.P. and K.L.; resources, G.R. and K.G.; data curation, A.C. and K.W.; writing—original draft preparation, A.C.; writing—review and editing, K.W., G.R. and K.L.; supervision, K.G.; project administration, G.R., K.G. and C.D. All authors have read and agreed to the published version of the manuscript.

Funding: This research received no external funding.

Institutional Review Board Statement: The study was conducted in accordance with the Declaration of Helsinki, and protocol was approved by the Board for Ethical issues of the University of Innsbruck, Austria (Certificate of Good Standing 73/2021), and the school authorities of the federal state as well as the school board of each participating school.

Informed Consent Statement: Informed consent was obtained from all subjects involved in the study.

Data Availability Statement: Data from this study are not public due to privacy policies and are available upon request to the corresponding author.

Conflicts of Interest: The authors declare no conflict of interest.

References

1. Namboothiri, G.N.; Sathyanath, M.S.; Baisil, S.; Gowthami, P.; Rashmi, A.; Kundapur, R.; Vidya, R.; Alex, P.; Shameena, A.U.; George, G.M.; et al. Module based health education on stress and depression—Effectiveness and feasibility study among schools in Dakshina Kannada: A pilot study. *J Indian Assoc. Child Adolesc. Ment. Health* **2021**, *17*, 37–56.
2. Carreras, M.; Puig, G.; Sánchez-Pérez, I.; Inoriza, J.M.; Coderch, J.; Gispert, R. Morbidity and self-perception of health, two different approaches to health status. *Gac. Sanit.* **2020**, *34*, 601–607. [CrossRef]
3. Bermejo-Cantarero, A.; Alvarez-Bueno, C.; Martinez-Vizcaino, V.; Redondo-Tebar, A.; Pzuelo-Carrascosa, D.P.; Sanchez-Lopez, M. Relationship between both cardiorespiratory and muscular fitness and health-related quality of life in children and adolescents: A systematic review and meta-analysis of observational studies. *Health Qual. Life Outcomes* **2021**, *19*, 127. [CrossRef] [PubMed]
4. Yi, X.R.; Fu, Y.; Burns, R.; Ding, M. Weight status, physical fitness, and health-related quality of life among Chinese adolescents: A cross-sectional study. *Int. J. Environ. Res. Public Health* **2019**, *16*, 2271. [CrossRef]
5. Eime, R.M.; Harvey, J.T.; Brown, W.J.; Payne, W.R. Does sport club participation contribute to health-related quality of life? *Med Sci. Sports. Exerc.* **2010**, *42*, 1022–1028. [CrossRef] [PubMed]
6. Balish, S.M.; Conacher, D.; Dithurbide, L. Sport and recreation are associated with happiness across countries. *Res. Q. Exerc. Sport* **2016**, *87*, 382–388. [CrossRef]
7. Motamed-Gorji, N.; Heshmat, R.; Qorbani, M.; Motlagh, M.; Soltani, A.; Shafiee, G.; Asayesh, H.; Ardalan, G.; Matin, N.; Mahdavi Gorabi, A.; et al. Is the association of weight disorders with perceived health status and life satisfaction independent of physical activity in children and adolescents? The CASPIAN-IV study. *J. Trop. Pediatr.* **2019**, *65*, 249–263. [CrossRef]
8. Ovaskainen, M.L.; Tapanainen, H.; Laatikainen, T.; Männistö, S.; Heinonen, H.; Vartiainen, E. Perceived health-related self-efficacy associated with BMI in adults in a population-based survey. *Scand. J. Public Health* **2015**, *43*, 197–203. [CrossRef]
9. Moral-García, J.E.; Agraso-López, A.D.; Ramos-Morcillo, A.J.; Jiménez, A.; Jiménez-Eguizábal, A. The influence of physical activity, diet, weight status and substance abuse on students' self-perceived health. *Int. J. Environ. Public Health* **2020**, *17*, 1387. [CrossRef]
10. Zhang, T.; Lu, G.; Wu, X.Y. Association between physical activity, sedentary behaviour and self-rated health among the general population of children and adolescents: A systematic review and meta-analysis. *BMC Public Health* **2020**, *20*, 1343. [CrossRef]
11. Ahmed, U.A.; Maharaj, S.S.; Van Oosterwijck, J. Effects of dynamic stabilization exercises and muscle energy technique on selected biopsychosocial outcomes for patients with chronic non-specific low back pain: A double-blind randomized controlled trial. *Scand. J. Pain* **2021**, *21*, 495–511. [CrossRef]
12. Tebar, W.R.; Werneck, A.O.; Silva, D.; de Souza, J.; Stubbs, B.; da Silva, C.; Ritti-Dias, R.; Christofaro, D. Poor self-rated health is associated with sedentary behavior regardless of physical activity in adolescents-PeNSE study. *Ment. Health Phys. Act.* **2021**, *20*, 100384. [CrossRef]
13. Kedra, A. Non-specific low back pain: Cross-sectional study of 11.423 children and youth and the association with the perception of heaviness in carrying of schoolbags. *PeerJ* **2021**, *9*, e11220. [CrossRef] [PubMed]

14. Santos, E.D. Prevalence of Low Back Pain and Associated Risks in School-Age Children. *Pain Manag. Nurs.* **2021**, *22*, 459–464. [CrossRef] [PubMed]
15. Yang, C.Y.; Tsai, Y.; Wu, P.; Ho, S.; Chou, C.; Huang, S. Pilates-based core exercise improves health-related quality of life in people living with chronic low back pain: A pilot study. *J. Bodyw. Mov. Ther.* **2021**, *27*, 294–299. [CrossRef]
16. Greier, K.; Drenowatz, C.; Ruedl, G.; Riechelmann, H. Association between daily TV time and fitness in 6- to 14-year old Austrian youth. *Transl. Pediatr.* **2019**, *8*, 371–377. [CrossRef]
17. Ruedl, G.; Greier, K.; Niedermeier, M.; Posch, M.; Prünster, V.; Faulhaber, M.; Burtscher, M. Factors associated with physical fitness among overweight and non-overweight Austrian secondary school students. *Int. J. Environ. Res. Public Health* **2019**, *16*, 4117. [CrossRef] [PubMed]
18. Kromeyer-Hauschild, K.; Wabitsch, M.; Kunze, D. Perzentile für den Body-mass-Index für das Kindes- und Jugendalter unter Heranziehung verschiedener deutscher Stichproben. *Monatsschr. Kinderheilkd.* **2001**, *49*, 807–818. [CrossRef]
19. Hodacova, L.; Hlavackova, E.; Sigmundova, D.; Kalman, M.; Kopcakova, J. Trends in life satisfaction and self-rated health in Czech school-aged children: HBSC study. *Cent. Eur. J. Public Health* **2017**, *25* (Suppl. S1), S51–S56. [CrossRef]
20. Paakkari, L.; Torppa, M.; Mazur, J.; Boberova, Z.; Sudeck, G.; Kalman, M.; Paakkari, O. A comparative study on adolescents' health literacy in Europe: Findings from the HBSC study. *Int. J. Environ. Res. Public Health* **2020**, *17*, 3543. [CrossRef]
21. Bös, K.; Schlenker, L.; Büsch, D.; Lämmle, L.; Müller, H.; Oberger, J.; Seidel, I.; Tittlbach, S. *Deutscher Motorik Test 6–18 (DMT 6–18) [German Motor Performance Test 6–18 (DMT 6–18)]*; Czwalina: Hamburg, Germany, 2009.
22. Federal Ministry of Social Affairs, Health, Care and Consumer Protection. *Austrian Health Interview Survey 2019*; Statistik Austria: Wien, Austria, 2019.
23. Pace, F.; Sciotto, G. Gender Differences in the Relationship between Work–Life Balance, Career Opportunities and General Health Perception. *Sustainability* **2022**, *14*, 357. [CrossRef]
24. Okunrintemi, V.; Valero-Elizondo, J.; Patrick, B.; Salami, J.; Tibuakuu, M.; Ahmad, S.; Ogunmoroti, O.; Mahajan, S.; Khan, S.U.; Gulati, M.; et al. Gender Differences in Patient-Reported Outcomes Among Adults with Atherosclerotic Cardiovascular Disease. *J. Am. Heart Assoc.* **2018**, *7*, e010498. [CrossRef] [PubMed]
25. Sood, R.; Jenkins, S.; Sood, A.; Clark, M. Gender Differences in Self-perception of Health at a Wellness Center. *Am. J. Health Behav.* **2019**, *43*, 1129–1135. [CrossRef]
26. Liu, H.; Liu, Y.; Li, B. Predictive Analysis of Health/Physical Fitness in Health-Promoting Lifestyle of Adolescents. *Front. Public Health* **2012**, *18*, 691669. [CrossRef] [PubMed]
27. Cadenas Sanchez, C.; Mena Molina, A.; Torres Lopez, L.; Migueles, J.H.; Rodriguez-Ayllon, M.; Lubans, D.R.; Ortega, F.B. Healthier Minds in Fitter Bodies: A Systematic Review and Meta-Analysis of the Association between Physical Fitness and Mental Health in Youth. *Sports Med.* **2021**, *51*, 2571–2605. [CrossRef] [PubMed]
28. Mantilla, C.; Jones, T.; Decker, K.M.; Jacobo, A.M.; Sontheimer, S.Y.; Mirro, M.R.; Hare, M.E.; Han, J.C. Diabetes Prevention Program in Youth (Insulin Superheroes Club) Pilot: Improvement in Metabolic Parameters and Physical Fitness After 16 Weeks of Lifestyle Intervention. *Diabetes Care* **2017**, *40*, e63–e64. [CrossRef]
29. Lemes, V.; Gaya, A.R.; Sadarangani, K.P.; Aguilar-Farias, N.; Rodriguez-Rodriguez, F.; Martins, C.M.D.L.; Fochesatto, C.; Cristi-Montero, C. Physical Fitness Plays a Crucial Mediator Role in Relationships Among Personal, Social, and Lifestyle Factors With Adolescents' Cognitive Performance in a Structural Equation Model. The Cogni-Action Project. *Front. Pediatr.* **2021**, *9*, 656916. [CrossRef]
30. Dostálová, R.; Stillman, C.; Erickson, K.I.; Slepička, P.; Mudrák, J. The Relationship between Physical Activity, Self-Perceived Health, and Cognitive Function in Older Adults. *Brain Sci.* **2021**, *11*, 492. [CrossRef] [PubMed]
31. Gomes, M.L.; Tonrquist, L.; Tornquist, D.; Caputo, E.L. Body image is associated with leisure-time physical activity and sedentary behavior in adolescents: Data from the Brazilian National School-based Health Survey (PeNSE 2015). *Braz. J. Psychiatry* **2021**, *43*, 584–589. [CrossRef]
32. Sukys, S.; Tilindiene, I.; Trinkuniene, L. Association between health literacy and leisure time physical activity among Lithuanian adolescents. *Health Soc. Care Community* **2021**, *29*, e387–e395. [CrossRef]
33. Borraccino, A.; Lazzeri, G.; Kakaa, O.; Badura, P.; Bottigliengo, D.; Dalmasso, P.; Lemma, P. The Contribution of Organised Leisure-Time Activities in Shaping Positive Community Health Practices among 13-and 15-Year-Old Adolescents: Results from the Health Behaviours in School-Aged Children Study in Italy. *Int. J. Environ. Res. Public Health* **2020**, *17*, 6637. [CrossRef]
34. Leonard, H.; Khurana, A.; Hammond, M. Bedtime media use and sleep: Evidence for bidirectional effects and associations with attention control in adolescents. *Sleep Health* **2021**, *7*, 491–499. [CrossRef] [PubMed]
35. Rodrigues, D.; Gama, A.; Machado-Rodrigues, A.; Nogueira, H.; Rosado-Marques, V.; Silva, M.R.; Padez, C. Home vs. bedroom media devices: Socioeconomic disparities and association with childhood screen- and sleep-time. *Sleep Med.* **2021**, *83*, 230–234. [CrossRef] [PubMed]
36. Pirdehghan, A.; Khezmeh, E.; Panahi, S. Social Media Use and Sleep Disturbance among Adolescents: A Cross-Sectional Study. *Iran. J. Psychiatry* **2021**, *16*, 137–145. [CrossRef] [PubMed]
37. American Academy of Pediatrics. *Media and Children*. Available online: https://www.aap.org/en/patient-care/media-and-children/ (accessed on 5 March 2022).
38. Pan, C.; Maiano, C.; Morin, A.J.S. Physical self-concept and body dissatisfaction among Special Olympics athletes: A comparison between sex, weight status, and culture. *Res. Dev. Disabil.* **2018**, *76*, 1–11. [CrossRef] [PubMed]

39. David, O.; Predatu, R.; Cardos, R. Effectiveness of the REThink therapeutic online video game in promoting mental health in children and adolescents. *Internet Interv.* **2021**, *25*, 100391. [CrossRef] [PubMed]
40. Demetriou, C.; Uzun Ozer, B.; Essau, C. Self-Report Questionnaire. In *The Encyclopedia of Clinical Psychology*; Cautin, R.L., Lilienfeld, S.O., Eds.; Wiley and Sons: New York, NY, USA, 2015. [CrossRef]
41. Rolstad, S.; Adler, J.; Ryden, A. Response Burden and Questionnaire Length: Is Shorter Better? A Review and Meta-analysis. *Value Health* **2011**, *14*, 1101–1108. [CrossRef]
42. Sahlqvist, S.; Song, Y.; Bull, F.; Adams, E.; Preston, J.; Ogilvie, D.; iConnect Consortium. Effect of questionnaire length, personalisation and reminder type on response rate to a complex postal survey: Randomised controlled trial. *BMC Med. Res. Methodol.* **2011**, *11*, 62. [CrossRef] [PubMed]
43. Fisher, G.; Matthews, R.; Mitchell Gibbson, A. Developing and Investigating the Use of Single-Item Measures in Organizational Research. *J. Occup. Health Psychol.* **2015**, *21*, 3–23. [CrossRef]
44. Olivares, P.; Leyton, G.; Salazar, E. Personality factors and self-perceived health in Chilean elderly population. *Health* **2013**, *5*, 86–96. [CrossRef]
45. Jezewska-Zychowicz, M.; Wadolowska, L.; Kowalkowska, J.; Lonnie, M.; Czarnocinska, J.; Babicz-Zielinska, E. Perceived Health and Nutrition Concerns as Predictors of Dietary Patterns among Polish Females Aged 13–21 Years (GEBaHealth Project). *Nutrients* **2017**, *9*, 613. [CrossRef] [PubMed]
46. Sagone, E.; Stasolla, F.; Verrastro, V. Influence of Social Support Network and Perceived Social Support on the Subjective Wellbeing of Mothers of Children with Autism Spectrum Disorder. *Front. Psychol.* **2022**, *13*, 835110. Available online: https://www.frontiersin.org/article/10.3389/fpsyg.2022.835110 (accessed on 31 May 2022).
47. van Baak, M.A.; Pramono, A.; Battista, F.; Beaulieu, K.; Blundell, J.E.; Busetto, L.; Carraça, E.V.; Dicker, D.; Encantado, J.; Ermolao, A.; et al. Effect of different types of regular exercise on physical fitness in adults with overweight or obesity: Systematic review and meta-analyses. *Obes. Rev.* **2021**, *22*, e13239. [CrossRef] [PubMed]

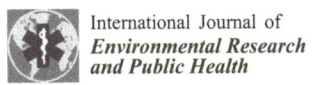

Article

Evaluation of Age Based-Sleep Quality and Fitness in Adolescent Female Handball Players

Mohamed Alaeddine Guembri [1,*,†], Ghazi Racil [2,†], Mohamed-Ali Dhouibi [3], Jeremy Coquart [4] and Nizar Souissi [1]

1. Research Unit: Physical Activity, Sport and Health (UR18JS01), National Observatory of Sports, Tunis 1003, Tunisia
2. Research Unit 17JS01 (Sport Performance, Health & Society), Higher Institute of Sport and Physical Education of Ksar Saîd, Manouba, Tunis 2010, Tunisia
3. Laboratory of Clinical Psychology: Intersubjectivity and Culture, Faculty of Humanities and Social Sciences, University of Tunis, Tunis 1007, Tunisia
4. Univ. Lille, Univ. Artois, Univ. Littoral Côte d'Opale, ULR 7369-URePSSS-Unité de Recherche Pluridisciplinaire Sport Santé Société, Lille, France
* Correspondence: alaaguembri@yahoo.fr
† These authors contributed equally to this work.

Abstract: The present study aimed to examine the differences in sleep hygiene, balance, strength, agility, and maximum aerobic speed (MAS) between two groups of female handball players aged under 14 (U14) and under 17 (U17) years. Seventy-two female handball players participated and were divided into two groups according to age: U14 (n = 36, age: 13.44 ± 0.5 years) and U17 (n = 36, age: 15.95 ± 0.76 years). Sleep hygiene was evaluated using three questionnaires: Sleep quality and sleepiness via the Pittsburgh (PSQI) and Epworth (ESS) questionnaires, and the insomnia questionnaire via the measurement of the insomnia severity index (ISI). Physical fitness was evaluated with the stork balance tests with eyes open (OEB) and closed (CEB), the vertical jump (SJ), horizontal jump (SBJ), and five jump (FJT) tests, the agility (t-test) and the maximum aerobic speed (MAS) tests. No significant differences were shown between U14 and U17 players in all PSQI, ISI, and ESS scores, and balance and strength performances. Meanwhile, the U17 players' performances were significant better in agility quality (p = 0.003 < 0.01) and MAS (p = 0.05) compared to the U14 players. Biological gender specificity during the maturation phase may inhibit the improvement of balance, and strength performances between the age of 13 and 17 years, while agility and MAS performances are more affected by age alterations.

Keywords: sleep quality; puberty; sleep disorders; physical condition; insomnia; sleepiness; body fat; lean body mass

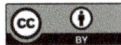

1. Introduction

Handball is a team sport with an intermittent nature involving several physical qualities such as balance [1,2], muscular strength [3,4], agility [5,6], and endurance [7,8]. Thus, improving these qualities is essential for development during childhood and adolescence [9].

Previous studies have shown the importance of this evaluation to distinguish the elite players from the sub-elite players of the same age category [10,11]. It was demonstrated, however, that the reactive agility quality presented, for example, a distinguishing factor for experienced versus amateur players [12]. Although basic motor abilities have been evaluated in women's handball [13], to the best of the authors' knowledge, no studies have examined the difference that may occur in some measures of physical condition in the young players.

Mostly, young athletes' training sessions are based on technical and tactical work and less on the development of physical abilities, which change with age and are affected by biological maturation [14]. It is important to mention that the stabilization of fitness is noted between the beginning and end of puberty [15], and that girls' morphological development is marked by a high intensity of fat mass accumulation at that phase, which represents an inhibiting factor for performance [16].

Understanding the effects of changes in girls during the transition from pre-puberty to post-puberty seems to be of interest for coaches to better plan and intervene, especially on the physical level, to optimize performance. Therefore, one of the objectives of our study was to focus on the differences in some measures of physical fitness in female handball players between the ages of under 14 and under 17. We hypothesized that performance is better for U17 compared to U14 for both anaerobic and aerobic tests. However, having 3 years' experience in practice, may present a good argument to distinguish this difference during maturation regardless of gender.

Indeed, having sleep disorders such as insomnia can inhibit the proper functioning of cognitive mechanisms such as attention, concentration, and memory, which are factors in sports performance. These troubles, which were suggested to be caused by fatigue and daytime sleepiness [17], are related to poor physical condition [18], including cardiorespiratory capacity [19]. This prompts us to focus on the evaluation of certain aspects of sleep in young athletes in their adolescent phase.

This period of adolescence undergoes dramatic changes in sleep [20,21]. In this context, two processes intervene in its regulation. The first one targets the intrinsic circadian system, and the second one targets the homeostatic sleep–wake system [22]. This context, however, explains the short sleep duration, during either the nights and even the day of sports training [23,24].

It was reported that many adolescents suffer from the prevalence of sleep disorders such as sleepiness [17] and insomnia [25,26]. As recently shown [27], more than 39% of adolescents suffered from poor sleep quality. In this regard, it is crucial to develop comprehensive sleep education in adolescents at first, and which should be respected in the school curriculum.

Furthermore, this finding leads us to evaluate the nature of sleep hygiene by establishing a comparison of the quality of sleep via the Pittsburgh questionnaire (PSQI), the insomnia questionnaire via the measurement of the insomnia severity index (ISI), and sleepiness via the Epworth questionnaire (ESS), between U14 and U17 female players.

However, the objectives of the present study were (1) to compare sleep parameters (PSQI, ISI, and ESS) between U14 and U17 female players and (2) to compare the differences in some fitness measures between these two different age groups.

2. Materials and Methods

2.1. Participants

Seventy-two healthy female handball players participated in this study. They were divided into two different age groups: U14 (36 players, age: 13.44 ± 0.5 years, height: 1.64 ± 0.04 m, BM: 57.83 ± 5.79 kg, BMI: 21.49 ± 1.52 kg m^{-2}) and U17 (36 players, age: 15.95 ± 0.76 years, height: 1.67 ± 0.05 m, BM: 59.21 ± 6.16 kg, BMI: 21.22 ± 1.63 kg m^{-2}). All of them belong to a regional local handball team, and they train for 1 h 30 min per session 4 times weekly. Before beginning the intervention, all participants and their parents signed an informed consent form in accordance with the international ethical standards, in particular the Declaration of Helsinki [28]. It should be noted that four participants withdrew before the start of the study for personal reasons (2 from each group) and their data were not accounted for in the statistical analysis.

2.2. Anthropometric Measurements

All anthropometric measurements were performed in the afternoon at the end of the week with the help of a specialized physician.

Body height was measured in centimeters with no shoes, heels together, and the back of the subject parallel to the stadiometer (Model 214 height rod; Seca, Hamburg, Germany).

Body mass (BM) was assessed to the nearest 0.1 kg with a digital scale (Tanita, Tokyo, Japan) and the body mass index (BMI = Mass [kg]/(Height [m])^2) was determined. The fat mass (FM), lean mass (LM), and body mass index (BMI) were measured for each participant by bioelectrical impedance analysis (BIA) (Tanita Body Composition Analyzer Mode TBF-300, Tokyo, Japan).

With the help of a qualified pediatrician, assessment of the pubertal stage was determined according to the Tanner classification [29] (Tanner and Whitehouse 1976): Pubertal children included Tanner stages II-III and post-pubertal children were in Tanner stages IV-V (refer to Table 1).

Table 1. Anthropometric parameters of the 2 groups of U14 and U17.

Group	U14 N = 36	U17 N = 36
PS (II–III/IV–V)	15/21	17/19
Height (m)	1.64 ± 0.04	1.67 ± 0.05 *
Body mass (kg)	57.83 ± 5.79	59.21 ± 6.16 *
Body mass index (kg m^{-2})	21.49 ± 1.52	21.22 ± 1.63 *
Body fat (%)	24.45 ± 1.5	22.27 ± 1.3
Lean body mass (kg)	43.95 ± 2.7	46.18 ± 3.1 *

Values are mean ± SD; PS: pubertal stage. Significantly different from U14: * $p < 0.05$.

2.3. Procedure

The experimental part of this study was spread over a vacation period of 3 days (Figure 1). Before the commencement of the experimentation, a physician made sure that the players were not sick, did not take any medication, and had not practiced any sport on that day. Thus, all tests were performed in a single session starting at 4:00 pm since performance peaks in the late afternoon for anaerobic tests and in accordance with the hours of the day in which most of the training sessions were regularly performed as determined by Chtourou et al [30], except for the VAMEVAL test, which was performed in the second session.

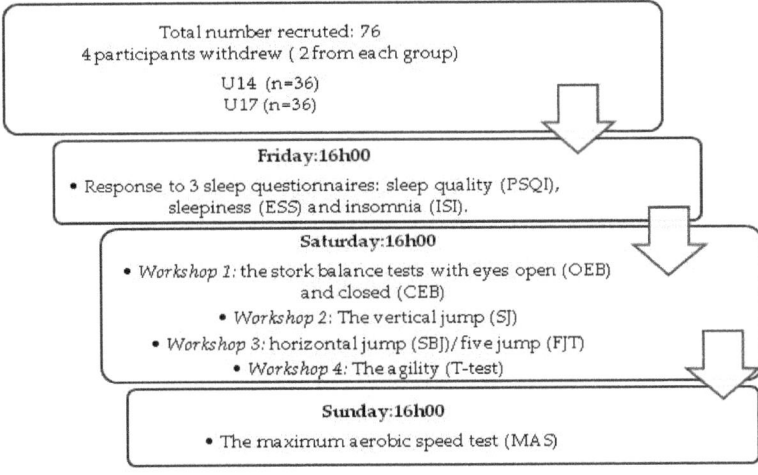

Figure 1. Study design for U14 and U17 female players.

Day1:

On the first day, the 2 groups completed the three sleep questionnaires. Thus, each participant had to answer questions about their sleep attitudes during the days and nights of the last month: The Pittsburgh Questionnaire (PSQI), the Insomnia Questionnaire (ISI), and the Sleepiness Questionnaire (ESS). Each of these is composed of several items. To answer the questionnaires, an explanation was presented by an examiner who gave a verbal signal to the participant who passed from one item to another.

The Pittsburgh sleep quality index (PSQI) [31] is a questionnaire for the subjective evaluation of sleep quality; it is composed of 19 questions combined into 7 scores. The 7 component scores are added together to obtain an overall score ranging from 0 to 21, and an increase in the score coincides with a decrease in sleep quality.

Moreover, the insomnia severity index (ISI) [32] is a self-reported subjective measure of insomnia symptoms and the levels of worry caused by sleep disorders, composed of seven items. When adding up the scores, it helps to give an overall score ranging from 0 to 28. Therefore, the scores between 0 and 7 = No insomnia; 8–14 = Subclinical insomnia (mild); 15–21 = Clinical insomnia (moderate); and 22–28 = Clinical insomnia (severe).

On the other side, the Epworth Sleepiness Scale (ESS) [33] is a self-administered questionnaire; it is composed of 8 items that measure the "usual probability of dozing or falling asleep" in common everyday situations. The ESS score ranges from 0 to 24, and when the score is higher than 10 it is an indicator of severe drowsiness.

Day2:

The second day of the intervention was dedicated to the realization of the tests in the indoor handball court. Each training session started with a warm-up of approximately 10-min based on running, joint mobilization, and stretching followed by five bursts of 20-m sprints [34].

Participants also performed the balance test "stork balance" with eyes open and eyes closed. This test consists of maintaining balance on one leg and on the sole of the foot for as long as possible.

Except for the test of the squat jump (SJ), which was performed in door a Handball court, the standing long jump (SBJ) and the five-jump tests (FJT) were performed outdoors on an athletic field. In the agility test "t-Test", the participant accelerated and decelerated with rapid changes of direction. When the players had completed all repetitions, they moved from one test to the other. The passive recovery time was fixed to 5-min. It is important to note that a familiarization test was performed at the beginning of the intervention to eliminate any learning factor that could bias the results. Four investigators assured the completion of all the tests. All participants were encouraged verbally. However, all measures were again collected and performed (in the same conditions) for comparison with baseline values.

2.3.1. Stork Balance Test

This test was performed as described by Sopa [35]. The participant was required to stand on a single leg of their choice, barefoot and on a flat surface. The other leg was raised so that the foot of that leg was glued next to the knee of the supporting leg. The participant had to put her hands on her hips. The clock started when the participant lifted the heel of the supporting leg. The participant had to maintain this position for as long as possible, and the timer stopped when she dropped the heel of the supporting leg, rotated the body in any direction, or lifted the hands from the hips. Each player had 3 attempts to practice balancing either with eyes open (OEB) or closed (CEB). The participant was allowed to practice their balance for one minute and the total time was recorded. The best result of the three attempts was taken into consideration.

2.3.2. Squat Jump (SJ)

This test involved evaluating the quality of jumps using an Opto-jump system [36]. Three trials were performed, and the best performance expressed in centimeters was retained for statistical analysis.

2.3.3. The Standing Broad Jump or the Horizontal Jump (SBJ)

This test was performed as indicated by [37].

From the standing position, both feet had to touch the starting line and the player had to jump as far as possible in a horizontal direction. The take-off and landing phases of the jump had to be performed with both feet. The distance from take-off to the heel of the nearest foot on landing was measured in centimeters. Three trials were performed, and the best performance was taken for later analysis.

2.3.4. Five Jump Test (FJT)

The participant performed five successive horizontal jumps [38], which started with their feet together and with an upright posture. The participant executed five bouncing strides on one leg, elevating the free knee and the opposite arm towards the front, and finished with both legs together. The distance covered was measured and expressed in meters. Three attempts were performed, and the best performance was taken into account.

2.3.5. The Agility *t* Test

This test was administered as described by [39]. At the signal, the participant sprinted forward 9.14 m, touched the end of the first cone with her right hand, then ran laterally to the left for 4.57 m to touch the end of the second cone with the left hand and continue to move again for 9.14 m to the right and touch the end of the third cone with the right hand. The participant made a lateral return of 4.57 m to the left to touch the cone in the middle with the left hand. The test ended with a backward run to the starting point (9.14 m). A photoelectric cell (Photocells, Microgate®, Bolzano, Italy) was used to measure the performance. Three attempts were performed, and the best performance was taken into account.

2.3.6. VAMEVAL Test

In order to assess the maximum aerobic speed (MAS), a running test was performed on a 200-m athletic track. This was administered as described by [34]. Blue cones were placed every 20-m at the lane line boundary of the track. Similarly, red cones were placed 2-m behind the blue cones. An examiner followed participants with a scoring table containing the beep times of the different levels, a stopwatch, and a whistle. The examiner made a short sound when the participant had to be next to the blue cone so that he could manage the running speed according to each level. At each whistle, the participant had to be within 2-m of the blue cones. When the participant did not follow the rhythm of the sound and was twice behind a red cone or when he stopped the race, the event was over. The maximum aerobic speed (MAS) corresponds to the level already finished. If the participant did not run the last stage for the full duration, then the method in [40] was used to calculate the MAS. The test started on the track at 8 km/h for 2 min, and for each stage of one minute, the speed increased by 0.5 km/h.

Maximum aerobic speed in km/h was recorded. VO_{2max} was calculated using the formula proposed by [41,42]: $VO_{2max} = 0.0324 \times v^2 + 2.143 \times v + 14.49$; where v is the speed of the last level expressed in km h^{-1} and VO_{2max} in mL kg^{-1} min^{-1}.

2.4. Statistical Analysis

Analyses of all data were performed using SPSS version 26.0 (SPSS, Inc., Chicago, IL, USA). Results were presented as mean ± standard deviation. The categorization of the 3 sleep variables (PSQI, ISI, and ESS) was presented as percentages for the U14 and U17 athletes. For all the studied variables, the normality of the data distribution was checked using the Kolmogorov–Smirnov method.

A student's *t*-test of independent samples was performed to compare the mean scores of PSQI, ISI, and ESS according to age (U14 and U17). Thereafter, the different measures of physical condition such as the average values of balance, strength, agility, and MAS between these 2 groups were also calculated. An alpha p value of less than 0.05 was used as a significance threshold.

3. Results

No significant differences were observed for the different sleep parameters (PSQI, ISI, and ESS) between the U14 and U17 players (Table 2).

Table 2. Comparison of the means of sleep quality, sleepiness, and insomnia between the two groups.

Group	PSQI	ISI	ESS
Group U14	5.44 ± 1.576	7.19 ± 2.649	6.36 ± 1.91
Group U17	5.47 ± 1.540	7.50 ± 2.49	6.31 ± 1.89

Values are mean ± SD; PSQI: Pittsburgh Sleep Quality Index; ISI: Insomnia Severity Index; ESS: Epworth Sleepiness Scale.

The prevalence of players with poor sleep quality (PSQI ≥ 5) was 61.1% for the U14 group and 63.8% for the U17 group of older participants; mild insomnia (ISI ≥ 11) was 8.3% for the U14 group and 8.4% for the U17 group; sleep debt (ESS > 8) was 19.4% for the U14 group and 22.3% for the second group (see Table 3).

Table 3. Percentages of sleep parameters of the U14 group and U17 group.

Variables	Group U14	Group U17	Average of the 2 Groups
PSQI ≥ 5	61.1%	63.8%	62.45%
PSQI < 5	38.9%	36.2%	37.55%
ISI ≥ 11	8.3%	8.4%	8.35%
ISI < 11	91.7%	91.6%	91.65%
ESS > 8	19.4%	22.3%	20.85%
ESS < 8	80.6%	77.7%	79.15%

PSQI ≥ 5: poor sleep quality; ISI ≥ 11: mild insomnia; ESS > 8: sleep debt or excessive daytime sleepiness.

Although it was not significant, the balance performance with eyes open and closed for the U14 group was better (0.59 and 0.31, respectively).

In the between-group comparison, the agility values were higher ($p < 0.01$) in favor of the U14 group compared to the U17 group. Therefore, we reject the null hypothesis of equality of variances, and a significant difference between the two groups regarding agility performances was noted. Concerning the vertical (SJ) and horizontal (SBJ) jump tests, no significant difference was noted ($p = 0.06$ and $p = 0.43$, respectively).

Although the difference was not significant (0.06 > 0.05), the performance of the five-jump test (FJT) of the younger U14 players was better than that of the others, with a difference of 2% between the two groups.

On the other hand, the mean performance of the maximum aerobic speed capacity of the older U17 players was significantly higher compared to the U14 players ($p < 0.05$) (see Table 4).

Table 4. Performance parameters of balance, agility, strength, and MAS in the two groups.

Group	OEB	CEB	SJ	SBJ	FJT	t-Test	VAMEVAL
U14	11.01 ± 8.52	2.88 ± 0.86	24.8 ± 5.38	1.59 ± 0.20	9.12 ± 0.54	12.8 ± 1.11	12.2 ± 1.35
U17	10.49 ± 9.75	2.24 ± 1.11	28.5 ± 4.04	1.66 ± 0.20	8.90 ± 0.98	11.7 ** ± 0.59	12.69 * ± 0.91

Values are mean ± SD; OEB: open-eye balance; CEB: closed-eye balance; SJ: squat jump; SBJ: squat broad jump; FJT: five jump test; t-Test: Agility t-Test; VAMEVAL: maximum aerobic capacity test. Significantly different from U14: * $p < 0.05$, ** $p < 0.01$.

4. Discussion

The current study examined the evaluation of the differences in PSQI, ISI, and ESS scores between U14 and U17 female players and of some measures of balance, strength, agility, and maximum aerobic speed.

Collectively, the main findings indicated, however, no significant differences in the different sleep parameters between the two groups of female players. However, significantly higher performances for the U17 category in agility quality and MAS, when compared to the U14 players, were noted.

Concerning the sleep parameters, this can be explained by the similarities in age between these two groups although they belong to different categories (U14: school A; U17: cadet B).

Furthermore, as the PSQI, ISI, and ESS scores increased in relation to the decreased sleep quality, this strengthens the idea of aptly targeting different participants' age categories in order to have better performance. When using different age categories, Davenne [43] also found that sleep disorders such as nocturnal awakenings, short durations of deep sleep with slow waves, and problems with early awakening were highly prevalent with advancing age.

Furthermore, Rasekhi et al. [44], noted several determinants of the appearance of poor sleep quality and increased ISI in adolescents, i.e., gender, BMI, nature of sport, coffee consumption, daily activity, diet, and skipping breakfast. A recent study by Bruce et al. [45] even noted the importance of the biological factor at this age range, which causes a biological delay in the time taken to fall asleep. In fact, to attend school, most young are obligated to wake up too early, as is the fact for our female players. Hence, a sleep debt during the school week as shown in the current study, resulted in an in-crease in the ISI, ESS, and PSQI scores. However, sleep disorders, comprising poor sleep quality that exceeded 61% (PSQI $\geq$ 5), mild insomnia (ISI $\geq$ 11) which was approximately 8.3%, and sleep deprivation (ESS > 8) which was 19.4% for the U14 group against 22.3% for the U17 group, might all be considered as stimulating negative factors. These corroborate the study of Bel et al. [46] conducted on adolescents, which showed that the prevalence of sleep disorders is the result of the accumulation of several factors such as the relationship between insufficient sleep and poor nutrition. It is therefore a necessity to adopt educational strategies that may develop a culture of healthy lifestyles in order to have mentally and physically balanced adolescents.

Furthermore, Ferranti et al. [47] noted in one study that only 47% of adolescents followed the recommendations for daily sleep hours, while Carvalho [27] showed that more than 39% of adolescents had poor sleep quality and this was related to poor quality of life, such as nutrition or daily activities. According to Figueiro [48], a sleep phase characterized by long sleep latencies relative to desired bedtimes resulted in significant sleep deprivation in subjects' daily activities.

From another perspective, we noted that the balance performance of the stork with eyes open and closed was better for the U14 group compared to the U17 group. We have to stress the fact that there were no previous studies having compared the unipodal balance quality of U17 and U14 female players in handball. Since unhealthy sleep habits increase with age, we suppose that this may be one of the factors that affected the behavior of the female players in the present study. In fact, the prevalence of sleep disorders has further been shown to affect the muscle strength of the lower limbs [49–51], which helped to maintain control of the posture through sensorimotor strategies. Maintained over a long period of time, this sleep disorder can deteriorate postural stability by acting on cognitive and biomechanical mechanisms [52–55]. According to Cerrah et al. [56], this requires may be the application of functional balance training for adolescents three times a week to improve static balance performance.

Concerning the participants' average BMI values, the results showed that in the U14 group, these were significantly elevated compared to the U17 group. In fact, Rusek et al. [57] focused on sedentary adolescents of both sexes and showed that the increase in BMI values corresponded to better balance performance. In the following study, the 3 years of experience in sports practice for the U17 group were supposed to be sufficient in showing better sensorimotor performances resulting in a better balance and good postural control. Those results seem to be in disagreement with what was reported by Caballero et al. [58], showing that the level of expertise related to handball practice was a factor that improved postural balance. It is important to mention that his study was based on male handball players, and it may be that the increased testosterone secretion affected the noted anthropometric changes.

Regarding the between-group jump comparison (SJ, SBJ, FJT), they were indicative of the quality of the explosive strength using the lower limbs, even though no significant differences were noted. This study showed however that no significant difference was obtained for the comparison of the different jump performances (SJ, SBJ, FJT) between the two groups. Previous studies [59,60] involved participants of both sexes, aged between 6 and 18 years, and indicated an increase in SBJ performance in girls to a plateau at age 12–13 years. In fact, the study by Chung et al. [61], conducted on 12.712 Chinese students between the ages of 8 and 18 years, generated standard SBJ test data and showed stability of SBJ performance for female players from the age of 12 years old, while these values continue to increase for males up to 18 years with a very significant difference between the two sexes. Similarly, Ramírez-Vélez et al. [62] found that SBJ scores increased from the age of 9 to 12.9 years and reached a plateau at an age between 13 and 15.9 years for girls.

In another study, Ramos-Sepúlveda et al. [63] found further, better performances for males and which depended on muscle strength. We presume, therefore, that in the growth phase, the distinction according to sex is necessary to improve the explosive strength of the lower limbs, because this age interval is characterized by the linear increase in muscular explosive strength for both sexes. This latter is related to mechanical and neurological factors as previously shown [64]. Moreover, male subjects possess a more rapid increase in gonadal steroid hormones, growth hormones, and muscle mass and bone mineral content favoring better muscular strength performance until late adolescence [61]. In contrast, girls have an intense accumulation of fat mass in the early pubertal phase [16], which presents an inhibiting factor for muscle strength.

Concerning the agility *t*-test in U17 and U14 female handball players, the results showed better performance for U17 players with a highly significant difference compared to U14 players ($p < 0.01$ with a difference of 9%). The morphological factors are supposed to be related to maturation, such as height, the amount of fat mass, and muscle tissue mass [60].

Furthermore, the increases noted in the agility performance between U14 and U17 may have occurred in relation to the intermittent nature of the practiced sport involving multidirectional changes. Thus, regular practice in such a sport optimizes the quality of agility that naturally improves throughout childhood and adolescence, albeit in a non-linear fashion [65,66].

Lastly, the different measures of maximum aerobic speed (MAS) showed significant results that were better in U17 players compared to U14. This result may explain the importance of regular and continuous physical activities practiced during the preparation period, leading to improved aerobic capacity as indicated by other authors [67,68]. However, other studies reported conflicting results. For example, Berthoin et al. [69] showed that the MAS increased from 6 to 11 years for girls and then remained constant until 17 years for both sexes. Therefore, it is essential to take into account certain particularities such as sex or the intervention of certain biological processes (i.e., testosterone, GH, etc.) with a better evaluation of the aerobic capacity during the maturation phase.

However, the present study also has limitations. First, the number of participants studied is relatively small, and some subjects refused to join the study at the beginning, which may have led to selection bias in the results of the study. Second, perhaps the presence of a third group older than those studied could have added other interpretations. This will be taken into consideration in the following study. Third, only girls were included in this study, which didn't allow us to better examine gender differences and show the effect of sleep on exercise performances.

5. Conclusions

In conclusion, our collected results suggest the need to focus several factors, to assess physical abilities. It is therefore essential to employ a program in the field of sports practice adapted to young players, taking into account the biological changes related to their muscular development, while targeting qualities such as balance and strength, which are less developed, especially between 13 and 17 years. However, other studies seem necessary to examine the impact of the prevalence of sleep disorders in a larger and more varied population in order to improve the quality of games and ensure better performances.

Author Contributions: Conceptualization, M.A.G. and G.R.; methodology, M.A.G. and G.R.; software, M.-A.D.; validation, M.A.G. and N.S.; formal analysis, M.-A.D.; investigation, M.A.G., G.R. and N.S.; resources, M.-A.D.; data curation, M.A.G. and G.R.; writing—original draft preparation, M.A.G., J.C. and G.R.; writing—review and editing, M.A.G., J.C., G.R. and N.S.; visualization, M.-A.D. and N.S.; supervision, N.S.; project administration, M.A.G.; funding acquisition, M.A.G. and G.R. All authors have read and agreed to the published version of the manuscript.

Funding: This research received no external funding.

Institutional Review Board Statement: The study was approved by the Manouba University Institutional Review Committee for the ethical use of human participants. Written informed consent to participate in this study was provided by the participants' legal guardian.

Informed Consent Statement: All subjects and their parents have provided written informed consent in accordance with international ethical standards and the Declaration of Helsinki.

Data Availability Statement: In this study, the data presented are available on request from the corresponding author.

Acknowledgments: The authors would like to thank all the players who voluntarily participated in this study. They also thank the staff and coaches for their help in collecting the data in appropriate conditions.

Conflicts of Interest: The authors declare that there is no conflict of interest regarding the manuscript and its preparation.

References

1. Daneshjoo, A.; Hoseinpour, A.; Sadeghi, H.; Kalantari, A.; Behm, D.G. The Effect of a Handball Warm-Up Program on Dynamic Balance among Elite Adolescent Handball Players. *Sports* **2022**, *10*, 18. [CrossRef] [PubMed]
2. Gioftsidou, A.; Malliou, P.; Sofokleous, P.; Pafis, G.; Beneka, A.; Godolias, G. The Effects of Balance Training on Balance Ability in Handball Players. *Exerc. Qual. Life* **2012**, *4*, 15–22. [CrossRef]
3. Ljubica, M.; Bjelica, B.; Aksović, N.; Cicović, V.; D'Onofrio, R. Estimation of Explosive Power of Lower Extremities in Handball. *Ital. J. Sport. Rehabil. Posturol.* **2021**, *10*, 2507–2617.
4. Oxyzoglou, N.; Kanioglou, A.; Rizos, S.; Mavridis, G.; Kabitsis, C. Muscular Strength and Jumping Performance after Handball Training versus Physical Education Program for Pre-Adolescent Children. *Percept. Mot. Ski.* **2007**, *104 Pt 2*, 1282–1288. [CrossRef] [PubMed]
5. Karcher, C.; Buchheit, M. On-Court Demands of Elite Handball, with Special Reference to Playing Positions. *Sport. Med.* **2014**, *44*, 797–814. [CrossRef] [PubMed]
6. Spasic, M.; Krolo, A.; Zenic, N.; Delextrat, A.; Sekulic, D. Reactive Agility Performance in Handball; Development and Evaluation of a Sport-Specific Measurement Protocol. *J. Sport. Sci. Med.* **2015**, *14*, 501–506.
7. Camacho-Cardenosa, A.; Camacho-Cardenosa, M.; Brazo-Sayavera, J. Endurance Assessment in Handball: A Systematic Review. *Eur. J. Hum. Mov.* **2019**, *43*, 13–39.
8. Wagner, H.; Finkenzeller, T.; Würth, S.; von Duvillard, S.P. Individual and Team Performance in Team-Handball: A Review. *J. Sport. Sci. Med.* **2014**, *13*, 808–816.
9. Zech, A.; Venter, R.; de Villiers, J.E.; Sehner, S.; Wegscheider, K.; Hollander, K. Motor Skills of Children and Adolescents Are Influenced by Growing up Barefoot or Shod. *Front. Pediatr.* **2018**, *6*, 115. [CrossRef]
10. Trecroci, A.; Longo, S.; Perri, E.; Iaia, F.M.; Alberti, G. Field-Based Physical Performance of Elite and Sub-Elite Middle-Adolescent Soccer Players. *Res. Sport. Med.* **2019**, *27*, 60–71. [CrossRef]
11. Waldron, M.; Murphy, A. A Comparison of Physical Abilities and Match Performance Characteristics among Elite and Sub-elite Under-14 Soccer Players. *Pediatr. Exerc. Sci.* **2013**, *25*, 423–434. [CrossRef]

12. Trajković, N.; Sporiš, G.; Krističević, T.; Madić, D.M.; Bogataj, Š. The Importance of Reactive Agility Tests in Differentiating Adolescent Soccer Players. *Int. J. Environ. Res. Public Health* **2020**, *17*, 3839. [CrossRef] [PubMed]
13. Srhoj, V.; Rogulj, N.; Zagorac, N.; Katić, R. A New Model of Selection in Women's Handball. *Coll. Antropol.* **2006**, *30*, 601–605. [PubMed]
14. Lloyd, R.S.; Oliver, J.L.; Faigenbaum, A.D.; Myer, G.D.; De Ste Croix, M.B.A. Chronological Age vs. Biological Maturation: Implications for Exercise Programming in Youth. *J. Strength Cond. Res.* **2014**, *28*, 1454–1464. [CrossRef] [PubMed]
15. Greier, K.; Drenowatz, C.; Ruedl, G.; Kirschner, W.; Mitmannsgruber, P.; Greier, C. Physical Fitness across 11- to 17-Year-Old Adolescents: A Cross-Sectional Study in 2267 Austrian Middle- and High-School Students. *Adv. Phys. Educ.* **2019**, *9*, 258–269. [CrossRef]
16. Vink, E.E.; van Coeverden, S.C.C.M.; van Mil, E.G.; Felius, B.A.; van Leerdam, F.J.M.; Delemarre-van de Waal, H.A. Changes and Tracking of Fat Mass in Pubertal Girls. *Obesity* **2010**, *18*, 1247–1251. [CrossRef]
17. Drake, C.; Nickel, C.; Burduvali, E.; Roth, T.; Jefferson, C.; Pietro, B. The Pediatric Daytime Sleepiness Scale (PDSS): Sleep Habits and School Outcomes in Middle-School Children. *Sleep* **2003**, *26*, 455–458.
18. Chasens, E.R.; Sereika, S.M.; Weaver, T.E.; Umlauf, M.G. Daytime Sleepiness, Exercise, and Physical Function in Older Adults. *J. Sleep Res.* **2007**, *16*, 60–65. [CrossRef]
19. Strand, L.B.; Laugsand, L.E.; Wisløff, U.; Nes, B.M.; Vatten, L.; Janszky, I. Insomnia Symptoms and Cardiorespiratory Fitness in Healthy Individuals: The Nord-Trøndelag Health Study (HUNT). *Sleep* **2013**, *36*, 99–108. [CrossRef]
20. Colrain, I.M.; Baker, F.C. Changes in Sleep as a Function of Adolescent Development. *Neuropsychol. Rev.* **2011**, *21*, 5–21. [CrossRef]
21. Carskadon, M.A.; Acebo, C.; Richardson, G.S.; Tate, B.A.; Seifer, R. An Approach to Studying Circadian Rhythms of Adolescent Humans. *J. Biol. Rhythm.* **1997**, *12*, 278–289. [CrossRef] [PubMed]
22. Crowley, S.J.; Acebo, C.; Carskadon, M.A. Sleep, Circadian Rhythms, and Delayed Phase in Adolescence. *Sleep Med.* **2007**, *8*, 602–612. [CrossRef]
23. Moore, M.; Meltzer, L.J. The Sleepy Adolescent: Causes and Consequences of Sleepiness in Teens. *Paediatr. Respir. Rev.* **2008**, *9*, 114–121. [CrossRef] [PubMed]
24. Sadeh, A.; Dahl, R.E.; Shahar, G.; Rosenblat-Stein, S. Sleep and the Transition to Adolescence: A Longitudinal Study. *Sleep* **2009**, *32*, 1602–1609. [CrossRef] [PubMed]
25. Johnson, E.O.; Roth, T.; Schultz, L.; Breslau, N. Epidemiology of DSM-IV Insomnia in Adolescence: Lifetime Prevalence, Chronicity, and an Emergent Gender Difference. *Pediatrics* **2006**, *117*, e247–e256. [CrossRef] [PubMed]
26. Roberts, R.E.; Roberts, C.R.; Duong, H.T. Chronic Insomnia and Its Negative Consequences for Health and Functioning of Adolescents: A 12-Month Prospective Study. *J. Adolesc. Health* **2008**, *42*, 294–302. [CrossRef]
27. Carvalho, A.S.; Fernandes, A.P.; Gallego, A.B.; Vaz, J.A.; Vega, M.S. The Relation of Sports with Sleep Quality and Anthropometric Measures at Secondary Schools. *J. Sport Health Res.* **2019**, *11*, 91–106.
28. Harriss, D.J.; Atkinson, G. Update—Ethical Standards in Sport and Exercise Science Research. *Int. J. Sport. Med.* **2011**, *32*, 819–821. [CrossRef]
29. Tanner, J.M.; Whitehouse, R.H. Clinical Longitudinal Standards for Height, Weight, Height Velocity, Weight Velocity, and Stages of Puberty. *Arch. Dis. Child.* **1976**, *51*, 170–179. [CrossRef]
30. Chtourou, H.; Souissi, N. The Effect of Training at a Specific Time of Day: A Review. *J. Strength Cond. Res.* **2012**, *26*, 1984–2005. [CrossRef]
31. Buysse, D.J.; Reynolds, C.F.; Monk, T.H.; Berman, S.R.; Kupfer, D.J. The Pittsburgh Sleep Quality Index: A New Instrument for Psychiatric Practice and Research. *Psychiatry Res.* **1989**, *28*, 193–213. [CrossRef] [PubMed]
32. Morin, C.M. *Insomnia: Psychological Assessment and Management*; Guilford Press: New York, NY, USA, 1993; pp. xvii, 238.
33. Johns, M.W. A New Method for Measuring Daytime Sleepiness: The Epworth Sleepiness Scale. *Sleep* **1991**, *14*, 540–545. [CrossRef] [PubMed]
34. Racil, G.; Ben Ounis, O.; Hammouda, O.; Kallel, A.; Zouhal, H.; Chamari, K.; Amri, M. Effects of High vs. Moderate Exercise Intensity during Interval Training on Lipids and Adiponectin Levels in Obese Young Females. *Eur. J. Appl. Physiol.* **2013**, *113*, 2531–2540. [CrossRef]
35. Sopa, I.S.; Szabo, D.A. Testing agility and balance in volleyball game. *Discobolul Phys. Educ. Sport Kinetother. J.* **2015**, *XII*, 167–174.
36. Bosco, C.; Luhtanen, P.; Komi, P.V. A Simple Method for Measurement of Mechanical Power in Jumping. *Eur. J. Appl. Physiol. Occup. Physiol.* **1983**, *50*, 273–282. [CrossRef]
37. Saint-Maurice, P.F.; Laurson, K.R.; Kaj, M.; Csányi, T. Establishing Normative Reference Values for Standing Broad Jump Among Hungarian Youth. *Res. Q. Exerc. Sport.* **2015**, *86* (Suppl. 1), S37–S44. [CrossRef] [PubMed]
38. Chamari, K.; Chaouachi, A.; Hambli, M.; Kaouech, F.; Wisløff, U.; Castagna, C. The Five-Jump Test for Distance as a Field Test to Assess Lower Limb Explosive Power in Soccer Players. *J. Strength Cond. Res.* **2008**, *22*, 944–950. [CrossRef]
39. Jlid, M.C.; Coquart, J.; Maffulli, N.; Paillard, T.; Bisciotti, G.N.; Chamari, K. Effects of in Season Multi-Directional Plyometric Training on Vertical Jump Performance, Change of Direction Speed and Dynamic Postural Control in U-21 Soccer Players. *Front. Physiol.* **2020**, *11*, 374. [CrossRef]
40. Kuipers, H.; Verstappen, F.T.; Keizer, H.A.; Geurten, P.; van Kranenburg, G. Variability of Aerobic Performance in the Laboratory and Its Physiologic Correlates. *Int. J. Sport. Med.* **1985**, *6*, 197–201. [CrossRef]

41. Pugh, L.G. Oxygen Intake in Track and Treadmill Running with Observations on the Effect of Air Resistance. *J. Physiol.* **1970**, *207*, 823–835. [CrossRef]
42. Shephard, R.J. A Nomogram to Calculate the Oxygen-Cost of Running at Slow Speeds. *J. Sport. Med. Phys. Fit.* **1969**, *9*, 10–16.
43. Davenne, D. Activité physique et sommeil chez les seniors. *Médecine Du Sommeil* **2015**, *12*, 181–189. [CrossRef]
44. Rasekhi, S.; Pour Ashouri, F.; Pirouzan, A. Effects of Sleep Quality on the Academic Performance of Undergraduate Medical Students. *Health Scope* **2016**, *5*, e31641. [CrossRef]
45. Bruce, E.S.; Lunt, L.; McDonagh, J.E. Sleep in Adolescents and Young Adults. *Clin. Med.* **2017**, *17*, 424–428. [CrossRef] [PubMed]
46. Bel, S.; Michels, N.; Vriendt, T.D.; Patterson, E.; Cuenca-García, M.; Diethelm, K.; Gutin, B.; Grammatikaki, E.; Manios, Y.; Leclercq, C.; et al. Association between self-reported sleep duration and dietary quality in European adolescents. *Br. J. Nutr.* **2013**, *110*, 949–959. [CrossRef] [PubMed]
47. Ferranti, R.; Marventano, S.; Castellano, S.; Giogianni, G.; Nolfo, F.; Rametta, S.; Matalone, M.; Mistretta, A. Sleep Quality and Duration Is Related with Diet and Obesity in Young Adolescent Living in Sicily, Southern Italy. *Sleep Sci.* **2016**, *9*, 117–122. [CrossRef]
48. Figueiro, M.G. Delayed Sleep Phase Disorder: Clinical Perspective with a Focus on Light Therapy. *Nat. Sci. Sleep.* **2016**, *8*, 91–106. [CrossRef]
49. Chen, Y.; Cui, Y.; Chen, S.; Wu, Z. Relationship between Sleep and Muscle Strength among Chinese University Students: A Cross-Sectional Study. *J. Musculoskelet. Neuronal Interact.* **2017**, *17*, 327–333.
50. Knowles, O.E.; Drinkwater, E.J.; Urwin, C.S.; Lamon, S.; Aisbett, B. Inadequate Sleep and Muscle Strength: Implications for Resistance Training. *J. Sci. Med. Sport* **2018**, *21*, 959–968. [CrossRef]
51. Morasso, P.G.; Sanguineti, V. Ankle Muscle Stiffness Alone Cannot Stabilize Balance during Quiet Standing. *J. Neurophysiol.* **2002**, *88*, 2157–2162. [CrossRef]
52. Ahrberg, K.; Dresler, M.; Niedermaier, S.; Steiger, A.; Genzel, L. The Interaction between Sleep Quality and Academic Performance. *J. Psychiatr. Res.* **2012**, *46*, 1618–1622. [CrossRef] [PubMed]
53. Avni, N.; Avni, I.; Barenboim, E.; Azaria, B.; Zadok, D.; Kohen-Raz, R.; Morad, Y. Brief Posturographic Test as an Indicator of Fatigue. *Psychiatry Clin. Neurosci.* **2006**, *60*, 340–346. [CrossRef] [PubMed]
54. Gomez, S.; Patel, M.; Berg, S.; Magnusson, M.; Johansson, R.; Fransson, P.A. Effects of Proprioceptive Vibratory Stimulation on Body Movement at 24 and 36h of Sleep Deprivation. *Clin. Neurophysiol.* **2008**, *119*, 617–625. [CrossRef] [PubMed]
55. Nakano, T.; Araki, K.; Michimori, A.; Inbe, H.; Hagiwara, H.; Koyama, E. Nineteen-Hour Variation of Postural Sway, Alertness and Rectal Temperature during Sleep Deprivation. *Psychiatry Clin. Neurosci.* **2001**, *55*, 277–278. [CrossRef] [PubMed]
56. Cerrah, A.O.; Bayram, İ.; Yildizer, G.; Uğurlu, O.; Şimşek, D.; Ertan, H. Effects of functional balance training on static and dynamic balance performance of adolescent soccer players. *Int. J. Sport Exerc. Train. Sci.—IJSETS* **2016**, *2*, 73–81. [CrossRef]
57. Rusek, W.; Adamczyk, M.; Baran, J.; Leszczak, J.; Inglot, G.; Baran, R.; Pop, T. Is There a Link between Balance and Body Mass Composition in Children and Adolescents? *Int. J. Environ. Res. Public Health* **2021**, *18*, 10449. [CrossRef]
58. Caballero, C.; Barbado, D.; Urbán, T.; García-Herrero, J.A.; Moreno, F.J. Functional Variability in Team-Handball Players during Balance Is Revealed by Non-Linear Measures and Is Related to Age and Expertise Level. *Entropy* **2020**, *22*, 822. [CrossRef]
59. Kolimechkov, S.; Petrov, L.; Alexandrova, A. Alpha-fit test battery norms for children and adolescents from 5 to 18 years of age obtained by a linear interpolation of existing european physical fitness references. *Eur. J. Phys. Educ. Sport Sci.* **2019**, *5*. [CrossRef]
60. Thomas, E.; Petrigna, L.; Tabacchi, G.; Teixeira, E.; Pajaujiene, S.; Sturm, D.J.; Sahin, F.N.; Gómez-López, M.; Pausic, J.; Paoli, A.; et al. Percentile Values of the Standing Broad Jump in Children and Adolescents Aged 6-18 Years Old. *Eur. J. Transl. Myol.* **2020**, *30*, 9050. [CrossRef]
61. Chung, L.M.Y.; Chow, L.P.Y.; Chung, J.W.Y. Normative Reference of Standing Long Jump Indicates Gender Difference in Lower Muscular Strength of Pubertal Growth. *Health* **2013**, *5*, 6. [CrossRef]
62. Ramírez-Vélez, R.; Martínez, M.; Correa-Bautista, J.E.; Lobelo, F.; Izquierdo, M.; Rodríguez-Rodríguez, F.; Cristi-Montero, C. Normative Reference of Standing Long Jump for Colombian Schoolchildren Aged 9–17.9 Years: The FUPRECOL Study. *J. Strength Cond. Res.* **2017**, *31*, 2083–2090. [CrossRef] [PubMed]
63. Ramos-Sepúlveda, J.A.; Ramírez-Vélez, R.; Correa-Bautista, J.E.; Izquierdo, M.; García-Hermoso, A. Physical Fitness and Anthropometric Normative Values among Colombian-Indian Schoolchildren. *BMC Public Health* **2016**, *16*, 962. [CrossRef] [PubMed]
64. Beunen, G.; Thomis, M. Muscular Strength Development in Children and Adolescents. *Pediatr. Exerc. Sci.* **2000**, *12*, 174–197. [CrossRef]
65. Eisenmann, J.C.; Malina, R.M. Age- and Sex-Associated Variation in Neuromuscular Capacities of Adolescent Distance Runners. *J. Sport. Sci.* **2003**, *21*, 551–557. [CrossRef] [PubMed]
66. Vänttinen, T.; Blomqvist, M.; Nyman, K.; Häkkinen, K. Changes in Body Composition, Hormonal Status, and Physical Fitness in 11-, 13-, and 15-Year-Old Finnish Regional Youth Soccer Players during a Two-Year Follow-Up. *J. Strength Cond. Res.* **2011**, *25*, 3342–3351. [CrossRef]
67. Racil, G.; Coquart, J.; Elmontassar, W.; Haddad, M.; Goebel, R.; Chaouachi, A.; Amri, M.; Chamari, K. Greater Effects of High- Compared with Moderate-Intensity Interval Training on Cardio-Metabolic Variables, Blood Leptin Concentration and Ratings of Perceived Exertion in Obese Adolescent Females. *Biol. Sport* **2016**, *33*, 145–152. [CrossRef]

68. Welde, B.; Morseth, B.; Handegård, B.H.; Lagestad, P. Effect of Sex, Body Mass Index and Physical Activity Level on Peak Oxygen Uptake Among 14-19 Years Old Adolescents. *Front. Sport. Act. Living* **2020**, *2*, 78. [CrossRef]
69. Berthoin, S.; Baquet, G.; Mantéca, F.; Lensel-Corbeil, G.; Gerbeaux, M. Maximal Aerobic Speed and Running Time to Exhaustion for Children 6 to 17 Years Old. *Pediatr. Exerc. Sci.* **1996**, *8*, 234–244. [CrossRef]

Disclaimer/Publisher's Note: The statements, opinions and data contained in all publications are solely those of the individual author(s) and contributor(s) and not of MDPI and/or the editor(s). MDPI and/or the editor(s) disclaim responsibility for any injury to people or property resulting from any ideas, methods, instructions or products referred to in the content.

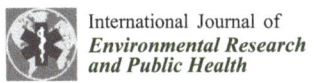

Article

Changes in Physical Fitness during the COVID-19 Pandemic in German Children

Tanja Eberhardt *, Klaus Bös and Claudia Niessner

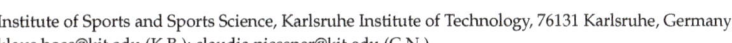

Institute of Sports and Sports Science, Karlsruhe Institute of Technology, 76131 Karlsruhe, Germany; klaus.boes@kit.edu (K.B.); claudia.niessner@kit.edu (C.N.)
* Correspondence: tanja.eberhardt@kit.edu

Citation: Eberhardt, T.; Bös, K.; Niessner, C. Changes in Physical Fitness during the COVID-19 Pandemic in German Children. *Int. J. Environ. Res. Public Health* **2022**, *19*, 9504. https://doi.org/10.3390/ijerph19159504

Academic Editors: Clemens Drenowatz and Klaus Greier

Received: 31 May 2022
Accepted: 28 July 2022
Published: 2 August 2022

Publisher's Note: MDPI stays neutral with regard to jurisdictional claims in published maps and institutional affiliations.

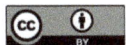

Copyright: © 2022 by the authors. Licensee MDPI, Basel, Switzerland. This article is an open access article distributed under the terms and conditions of the Creative Commons Attribution (CC BY) license (https://creativecommons.org/licenses/by/4.0/).

Abstract: With the beginning of the COVID-19 pandemic in December 2019, each country has developed strategies to try to control the virus. The restrictions and subsequent consequences also limited the possibilities and structures for being physically active. Therefore, the aim of this study was to examine changes in physical fitness in a cohort that was investigated over an extended period. Physical fitness testing was conducted with the IPPTP-R in a primary school from a small rural community annually since 2012. Mean values of test items were calculated for each cohort. We conducted an ANCOVA to examine the differences between cohorts PreCOVID and 2020 as the first year of the COVID-19 pandemic, and between PreCOVID and 2021 as the second year of the COVID-19 pandemic. Overall, no evidence for a negative effect of the COVID-19 pandemic on physical fitness in children between the ages of 7 and 9 years was found. In strength tests, performances increased when comparing the PreCOVID cohort and COVID-19 cohorts (Push-Ups: $p < 0.001$, $\eta_p^2 = 0.032$; $p = 0.017$, $\eta_p^2 = 0.006$). No evidence for a change was found for endurance (6-min Run: $p = 0.341$, $\eta_p^2 = 0.001$; $p = 0.267$, $\eta_p^2 = 0.001$). The rural community maintained physical fitness despite restrictions and limitations through the environmental circumstances. Considering this, it is a positive example of how adequate long-term efforts promoting physical fitness make an impact and an active friendly environment helps to overcome COVID-19 pandemics limiting the structures for being physically active.

Keywords: motor performance; motor development; youth; effects; influences; cross-sectional study

1. Introduction

The importance of physical fitness for the healthy development of children and the positive influence for a lifelong active lifestyle are well-known and documented [1,2]. The level of physical fitness predicts an individual's level of engaging in physical activity through given opportunities and limited capacities [3,4]. Physical fitness is the basis on which movement patterns are developed to be able to be physically active and, on the other hand, has a positive impact on psychosocial factors [5–8].

Nevertheless, the levels of physical activity and physical fitness in youth have declined over the last decades, along with other variables influencing an active lifestyle. Since the beginning of the twenty-first century, physical fitness has been stagnating at a low level worldwide. Overall, children are less fit than those of former generations [9–12]. Accordingly, the majority of children and adolescents do not meet the recommendations of the World Health Organization for daily physical activity [13,14]. Sedentary behavior of children and adolescents has increased and screen-time exceeds recommendations [15,16]. As a consequence, the prevalence of obesity and overweight has steadily increased in past years, especially in younger children [17].

With the beginning of the COVID-19 pandemic in December 2019, each country has developed a strategy to try to control the virus. In Germany, the first officially registered case of COVID-19 appeared at the end of January 2020. Nationwide school closures and contact restrictions were implemented for the first time in March 2020, and again in December 2020 until March 2021 [18]. These restrictions also affected sports clubs, fitness centers, and the cancellation of all sports in schools, i.e., physical education lessons, extracurricular sports groups, or being active during breaks in the schoolyard. The COVID-19 pandemic and the subsequent consequences therefore not only limited social life, but also the possibilities and structures for being physically active.

There are studies that have examined the influence of the COVID-19 pandemic on physical activity [19,20]. A meta-analysis revealed a slightly negative global change in physical activity for children and adolescents [19]. In Germany, the differentiated analysis of data from the Motorik–Modul (MoMo) study showed an increase of daily physical activity, such as playing outside or unstructured activities, during the first lockdown, but children could not maintain this level during the second lockdown [21]. In contrast, the time spent in organized sports and overall physical activity decreased over the study period [20–22].

There are also some studies that examined the influence of the COVID-19 pandemic and associated restrictions not only on physical activity, but also on the physical fitness construct [23–26]. Despite different measurement methods and study participants, the studies all reported a declining trend for endurance [23,24,27]. There appears to be less and inconclusive evidence for decreasing strength [24,25]. However, most of the studies have single measurement points before, during, or after the COVID-19 pandemic, but there is a lack of long-term monitoring. In our study, we conducted physical fitness testing in the same cohort over a period of eight years, plus 2020 and 2021, years in which the COVID-19 pandemic occurred. Therefore, these cohorts, which constitute the specific study population, provide the opportunity to draw conclusions based on a strong foundation of physical fitness data.

The aim of the study was to examine effects of the COVID-19 pandemic and changes in the different dimensions of physical fitness in a cohort that was investigated over an extended period.

2. Materials and Methods

This study used a cross-sectional cohort design with a population-based ad hoc sample. Overall, ten cohorts were followed yearly from 2012 until 2021. In the following, cohort always refers to the age group of 7–9-year-olds in the respective testing year. The International Physical Performance Test Profile—revised (IPPTP-R) was used to test the physical fitness in in the German federal state of Baden-Württemberg [28]. All data presented in this paper were from children from a small rural community with fewer than 5000 inhabitants located in the northeast of Baden-Württemberg that participated in the test procedure over the entire period of ten years.

2.1. Physical Fitness

The IPPTP-R is an effective and validated physical fitness assessment tool developed to be conducted in practical settings [28]. It is based on the approach of Bös and Mechling [29] and the German Motor-Test 6–18 [30]. It contains eight test items representing the five main dimensions of physical fitness endurance, strength, speed, coordination, and flexibility. Additionally, constitutional data including height, weight, and BMI were collected, and children's age and sex, as well as test date and other characteristics of data collection were recorded. Table 1 shows the different test items. The detailed and precise description of the test items can be found in the existing manuals [28,30].

2.2. Data Collection

The primary school in the community reported on here conducted the testing annually in October, except in 2020, when testing was limited due to the COVID-19 lockdown. Therefore, the 2020 tests were conducted in December. The teachers and volunteers were trained as multipliers using manuals, test material, and additional support and to execute the test tools. On a testing day, each child was tested in the school, sorted according to class. Parents provided informed consent forms through the primary school that conducted the testing. With informed consent, the test results were entered into the evaluation software and any personalized raw data on children's physical fitness were pseudonymized initially and checked for quality. The data set regarding this community was retrieved from the total data set using postal code as variable of allocation. The extracted data were then analyzed in a separate dataset.

Table 1. Test items of the IPPTP-R.

Dimension	Test Item	Unit
Endurance	6 min Run	Meter
Strength	Standing Long Jump	Centimeters
	Sit-Ups	Number in 40 s
	Push-Ups	Number in 40 s
Speed	20 m Dash	Seconds
Coordination	Balancing Backwards	Number of steps
	Jumping Sideways	Number of jumps in 15 s
Flexibility	Stand and Reach	Centimeters

2.3. Sample Description

As mentioned above, all data were from one community in the German state of Baden-Württemberg, which participated over the entire study period. Overall, 999 primary school children between the ages of 7 to 9 years (MV ± SD: age: 7.98 ± 0.82; weight: 29.0 ± 6.9 kg; height: 132.8 ± 7.5 cm) were included in the analysis. Among them, 55.6% (n = 555) were boys and 44.4% (n = 444) were girls. In the analysis, cohorts were compared to examine the effects and consequences of the COVID-19 pandemic on physical fitness levels. The different cohorts from the period between 2012 and 2019 were combined and considered representative of the physical fitness of children in the community before COVID-19. This cohort, called PreCOVID, comprised 801 children (MV ± SD: age: 7.97 ± 0.82; weight: 28.8 ± 7.0 kg; height: 132.7 ± 7.4 cm). The cohort from 2020, the first year of the COVID-19 pandemic, called COVID1, included 91 children in the analysis (MV ± SD: age: 7.93 ± 0.87; weight: 28.9 ± 5.7 kg; height: 132.7 ± 7.8 cm). The cohort from 2021 (COVID2) included 107 children (MV ± SD: age: 8.08 ± 0.77; weight: 30.2 ± 7.1 kg; height: 133.4 ± 8.1 cm). The exact number of children according to cohort and gender is shown in Table 2.

Table 2. Distribution of the sample.

Cohort	Year of Measurement	Boys (n)		Girls (n)		Overall (n)	
2012–2019 PreCOVID	2012	57		44		101	
	2013	62		39		101	
	2014	56		43		99	
	2015	39	n = 460	28	n = 341	67	n = 801
	2016	61	(57.4%)	33	(42.6%)	94	(100%)
	2017	57		45		102	
	2018	64		49		113	
	2019	64		60		124	
2020 COVID1	2020	43	n = 43 (47.3%)	48	n = 48 (52.7%)	91	n = 91 (100%)
2021 COVID2	2021	52	n = 52 (48.6%)	55	n = 55 (51.4%)	107	n = 107 (100%)
	Overall	555 (55.6%)		444 (44.4%)		n = 999 (100%)	

2.4. Statistical Analysis

Statistical analyses were performed using IBM SPSS Statistics 28 (IBM Corporation, Armonk, NY, USA). To obtain an overview of the distribution within the sample, frequency analyses and cross tables were conducted.

Descriptive statistics with mean values and 95% CI were calculated for each test item and cohort overall and separately for boys and girls to reflect the entire measurement period. Missing data were not interpolated. The analysis was controlled for age and BMI. We conducted a univariate analysis of covariance (ANCOVA) to examine the differences between the cohorts PreCOVID and COVID1, and between PreCOVID and COVID2 adjusted for gender. The PreCOVID cohort value was formed using the mean value of individual cohorts from 2012–2019. The level of significance was set at $p < 0.05$. Effects were assessed with partial eta squared (η_p^2). Pairwise comparisons with Bonferroni correction were performed to determine differences between the cohorts.

3. Results

Overall, 999 primary school children aged 7 to 9 years from a small rural community in the German state of Baden-Württemberg were included in the study (PreCOVID $n = 801$; COVID1: $n = 91$; COVID2: $n = 107$). There were no significant differences for age and BMI between the ten cohorts, but gender-specific differences in mean values in the test items.

Figure 1 shows the trends in test items for all measurement years overall and separately by gender (see Table A1).

There was a linear, consistent level of performance for the 20 m dash through 2017 in boys and girls. In 2018, an increase was observed for either gender, and this level of speed remained stable until the last measurement in 2021. The ANCOVA for the test item 20 m dash revealed that children in the cohort COVID1 were 0.20 s slower than in the PreCOVID cohort ($F(1,859) = 15.89$; $p < 0.001$; $\eta_p^2 = 0.018$). The comparison with cohort COVID2 showed a significant difference of 0.23 s ($F(1,861) = 18.69$; $p < 0.001$; $\eta_p^2 = 0.021$). The influence of the covariate gender was significant for both ANCOVAs ($p < 0.001$; $p < 0.001$).

The analysis of the test item balancing backwards showed an opposite gender-specific trend until 2015, followed by a peak in 2016 for both boys and girls. This increase stopped abruptly and tended to remain stable until 2019. No significant difference was found in the ANCOVA, with 0.22 steps between cohort PreCOVID and COVID1 ($F(1,874) = 0.06$; $p = 0.813$; $\eta_p^2 = 0.000$). However, children in cohort COVID2 performed 2.03 steps better than cohort PreCOVID ($F(1,893) = 5.67$; $p = 0.017$; $\eta_p^2 = 0.006$). The covariate gender had no significant influence on the analysis ($p = 0.232$; $p = 0.215$).

The mean values for jumping sideways revealed no trend. There were ups and downs through all cohorts, with a peak in 2020 and a minimum of performance in 2012 and 2017. There were inverse performance levels for boys and girls for the cohorts 2014 through 2016. Analyzing the differences for the test item jumping sideways showed that there was a difference of 4.32 fewer steps in PreCOVID compared with COVID1 ($F(1,874) = 27.05$; $p < 0.001$; $\eta_p^2 = 0.030$). There was no significant difference found between PreCOVID and COVID2, with 1.24 fewer steps measured for PreCOVID ($F(1,892) = 2.71$; $p = 0.100$; $\eta_p^2 = 0.003$). The influence of the covariate gender was not significant ($p = 0.423$; $p = 0.353$).

A steadily declining trend was found for the test item stand and reach, with its minimum in 2018. The level of flexibility subsequently increased. This development was found for boys and girls equally, but with clear differences in the measured values. The ANCOVA revealed 0.88 cm more in COVID1 than in cohort PreCOVID, but the difference was not significant ($F(1,871) = 1.44$; $p = 0.230$; $\eta_p^2 = 0.002$). PreCOVID had 1.00 cm less for stand and reach than COVID2, but this difference was also not significant ($F(1,888) = 2.16$; $p = 0.142$; $\eta_p^2 = 0.002$). The covariate was statistically significant in both cohort comparisons ($p < 0.001$; $p < 0.001$).

Push-up performance was consistent over the cohorts before increasing in 2017 and peaking in 2019. A significant difference was found in COVID1 with 2.29 more performed push-ups compared with PreCOVID ($F(1,875) = 28.63$; $p < 0.001$; $\eta_p^2 = 0.032$). There was a significant positive difference between PreCOVID and COVID2 of 0.94 (F(1,892) = 5.69; $p = 0.017; \eta_p^2 = 0.006$). The covariate gender had no significant influence on either ANCOVA ($p = 0.855; p = 0.924$).

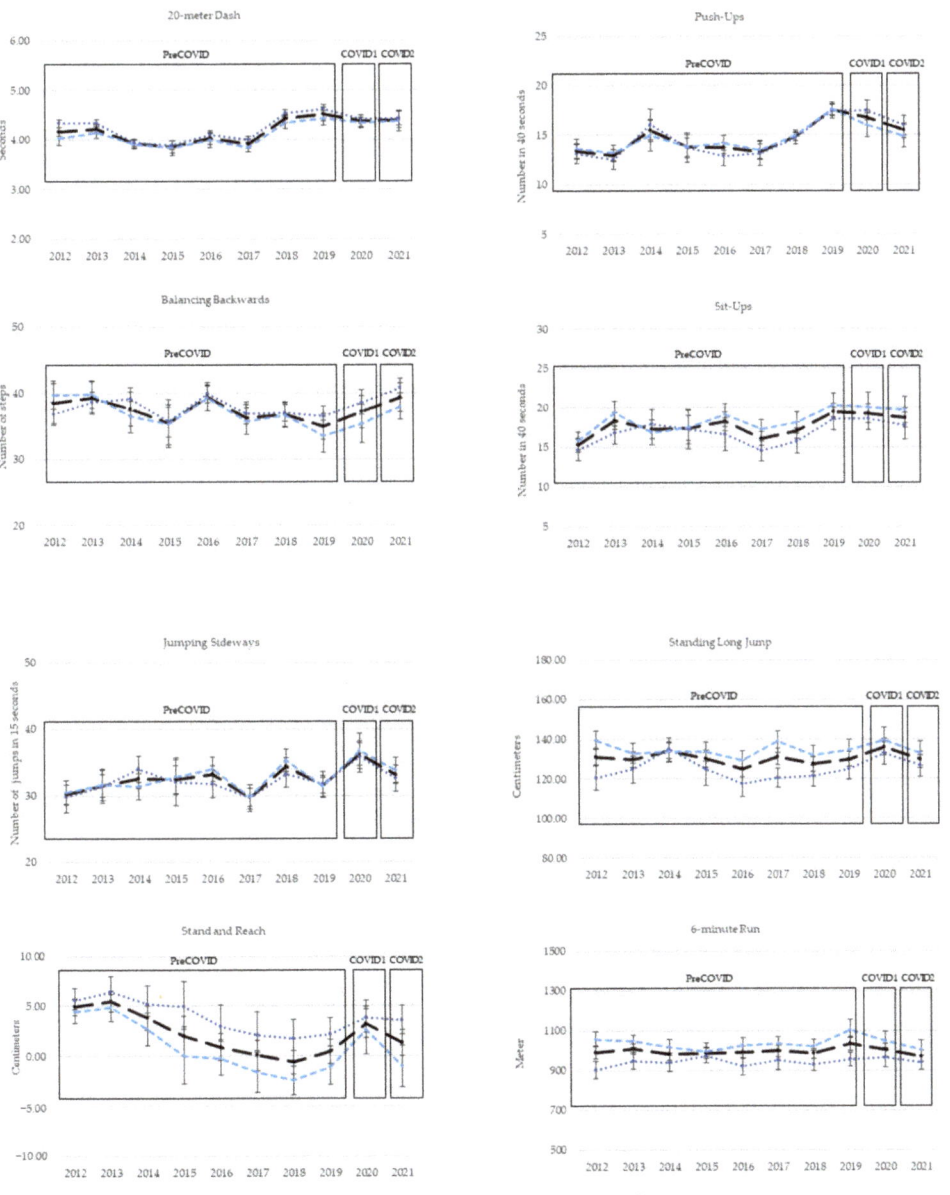

Figure 1. Trends for test items over each year of measurement overall, and for boys and girls separately.

The test item sit-ups improved consistently, but showed an apparent reversal in gender-specific performance for 2014 and the highest levels up to 2019. Analyzing cohort differences with the ANCOVA, the performance differed significantly with 1.95 more sit-ups in COVID1 than in PreCOVID ($F(1,863) = 9.87$; $p = 0.002$; $\eta_p^2 = 0.011$). In addition, with 1.36 more sit-ups, COVID2 was significantly better than PreCOVID ($F(1,881) = 5.50$; $p = 0.019$; $\eta_p^2 = 0.006$). The covariate gender had a significant influence on the differences ($p < 0.001$; $p < 0.001$).

For standing long jump, initial measurements already showed significant differences between boys and girls. This difference was found for all cohorts with no apparent trend. However, the analysis revealed that children in COVID1 jumped 7.24 cm farther than children in PreCOVID ($F(1,873) = 11.13$; $p < 0.001$; $\eta_p^2 = 0.013$). However, the comparison between PreCOVID and COVID2 showed no significant difference, with 0.56 cm more for COVID2 ($F(1,890) = 0.08$; $p = 0.782$; $\eta_p^2 = 0.000$). The covariate gender was statistically significant for both cohort comparisons ($p < 0.001$; $p < 0.001$).

The mean values for 6 min run in the 2012 cohort differed significantly for boys and girls. Performance differed by gender over the measurement period, but the development of the overall sample revealed no trend. No significant differences were found between COVID1 and PreCOVID for the 6 min run, with COVID1 running only 15.31 m more than PreCOVID ($F(1,857) = 0.91$; $p = 0.341$; $\eta_p^2 = 0.001$). The children in PreCOVID ran 16.94 m less than COVID2, but these differences were also not significant ($F(1,866) = 1.23$; $p = 0.267$; $\eta_p^2 = 0.001$). The covariate gender had a significant influence on the measured differences ($p < 0.001$; $p < 0.001$). See Tables A2 and A3 for the adjusted mean values of the ANCOVA in each test item and cohort.

4. Discussion

The aim of the study was to examine COVID-19 effects on the physical fitness of primary school children in a rural community in Baden-Württemberg with fewer than 5000 inhabitants. We conducted measurements over a long-term period and therefore have strong evidence for the overall levels and changes of physical fitness in the sample.

4.1. Summary and Evaluation of the Results

For the test item 20 m dash, the statistically significant differences had no practical relevance. Speed levels remained stable in the COVID-19 cohorts. Comparing the results for balancing backwards, we see that the previously constant performance increased in the measurement for COVID2, but remained the same in COVID1. In addition, representing the dimension coordination, jumping sideways also had a peak in COVID1, but the same stable level before and after. Thus, no evidence for an effect was found. Pombo et al. [31] also reported no inferior results for jumping sideways in 6–9-year-old Portuguese children tested before and after the COVID-19 lockdown. However, from December 2019 to September 2020, there was an overall general trend of shifting to a lower quartile [31]. An increase in children's performance categorized as "very low" in the 20 m shuttle run was also observed by Basterfield et al. for participants in a primary school in England [25]. Flexibility performance in the stand-and-reach test did not differ significantly between the three cohorts. The rising trend of recent years was not stopped by the pandemic. In contrast, there was a negative effect in the study in England, which measured a decrease of 1.8 cm between October 2019 and November 2020 for 8–10-year-old children [25].

The number of performed push-ups was significantly higher in both COVID cohorts compared to the overall 2012–2019 pre-pandemic cohort, which was also reflected in the results of the sit-ups test. There was no evidence that upper body strength levels were influenced negatively by COVID-19 restrictions and consequences. While Wahl-Alexander and Camic [27] found a decrease of 35.6% for push-ups and 19.4% for sit-ups in children with a mean age of 9.6 years between summer 2019 and 2020, other results are consistent with our findings. The same was found for leg strength, which was measured using the standing long jump test. Performance levels increased significantly in the COVID1 cohort, but then remained stable again compared to the PreCOVID cohort, and showed no evidence of negative effects. Basterfield et al. [25] and Wessely et al. [32] also reported a performance increase for standing long jump. This suggests that strength is more resilient to negative effects of COVID-19 than other dimensions of physical fitness [25]. However, Chambonnière et al. [24] measured the standing long jump performance of 3rd and 4th graders in France for the period between 2020 and 2021 and found a decrease of 34.7 cm. This is consistent with another study examining the same age between 2019 and 2020 [31].

The analysis for endurance revealed no significant difference between the cohorts and no effect of the COVID-19 pandemic. The performance levels for the 6 min run were stable across the measured cohorts. Other studies that analyzed endurance found different effects [23,25,27,31]. Jarnig et al. [23], who also implemented the 6 min run, reported a decrease of 102 m in children aged 7-to-10 years old between September 2019 and September 2020 [23]. Two other studies performed the 20 m shuttle run to measure effects for endurance and reported 2.39 [24] and 3 [25] fewer shuttles in their second measurement point.

4.2. Explanation Approaches

Overall, our results show no evidence for a negative effect of the COVID-19 pandemic on physical fitness in children between the ages of 7 and 9 years, but changes varied for the different test items and dimensions. Especially, performances of the COVID cohorts in test items for strength increased. It seems that alternative options of exercising physical fitness like online and indoor workouts mitigate some effects of COVID-19 pandemic. However, due to the restrictions and closures of organized forms in sports clubs or schools, we conclude that dimensions where high intensities and stimuli are needed could not benefit. This could suggest the relevant role of physical activity with peers and within an institution to maintain a global and comprehensive development in all dimensions of physical fitness.

When classifying the data into gender and age-specific percentiles of a nationwide reference sample, the children in this specific community represent a very high level of physical fitness above the average [33,34]. The community has various specific initiatives and commitments to promote physical activity. For example, the primary school curriculum emphasizes the importance of physical fitness and appropriate promotion is determined in the preamble. The community is also a part of the project "Bewegte Kommune-Kinder" which aims to enable a sufficient and adequate development of physical fitness for all children in the community. It seems that children who had higher levels of physical fitness before COVID-19 are more resilient with regard to restrictions and limitations affecting physical activity. Similary, Jarnig et al. [23] reported that children who were members of sports clubs had better cardiorespiratory fitness measures at all time points. However, a higher level in the beginning leads to a higher level after the pandemic [23]. Adequate levels of physical fitness appear to increase resilience to limited physical activity due to external circumstances, such as the lockdowns during the COVID-19 pandemic.

Furthermore, there is evidence that total physical activity did not decline globally during the COVID-19 pandemic but that the form of being physically active changed [19–21,35]. While organized physical activity decreased, time spent in habitual physical activity and unstructured forms such as playing outside increased [20,22,35]. Schmidt et al. [22] found an increase from 75 min per day before the COVID-19 pandemic to 105 min per day playing outside during lockdown in spring 2020 for 6-to-10-year-old children in Germany. Most notably, socioeconomic background and place of residence are influencing determinants of levels of physical activity and physical fitness [19,20,32,35]. We also analyzed physical activity changes in our sample and can confirm these findings. Children indicated that they spent less minutes for physical activity in sports clubs, while time for physical activity in leisure time increased during the COVID-19 pandemic [36].

Wessely et al. [32] reported decreasing results for measurements of physical fitness during the COVID-19 pandemic, whereby children with a high social burden showed lower performance levels. Children with low socioeconomic status also showed lower levels of physical activity, but the home and living environment had a particular influence [19,20]. In our study, we have no data on socioeconomic status of the study subjects, but we consider community structure data. The community has less than 5000 inhabitants and is located in the north-east of Baden-Württemberg in Germany. The environment is known as rural with access to green areas and playgrounds. For the children in this community, the environment might have provided easy opportunities to be physically active during the COVID-19 pandemic and thus possibly prevented a negative effect on physical fitness. For rural children, the impact of COVID-19 policies and restrictions was limited, but results may differ in urban children. Asked with whom they were physically active, more children in this community named their parents, when restrictions were issued [36].

4.3. Limitations

There are limitations regarding sample and selection bias since we investigated an ad hoc sample with a cross-sectional cohort design of children from one primary school in a rural community of the German federal state Baden-Württemberg. The sample is not representative and its results show a selection effect concerning a higher physical activity and fitness compared with the whole of Germany. However, the long study period and the number of cohort measurements before and during the COVID-19 pandemic ensure that children's physical fitness is considered globally and not just a one-point statement based on a one-point measurement.

Moreover, in this study were some confounding factors, e.g., socio-economic status, educational level of parents, and level of testosterone, which may affect the results, but were not controlled. However, we can use some physical activity data to classify. For future investigations, the methodology should be improved and possible cofounding data collected.

4.4. Practical Implications

The results showed that this particular community, which has been testing and supplementing physical fitness promotion with additional projects for ten years, has an above-average level of physical fitness. The data thus suggest that a variety of long-term physical fitness programs really do help a lot when it comes to promoting an active and healthy lifestyle. The programs should be anchored sustainably in the community and target people's behavior and the conditions. Because not every child had the same opportunities to be physically active [18,32], especially in times when restrictions and limitations influence regular and structured physical activity, policy makers, communities, and other relevant stakeholders must provide children with access to environments that are conducive to and supportive of physical activity. Parents should operate as role models for an active lifestyle. Further research needs to examine larger cohort data to determine generalizable effects of the COVID-19 pandemic on physical fitness in children. In addition, these cohorts need to be monitored for additional years to establish long-term effects and influences. Pooling data, for example with the MO|RE data repository, from many small samples tested with a uniform and standardized measurement tool helps provide a wide range of participants and increases the comparability of findings across studies [37].

5. Conclusions

In conclusion, this study examined effects of the COVID-19 pandemic and changes in various dimensions of physical fitness in a cohort investigated over a long-term period of ten years. We found no evidence for an overall negative effect, but results differed between test items and dimensions. The rural community presented in this study is well aware of the importance of physical fitness. Physical fitness was maintained despite restrictions and limitations through the environmental circumstances. Considering this, this sample is a positive example of maintaining physical fitness throughout the COVID-19 pandemic. Adequate interventions and long-term efforts make an impact, but should address each child.

Author Contributions: Conceptualization, T.E., K.B. and C.N.; methodology, T.E. and C.N.; formal analysis, T.E.; investigation, T.E., K.B. and C.N.; data curation, T.E.; writing—original draft preparation, T.E.; writing—review and editing, K.B. and C.N.; visualization, T.E.; supervision, K.B. and C.N.; project administration, T.E., K.B. and C.N. All authors have read and agreed to the published version of the manuscript.

Funding: This research received no funding.

Institutional Review Board Statement: The study was conducted in accordance with the Declaration of Helsinki, and approved by the Karlsruhe Institute of Technology.

Informed Consent Statement: Informed consent was obtained from all subjects involved in the study through the primary school, which conducted the testing.

Data Availability Statement: The datasets presented in this study will be publicly archived at: http://motor-researchdata.org/.

Acknowledgments: We acknowledge support by the KIT-Publication Fund of the Karlsruhe Institute of Technology. We would like to thank the participating primary school for conducting the testing and all children for participating. Also, we would like to thank the mayor of the community for making the cooperation possible.

Conflicts of Interest: The authors declare no conflict of interest. The funders had no role in the design of the study; in the collection, analysis, or interpretation of data; in the writing of the manuscript, or in the decision to publish the results.

Appendix A

Table A1. Mean values for each test item and cohort overall and separately for boys and girls.

Test Item	Cohort	Mean Value (95% CI)		
		Male	Female	Overall
20 m	2012	4.03 (3.94–4.11)	4.33 (4.19–4.48)	4.16 (4.08–4.24)
	2013	4.15 (4.07–4.24)	4.35 (4.22–4.47)	4.23 (4.15–4.30)
	2014	3.91 (3.83–4.00)	3.94 (3.85–4.02)	3.92 (3.86–3.98)
	2015	3.83 (3.71–3.96)	3.89 (3.75–4.04)	3.86 (3.77–4.00)
	2016	3.99 (3.88–4.10)	4.10 (3.94–4.26)	4.02 (3.93–4.12)
	2017	3.85 (3.75–3.94)	4.00 (3.90–4.09)	3.91 (3.85–3.98)
	2018	4.34 (4.26–4.41)	4.54 (4.43–4.65)	4.42 (4.36–4.49)
	2019	4.43 (4.30–4.57)	4.62 (4.47–4.76)	4.52 (4.42–4.62)
	2020	4.34 (4.21–4.47)	4.41 (4.30–4.52)	4.38 (4.29–4.46)
	2021	4.38 (4.20–4.55)	4.43 (4.22–4.63)	4.40 (4.27–4.53)
BalBw	2012	39.74 (37.60–41.87)	36.86 (33.85–39.88)	38.49 (36.71–40.26)
	2013	39.80 (37.80–41.81)	38.64 (36.10–41.18)	39.35 (37.80–40.90)
	2014	36.39 (33.96–38.82)	39.14 (36.56–41.72)	37.61 (35.85–39.37)
	2015	35.23 (32.16–38.30)	35.61 (31.99–39.22)	35.39 (33.11–37.67)
	2016	39.27 (37.38–41.16)	39.91 (37.78–42.04)	39.50 (38.09–40.91)
	2017	35.73 (33.68–37.78)	36.79 (34.33–39.24)	36.18 (34.63–37.73)
	2018	36.61 (34.71–38.51)	36.98 (35.15–38.81)	36.77 (35.45–38.09)
	2019	33.43 (31.04–35.82)	36.41 (34.42–38.39)	34.87 (33.30–36.43)
	2020	35.33 (32.42–38.24)	38.56 (36.08–41.05)	37.11 (35.23–39.00)
	2021	37.90 (35.88–39.93)	40.72 (38.51–42.94)	39.34 (37.84–40.84)
JumpSw	2012	30.48 (28.64–32.32)	29.90 (27.50–32.30)	30.23 (28.78–31.68)
	2013	31.62 (29.37–33.86)	31.45 (28.96–33.94)	31.55 (29.90–33.20)
	2014	31.35 (29.41–33.29)	34.01 (32.04–35.98)	32.53 (31.14–33.92)
	2015	32.78 (30.20–35.37)	32.09 (28.49–35.69)	32.49 (30.42–34.56)
	2016	33.95 (32.14–35.76)	31.80 (29.77–33.84)	33.18 (31.81–34.55)
	2017	29.84 (27.98–31.71)	29.67 (27.64–31.70)	29.77 (28.42–31.13)
	2018	35.29 (33.59–36.98)	33.17 (31.23–35.10)	34.38 (33.11–35.53)
	2019	31.33 (29.70–32.97)	31.77 (29.90–33.64)	31.54 (30.32–32.76)

Table A1. Cont.

Test Item	Cohort	Mean Value (95% CI)		
		Male	Female	Overall
	2020	36.68 (34.03–39.34)	35.83 (33.53–38.14)	36.23 (34.51–37.94)
	2021	33.77 (31.86–35.68)	32.56 (30.59–34.54)	33.15 (31.79–34.51)
St&R	2012	4.48 (3.34–5.62)	5.54 (4.32–6.76)	4.94 (4.11–5.77)
	2013	4.84 (3.49–6.20)	6.40 (4.85–7.95)	5.45 (4.43–6.47)
	2014	2.70 (1.05–4.35)	5.20 (3.39–7.02)	3.81 (2.58–5.03)
	2015	−0.02 (−2.73–2.69)	4.94 (2.41–7.47)	2.01 (0.06–3.96)
	2016	−0.21 (−1.89–1.48)	2.97 (0.82–5.12)	0.90 (−0.44–2.24)
	2017	−1.60 (−3.59–0.39)	2.09 (−0.22–4.40)	0.07 (−1.46–1.60)
	2018	−2.43 (−3.84–−1.02)	1.74 (−0.16–3.63)	−0.62 (−1.81–0.57)
	2019	−1.13 (−2.82–0.56)	2.17 (0.55–3.79)	0.47 (−0.73–1.66)
	2020	2.57 (0.17–4.97)	3.82 (2.08–5.57)	3.25 (1.82–4.68)
	2021	−0.99 (−3.06–1.08)	3.54 (2.04–5.04)	1.32 (−0.01–2.64)
PU	2012	13.61 (12.63–14.60)	13.14 (12.13–14.15)	13.41 (12.71–14.10)
	2013	13.18 (12.39–13.98)	12.54 (11.55–13.53)	12.93 (12.32–13.54)
	2014	14.96 (13.37–16.56)	16.09 (14.56–17.63)	15.46 (14.36–16.57)
	2015	13.85 (12.68–15.01)	13.71 (12.21–15.21)	13.79 (12.89–14.69)
	2016	14.19 (13.43–14.94)	12.85 (11.92–13.77)	13.71 (13.11–14.30)
	2017	13.47 12.50–14.45)	13.14 (11.93–14.34)	13.33 (12.58–14.07)
	2018	14.94 (14.40–15.48)	14.67 (14.07–15.27)	14.82(14.42–15.22)
	2019	17.65 (16.93–18.37)	17.45 (16.73–18.17)	17.55 (17.05–18.06)
	2020	15.98 (14.75–17.20)	17.49 (16.48–18.50)	16.78 (16.00–17.57)
	2021	14.88 (13.77–16.00)	15.96 (14.99–16.93)	15.44 (14.71–16.17)
SU	2012	15.88 (14.75–17.00)	14.70 (13.34–16.06)	15.36 (14.50–16.23)
	2013	19.32 (17.76–20.87)	16.84 (15.41–18.27)	18.36 (17.24–19.47)
	2014	16.87 (15.29–18.44)	17.90 (16.06–19.75)	17.32 (16.14–18.50)
	2015	17.54 (15.41–19.67)	17.26 (14.73–19.78)	17.42 (15.84–19.01)
	2016	19.09 (17.60–20.57)	16.65 (14.61–18.68)	18.23 (17.03–19.43)
	2017	17.25 (16.01–18.49)	14.55 (13.29–15.81)	16.09 (15.18–17.01)
	2018	18.11 (16.79–19.43)	15.78 (14.19–17.36)	17.10 (16.08–18.12)
	2019	20.32 (18.76–21.88)	18.59 (17.22–19.97)	19.48 (18.44–20.52)
	2020	20.00 (18.08–21.92)	18.60 (17.18–20.01)	19.25 (18.09–20.41)
	2021	19.71 (18.02–21.40)	17.70 (16.03–19.37)	18.69 (17.51–19.87)
SLJ	2012	139.54 (134.95–144.13)	120.59 (114.53–126.65)	131.29 (127.21–135.37)
	2013	132.90 (127.89–137.92)	124.92 (118.14–131.71)	129.79 (125.74–133.84)
	2014	133.58 (128.50–138.67)	134.84 (128.92–140.76)	134.13 (130.34–137.92)
	2015	133.90 (129.10–138.70)	125.00 (116.76–133.24)	130.26 (125.85–134.66)
	2016	129.37 (124.65–134.09)	117.67 (110.92–124.42)	125.17 (121.20–129.15)
	2017	138.72 (133.39–144.05)	120.53 (115.73–125.32)	131.22 (127.15–135.29)
	2018	131.91 (129.87–136.94)	121.63 (116.18–127.07)	127.50 (123.73–131.27)
	2019	134.44 (129.30–139.59)	125.14 (119.90–130.37)	129.98 (126.27–133.70)
	2020	139.41 (133.13–145.70)	133.04 (127.39–138.70)	135.98 (131.80–140.15)
	2021	132.75 (126.53–138.97)	126.57 (121.29–131.86)	129.60 (125.56–133.65)
6 min	2012	1056.79 (1019.57–1094.01)	903.60 (859.31–947.90)	990.92 (959.09–1022.75)
	2013	1044.85 (1010.55–1079.14)	948.78 (907.96–989.61)	1007.82 (980.29–1035.35)
	2014	1016.37 (975.45–1057.28)	936.19 (893.23–979.15)	980.54 (950.28–1010.80)
	2015	996.31 (953.16–1039.46)	974.18 (936.37–1011.99)	987.06 (957.98–1016.14)
	2016	1026.43 (988.75–1064.10)	919.73 (876.69–962.76)	988.97 (958.83–1019.11)
	2017	1032.39 (996.43–1068.34)	950.41 (905.34–995.49)	997.01 (968.11–1025.91)
	2018	1022.42 (990.24–1054.60)	931.18 (900.59–961.77)	983.82 (959.87–1007.77)
	2019	1103.38 (1052.19–1154.57)	955.44 (920.26–990.62)	1031.84 (998.10–1065.57)
	2020	1045.39 (996.26–1094.52)	963.89 (918.40–1009.38)	1001.86 (968.03–1035.70)
	2021	1004.31 (956.22–1052.41)	939.65 (904.93–974.37)	969.65 (940.40–998.90)

20-m Dash: 20 m; Balancing Backwards: BalBw; Jumping Sideways: JumpSw; Stand and Reach: St&R; Push-Ups: PU; Sit-Ups: SU; Standing Long Jump: SLJ; 6-min Run: 6 min.

Table A2. Adjusted mean values of the ANCOVA in each test item- PreCOVID vs. COVID1.

Test Item	PreCOVID Mean Value (95% CI)	COVID1 Mean Value (95% CI)	Pairwise Comparisons Δ Mean Value (SD)
20 m	4.16 (4.13–4.19)	4.36 (4.27–4.46)	Δ +0.20 (0.05) $p < 0.001$
BalBw	37.26 (36.68–37.84)	37.04 (35.28–38.80)	Δ −0.22 (0.95) $p = 0.813$
JumpSw	31.95 (31.43–32.47)	36.27 (34.72–37.81)	Δ +4.32 (0.83) $p < 0.001$
St&R	2.09 (1.63–2.55)	2.98 (1.61–4.34)	Δ +0.88 (0.74) $p = 0.230$
PU	14.49 (14.23–14.76)	16.78 (15.98–17.58)	Δ +2.29 (0.43) $p < 0.001$
SU	17.45 (17.06–17.84)	19.40 (18.25–20.56)	Δ +1.95 (0.62) $p = 0.002$
SLJ	129.80 (128.43–131.14)	137.02 (132.99–141.06)	Δ +7.24 (2.17) $p = 0.001$
6 min	996.33 (986.26–1006.40)	1011.64 (981.75–1041.53)	Δ +15.31 (16.08) $p = 0.341$

20-m Dash: 20 m; Balancing Backwards: BalBw; Jumping Sideways: JumpSw; Stand and Reach: St&R; Push-Ups: PU; Sit-Ups: SU; Standing Long Jump: SLJ; 6-min Run: 6 min.

Table A3. Adjusted mean values of the ANCOVA in each test item- PreCOVID vs. COVID2.

Test Item	PreCOVID Mean Value (95% CI)	COVID2 Mean Value (95% CI)	Pairwise Comparisons Δ Mean Value (SD)
20 m	4.19 (4.13–4.19)	4.39 (4.29–4.49)	Δ +0.23 (0.05) $p < 0.001$
BalBw	37.26 (36.69–37.83)	39.29 (37.72–40.86)	Δ +2.03 (0.85) $p = 0.017$
JumpSw	31.95 (31.44–32.46)	33.19 (31.80–34.57)	Δ +1.24 (0.75) $p = 0.100$
St&R	2.09 (1.64–2.55)	1.10 (−0.15–2.34)	Δ −1.00 (0.68) $p = 0.142$
PU	14.49 (14.23–14.76)	15.44 (14.71–16.17)	Δ +0.94 (0.40) $p = 0.017$
SU	17.45 (17.06–17.84)	18.81 (17.74–19.88)	Δ +1.36 (0.58) $p = 0.019$
SLJ	129.80 (128.44–131.17)	130.36 (126.64–134.08)	Δ +0.56 (2.02) $p = 0.782$
6 min	996.23 (986.25–1006.22)	979.29 (951.07–1007.51)	Δ −16.94 (15.26) $p = 0.267$

20-m Dash: 20 m; Balancing Backwards: BalBw; Jumping Sideways: JumpSw; Stand and Reach: St&R; Push-Ups: PU; Sit-Ups: SU; Standing Long Jump: SLJ; 6-min Run: 6 min.

References

1. Ortega, F.B.; Ruiz, J.R.; Castillo, M.J.; Sjöström, M. Physical fitness in childhood and adolescence: A powerful marker of health. *Int. J. Obes.* **2008**, *32*, 1–11. [CrossRef] [PubMed]
2. Robinson, L.E.; Stodden, D.F.; Barnett, L.M.; Lopes, V.P.; Logan, S.W.; Rodrigues, L.P.; D'Hondt, E. Motor Competence and its Effect on Positive Developmental Trajectories of Health. *Sports Med.* **2015**, *45*, 1273–1284. [CrossRef] [PubMed]
3. Lubans, D.R.; Morgan, P.J.; Cliff, D.P.; Barnett, L.M.; Okely, A.D. Fundamental movement skills in children and adolescents: Review of associated health benefits. *Sports Med.* **2010**, *40*, 1019–1035. [CrossRef] [PubMed]
4. Utesch, T.; Bardid, F.; Büsch, D.; Strauss, B. The Relationship Between Motor Competence and Physical Fitness from Early Childhood to Early Adulthood: A Meta-Analysis. *Sports Med.* **2019**, *49*, 541–551. [CrossRef]
5. Stiller, J.; Würth, S.; Alfermann, D. Die Messung des physischen Selbstkonzepts (PSK). *Z. Für Differ. Und Diagn. Psychol.* **2004**, *25*, 239–257. [CrossRef]
6. Hänsel, F. Kognitive Aspekte. In *Sport und Selbstkonzept: Struktur, Dynamik und Entwicklung*; Conzelmann, A., Hänsel, F., Eds.; Hofmann: Schorndorf, Germany, 2008; pp. 26–44.

7. Clark, J.E. The Mountain of Motor Development: A Metaphor. In *Motor Development: Research and Reviews*; Clark, J.E., Humphrey, J., Eds.; NASPE Publications: Reston, VA, USA, 2002; pp. 163–190.
8. Utesch, T.; Dreiskämper, D.; Naul, R.; Geukes, K. Understanding physical (in-) activity, overweight, and obesity in childhood: Effects of congruence between physical self-concept and motor competence. *Sci. Rep.* **2018**, *8*, 5908. [CrossRef]
9. Führer, T.; Kliegl, R.; Arntz, F.; Kriemler, S.; Granacher, U. An Update on Secular Trends in Physical Fitness of Children and Adolescents from 1972 to 2015: A Systematic Review. *Sports Med.* **2021**, *51*, 303–320. [CrossRef]
10. Eberhardt, T.; Niessner, C.; Oriwol, D.; Buchal, L.; Worth, A.; Bös, K. Secular Trends in Physical Fitness of Children and Adolescents: A Review of Large-Scale Epidemiological Studies Published after 2006. *Int. J. Environ. Res. Public Health* **2020**, *17*, 5671. [CrossRef]
11. Niessner, C.; Hanssen-Doose, A.; Eberhardt, T.; Oriwol, D.; Worth, A.; Bös, K. Motorische Leistungsfähigkeit. In *Vierter Deutscher Kinder-Und Jugendsportbericht: Gesundheit, Leistung und Gesellschaft, 1. Auflage*; Breuer, C., Josten, C., Schmidt, W., Eds.; Hofmann-Verlag GmbH & Co. KG: Schorndorf, Germany, 2020; pp. 51–63. ISBN 9783778091807.
12. Hanssen-Doose, A.; Niessner, C.; Oriwol, D.; Bös, K.; Woll, A.; Worth, A. Population-based trends in physical fitness of children and adolescents in Germany, 2003–2017. *Eur. J. Sport Sci.* **2021**, *21*, 1204–1214. [CrossRef]
13. Woll, A.; Oriwol, D.; Anedda, B.; Burchartz, A.; Hanssen-Doose, A.; Kopp, M.; Niessner, C.; Schmidt, S.C.E.; Bös, K.; Worth, A. *Körperliche Aktivität, Motorische Leistungsfähigkeit und Gesundheit in Deutschland: Ergebnisse aus der Motorik-Modul-Längsschnittstudie (MoMo)*; Kit Scientific Working Papers: Karlsruhe, Germany, 2019; No. 121.
14. Finger, J.D.; Varnaccia, G.; Borrmann, A.; Lange, C.; Mensink, G. Körperliche Aktivität von Kindern und Jugendlichen in Deutschland—Querschnittergebnisse aus KiGGS Welle 2 und Trends. *J. Health Monit.* **2018**, *3*, 24–31. [CrossRef]
15. LeBlanc, A.G.; Gunnell, K.E.; Prince, S.A.; Saunders, T.J.; Barnes, J.D.; Chaput, J.-P. The Ubiquity of the Screen: An Overview of the Risks and Benefits of Screen Time in Our Modern World. *Transl. J. Am. Coll. Sports Med.* **2017**, *2*, 104–113.
16. Greier, K.; Drenowatz, C.; Ruedl, G.; Lackner, C.; Kroell, K.; Feurstein-Zerlauth, V. Differences in Motor Competence by TV Consumption and Participation in Club Sports in Children Starting Elementary School. *Int. J. School Health* **2018**, in press. [CrossRef]
17. Fang, K.; Mu, M.; Liu, K.; He, Y. Screen time and childhood overweight/obesity: A systematic review and meta-analysis. *Child Care Health Dev.* **2019**, *45*, 744–753. [CrossRef]
18. Schilling, J.; Tolksdorf, K.; Marquis, A.; Faber, M.; Pfoch, T.; Buda, S.; Haas, W.; Schuler, E.; Altmann, D.; Grote, U.; et al. Die verschiedenen Phasen der COVID-19-Pandemie in Deutschland: Eine deskriptive Analyse von Januar 2020 bis Februar 2021. *Bundesgesundheitsblatt Gesundh. Gesundh.* **2021**, *64*, 1093–1106. [CrossRef]
19. Wunsch, K.; Kienberger, K.; Niessner, C. Changes in Physical Activity Patterns Due to the Covid-19 Pandemic: A Systematic Review and Meta-Analysis. *Int. J. Environ. Res. Public Health* **2022**, *19*, 2250. [CrossRef]
20. Rossi, L.; Behme, N.; Breuer, C. Physical Activity of Children and Adolescents during the COVID-19 Pandemic-A Scoping Review. *Int. J. Environ. Res. Public Health* **2021**, *18*, 11440. [CrossRef]
21. Schmidt, S.; Burchartz, A.; Kolb, S.; Niessner, C.; Oriwol, D.; Hanssen-Doose, A.; Worth, A.; Woll, A. *Zur Situation der Körperlich-Sportlichen Aktivität von Kindern und Jugendlichen Während der COVID-19 Pandemie in Deutschland: Die Motorik-Modul Studie (MoMo)*; Kit Scientific Working Papers: Karlsruhe, Germany, 2021; No. 165.
22. Schmidt, S.C.E.; Anedda, B.; Burchartz, A.; Eichsteller, A.; Kolb, S.; Nigg, C.; Niessner, C.; Oriwol, D.; Worth, A.; Woll, A. Physical activity and screen time of children and adolescents before and during the COVID-19 lockdown in Germany: A natural experiment. *Sci. Rep.* **2020**, *10*, 21780. [CrossRef]
23. Jarnig, G.; Jaunig, J.; van Poppel, M.N.M. Association of COVID-19 Mitigation Measures With Changes in Cardiorespiratory Fitness and Body Mass Index Among Children Aged 7 to 10 Years in Austria. *JAMA Netw. Open* **2021**, *4*, e2121675. [CrossRef]
24. Chambonnière, C.; Fearnbach, N.; Pelissier, L.; Genin, P.; Fillon, A.; Boscaro, A.; Bonjean, L.; Bailly, M.; Siroux, J.; Guirado, T.; et al. Adverse Collateral Effects of COVID-19 Public Health Restrictions on Physical Fitness and Cognitive Performance in Primary School Children. *Int. J. Environ. Res. Public Health* **2021**, *18*, 11099. [CrossRef]
25. Basterfield, L.; Burn, N.L.; Galna, B.; Batten, H.; Goffe, L.; Karoblyte, G.; Lawn, M.; Weston, K.L. Changes in children's physical fitness, BMI and health-related quality of life after the first 2020 COVID-19 lockdown in England: A longitudinal study. *J. Sports Sci.* **2022**, *40*, 1088–1096. [CrossRef]
26. Greier, K.; Drenowatz, C.; Bischofer, T.; Petrasch, G.; Greier, C.; Cocca, A.; Ruedl, G. Physical activity and sitting time prior to and during COVID-19 lockdown in Austrian high-school students. *AIMS Public Health* **2021**, *8*, 531–540. [CrossRef] [PubMed]
27. Wahl-Alexander, Z.; Camic, C.L. Impact of COVID-19 on School-Aged Male and Female Health-Related Fitness Markers. *Pediatr. Exerc. Sci.* **2021**, *33*, 61–64. [CrossRef] [PubMed]
28. Bös, K.; Mechling, H.; Schlenker, L.; Eberhardt, T.; Abdelkarim, O. *International Physical Performance Test Profile for Boys and Girls from 9–17 Years-Revised: IPPTP-R*; Feldhaus Edition Czwalina: Hamburg, Germany, 2021; ISBN 9783880206953.
29. Bös, K.; Mechling, H. *Dimensionen Sportmotorischer Leistungen*; Hofmann: Schorndorf, Germany, 1983.
30. Bös, K. *Deutscher Motorik Test 6-18 (DMT 6-18): Manual und Internetbasierte Auswertungsplattform*; Feldhaus Edition Czwalina: Hamburg, Germany, 2016.
31. Pombo, A.; Luz, C.; de Sá, C.; Rodrigues, L.P.; Cordovil, R. Effects of the COVID-19 Lockdown on Portuguese Children's Motor Competence. *Children* **2021**, *8*, 199. [CrossRef] [PubMed]

32. Wessely, S.; Ferrari, N.; Friesen, D.; Grauduszus, M.; Klaudius, M.; Joisten, C. Changes in Motor Performance and BMI of Primary School Children over Time-Influence of the COVID-19 Confinement and Social Burden. *Int. J. Environ. Res. Public Health* **2022**, *19*, 4565. [CrossRef]
33. Niessner, C.; Utesch, T.; Oriwol, D.; Hanssen-Doose, A.; Schmidt, S.C.E.; Woll, A.; Bös, K.; Worth, A. Representative Percentile Curves of Physical Fitness From Early Childhood to Early Adulthood: The MoMo Study. *Front. Public Health* **2020**, *8*, 458. [CrossRef]
34. Kloe, M.; Oriwol, D.; Niessner, C.; Worth, A.; Bös, K. Wie leistungsfähig sind meine Schüler_innen? Leistungsbeurteilung mittels Referenzperzentilen zu den Testaufgaben 20-m-Sprint und 6-Minuten-Lauf. *Sportunterricht* **2020**, *69*, 386–392.
35. Schmidt, S.C.E.; Burchartz, A.; Kolb, S.; Niessner, C.; Oriwol, D.; Woll, A. Influence of socioeconomic variables on physical activity and screen time of children and adolescents during the COVID-19 lockdown in Germany: The MoMo study. *Ger. J. Exerc. Sport Res.* **2021**. [CrossRef]
36. Betz, J. Physical Activity and Motor Performance of Children during the COVID-19-Pandemic Using the Example of the Community of Michelfeld. Unpublished. Master's Thesis, Karlsruhe Institute of Technology, Karlsruhe, Germany, 2022.
37. Kloe, M.; Niessner, C.; Woll, A.; Bös, K. Open Data im sportwissenschaftlichen Anwendungsfeld motorischer Tests. *Ger. J. Exerc. Sport Res.* **2019**, *49*, 503–513. [CrossRef]

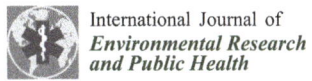

International Journal of
Environmental Research and Public Health

Article

Puberal and Adolescent Horse Riders' Fitness during the COVID-19 Pandemic: The Effects of Training Restrictions on Health-Related and Functional Motor Abilities

Sabrina Demarie [1,*], Emanuele Chirico [1], Cecilia Bratta [2] and Cristina Cortis [2]

1 Department of Movement, Human and Health Sciences, University of Rome "Foro Italico", Piazza de Bosis 6, 00135 Rome, Italy; e.chirico@studenti.uniroma4.it
2 Department of Human Sciences, Society and Health, University of Cassino and Lazio Meridionale, 03043 Cassino, Italy; cecilia.bratta@studenti.unicas.it (C.B.); c.cortis@unicas.it (C.C.)
* Correspondence: sabrina.demarie@uniroma4.it; Tel.: +39-333-8547757 or +39-06-36733260

Abstract: The aim of the study was to analyse the fitness level of young horse riders before and after 12 weeks of training restrictions instituted due to the COVID-19 emergency. Anthropometrical measure assessment and an eight-items fitness test battery were administered to 61 puberal and adolescent female amateur horse riders. Subjects were evaluated within 3 weeks before (pre-tests) the period of training restrictions and on the first day of normal training after it (post-tests). Post-test results showed significant increases in body weight (Z: −1.732; p value: 0.001; ES: −0.157) and BMI (F: 9.918; p value: 0.003; ES: 0.146), whilst the performance in hand grip and abdominal strength, hip mobility, and 10×5 m Shuttle and Cooper 12 min tests' outcomes significantly decreased (F: 29.779; p value: 0.001 F: 29.779; p value: 0.001 F: 29.779; p value: 0.001 F: 29.779; p value: 0.001 F: 29.779; p value: 0.001, respectively). Correlation analysis revealed that riders' experience was significantly correlated with hand grip ($p < 0.01$), leg strength ($p < 0.01$), hip mobility ($p < 0.05$), and 5×10 m Shuttle ($p < 0.01$) and the Cooper 12 min ($p < 0.01$) test results. It could be suggested that equestrian activities could produce a higher fitness level in puberal and adolescent riders, whilst home-based, unsupervised, and unattentively planned training during the twelve weeks of training restrictions might be insufficient to maintain it.

Keywords: SARS-CoV-2; adolescent fitness; young athletes; outdoor sport; horse riding

Citation: Demarie, S.; Chirico, E.; Bratta, C.; Cortis, C. Puberal and Adolescent Horse Riders' Fitness during the COVID-19 Pandemic: The Effects of Training Restrictions on Health-Related and Functional Motor Abilities. *Int. J. Environ. Res. Public Health* **2022**, *19*, 6394. https://doi.org/10.3390/ijerph19116394

Academic Editors: Clemens Drenowatz and Klaus Greier

Received: 3 April 2022
Accepted: 23 May 2022
Published: 24 May 2022

Publisher's Note: MDPI stays neutral with regard to jurisdictional claims in published maps and institutional affiliations.

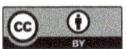

Copyright: © 2022 by the authors. Licensee MDPI, Basel, Switzerland. This article is an open access article distributed under the terms and conditions of the Creative Commons Attribution (CC BY) license (https://creativecommons.org/licenses/by/4.0/).

1. Introduction

Evidence that programmes promoting organised physical activities and sports amongst children and adolescents may contribute to the improvement of health-related quality of life has been systematically reported [1–8]. Horseback riding can be seen as an appropriate organised recreational physical activity, and indeed, it is practised by many young people. It is a sport which requires a high level of dexterity and postural muscular effort, with an emphasis on excellent fine motor skills and balance, in order for the rider to practise an ethological equitation [9]. It recruits aerobic and anaerobic energy systems with increasing energy cost as the horse progresses through the gaits; it improves postural control by coordinating one's body movements with those of the horse, and it has been proven to produce effective physical fitness changes ranging over various aspects such as muscle strength and muscle mass, total and regional body composition, cardiorespiratory endurances, agility, and balance enhancement [10–16]. Amongst the most suitable equestrian disciplines for children and adolescents are endurance, pony games and show jumping. Endurance is a long-distance competition against the clock which tests the speed and endurance of a horse and challenges the rider's effective use of pace. It requires a synergetic horse and rider combination to successfully complete a marked course within a specified time that is specifically designed to test their stamina and fitness on the track with distance, terrain, climate, and clock constraints without compromising the welfare of the horse. Although the rides are timed, the emphasis is on finishing the race in good condition rather than coming in first. Each course is divided into phases with a compulsory halt for a veterinary inspection which determines whether the horse is fit to continue or not. At the beginner's level, horses complete courses that vary from 15 km to 19 km long, either at walking or trotting speed. Pony games is a team sport that combines the love of ponies and friends with various races. Teams of four or five riders and ponies take part in a series of exciting races that involve a mix of turns, handovers, skill, vaulting, and galloping against other teams. Competitions are comprised of several relay-style races, requiring riders to pick up objects from the ground while remaining in the saddle, weave through a series of poles at high speeds, hand items to teammates without slowing their ponies, and dunking objects into buckets; beginners usually compete at the walking and trotting gaits. Show jumping is a competitive equestrian sport in which the horse and rider are required to jump over all of the fences in a course that has been designed for a particular show without knocking them down and within a set time limit. Competitors compete one by one, and judges determine whether the fences are successfully cleared and assign penalties and points; then, the times and scores are compared to determine the winner.

In Italy, where the study was conducted, after the first period of the SARS-CoV-2 pandemic when physical activities were restricted to home-based training and individual outdoor jogging and running, competitive horse riders have attempted other forms of training besides those on the horse; nonetheless, they suffered from significantly decreased performance with a substantial contribution of cognitive distress to the overall perception of effort [17]. It is worth noting that in Italy, high-level athletes and horse owners have been allowed to resume training after eight weeks of lockdown, while recreational athletes were kept from sport activities for four weeks longer. This led to concerns about the impact of detraining on young athletes' health, performance, and injury risk at the resumption of regular physical activity [18–20].

To this purpose, a detailed profile of athletes' physical fitness allowed not only the determination of the underlying performance qualities for training-planning purposes, but also a wide range of health-related attributes associated with the quality of life. Many studies investigated fitness- and health-related changes after the COVID-19 confinement in healthy or diseased school children and adolescents [21,22]. However, young athletes could suffer a major impact during confinement due to their greatly modified lifestyle. Most athletes will find themselves searching for an optimal solution to maintain their physical, physiological, and psychological levels as close as possible to their original ones. Many studies collected questionnaires and interview data on young athletes' confinement and on its outcomes, and general guidelines have been provided for athletes to optimally maintain physical and mental fitness whilst respecting the measures taken during the COVID-19 confinement period [23]. However, to the best of our knowledge, no studies collected objective measures of physical activity and fitness level changes in young, healthy athletes during the first strict confinement period that could be useful for planning the activities to be implemented in youth sports settings if a new wave of confinements were to occur in the future.

To quantitatively assess the physical attributes of the young and children, field fitness test batteries can be administered with inexpensive and easy-to-use equipment, being therefore useful for the continuous monitoring of training effects and fitness levels as well as for the comparison amongst different populations [24–26].

To assess the effect of twelve weeks of training restrictions due to the COVID-19 pandemic on young recreational horse riders of different equitation disciplines, the aim of the study was to analyse their fitness level by administering a motor fitness test battery before and after the emergency period and to compare their results with reference values of healthy, active, age-matched athletes of the same geographical region.

2. Materials and Methods

Sixty-six female puberal and adolescent (age range 9 to 18 with a mean age of 13.87 ± 0.34) recreational horse riders practicing endurance, pony games and show jumping equestrian disciplines were recruited for the study. Inclusion criteria were participating regularly and continuously and taking equestrian classes at least twice a week for 12 or more months. Exclusion criteria were noncomplying with home-based training during all of the 12 weeks of training restrictions, testing positive for SARS-CoV-2, or suffering injuries or illnesses during the test period or in the 3 preceding months. Three of the subjects either tested positive for SARS-CoV-2 or suffered injuries or illnesses during the test period or in the 3 preceding months, and 2 of them did not practice horse riding continuously in the previous year. This led to the exclusion of 5 riders and left 61 participants equally distributed amongst the three equestrian disciplines (Endurance, $n = 20$; Pony Games, $n = 20$; Show Jumping $n = 21$). Participants' equitation experience was assessed as the number of months ranging from the first time they rode a horse to the pre-test date, with a mean value of 13 ± 3.1 months. During the 6 months before the study, the subjects had regularly completed 2 ± 0.3 training sessions per week, each lasting 45–50 min each on the horse.

All riders and their legal tutors received written and oral information about the purpose of the study, of their rights as study participants, and of the anonymity of their data and provided written informed consent. The project received approval from the institutional review board (protocol code CAR-14/2019).

As depicted in Figure 1, fitness test batteries were part of the regular training program and were usually administered every 8 weeks by the coaches of the clubs involved. Since subjects were familiar with all test protocols long before data collection, a learning effect impact on the post-test outcome should not be likely. Tests were administered throughout the 3 weeks preceding the pandemic period and immediately after the resumption of physical activity after the 12 weeks of training restrictions. The motor fitness test battery comprised 8 items performed as previously described [24,26].

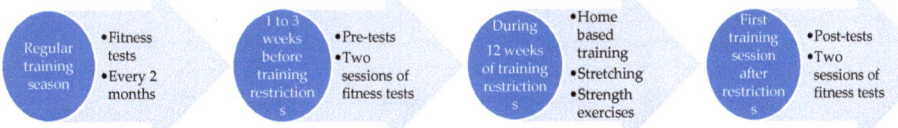

Figure 1. Training and test sessions timeline.

During the 12 weeks of the training restriction period, athletes trained on their own, on a regular basis, for approximately 45–50 min 2 days per week; the routine comprised stretching warm-up, no-load isometric and elastic-band-resisted exercises for the core, and upper and lower limb muscle strength training, as depicted in Figure 2. Home-based training was initially programmed for 8 weeks; one set and one repetition were added for every exercise every 2 weeks. From the first to the eighth and from the ninth to the twelfth week, the training programme remained unchanged [27].

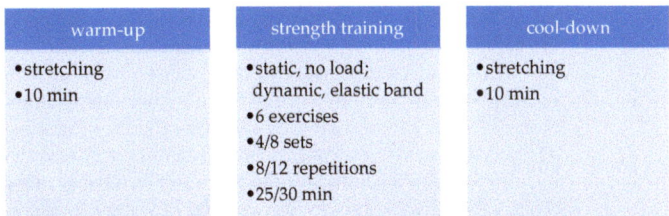

Figure 2. Description of the home based training sessions.

Compliance with the home-based training programme was ascertained by text messages to the coaches listing the number of exercises, sets, and repetitions completed during each week. The weekly training programme was considered completed if at least 80% of the maximal repetitions and sets were accomplished for each exercise.

2.1. Anthropometric Measures

To measure height, the athlete stood on the stadiometer platform with their shoes off. Their feet were together, and the heels were supported on the base of the device with the arms along the body. The participant was instructed to gaze outward, and the measurement was rounded to the nearest 0.5 cm. We assessed the body weight simultaneously by instructing the athlete to step on the scale (with their shoes off). The results were recorded in kilograms and centimetres (HE HEM Medical Weight Scale with Stadiometer, HIWEIGH, Shanghai, China). All anthropometric measurements were taken by the same medical doctor in charge of all of the clubs involved. Body mass index (BMI) was calculated as weight in kilograms/height meters squared [28].

2.2. Motor Fitness Test Batteries

Motor fitness tests are comprised in the Eurofit and ALPHA test batteries that have been widely used throughout Europe with children and adolescents [29]. They have been developed as a standardised European fitness test battery used to assess the effectiveness of physical education and to measure the health-related fitness of schoolchildren [30]. The fitness test battery's inter-rater reliability and test-retest reliability are considered adequate to support their clinical use; indeed, they have been successfully used with primary, middle, and high school students, providing reference data bases [26,31]. The same test items have been used in the school districts of our children and adolescents, ensuring that subjects may have come from similar ethnic, cultural, socio-economic, and socio-demographic groups. Physical education schoolteachers provided the results of their last collection, which served as reference values for comparison with our subjects.

The sit-and-reach test was employed to assess hip mobility since it has been suggested that hip flexibility is the main determinant of the back-saver sit-and-reach test in adolescents, and no significant differences in inter-method agreement were observed between the back-saver sit-and-reach test and the sit-and-reach test, implying that they are comparable [32]. The flamingo test was demonstrated to be suitable for measuring youth aged 9 to 17 years [33]. Amongst the balance tests, the flamingo test results were mostly predicted by strength of the abdominal muscle in pre-adolescent girls [34]; therefore, it seemed to be the most suitable for horse riders that centre their motor control in the core area. Moreover, the flamingo test showed the highest associations with the other motor abilities and correlated the best with endurance running as compared to the one-leg stance on a low beam and the low-beam walking test. Amongst the three tests, it also showed the highest reliability score (0.910) in pre-adolescent children [35].

In the flamingo test for balance, participants stood upright on a special wooden beam ($50 \times 3 \times 4$ cm). The leg they stood on was fully extended, whilst the free leg was bent at the knee, and the foot of that leg was held with the hand on the same side of the body. The timekeeper helped the participant assume the correct position and started taking the time when the subject released the timekeeper's hand. The result was the maximum number of attempts in 1 min, which was limited to 30. If the subject exceeded this number 15 times in the first 30 s, the subject's result was recorded as 31 [35].

The sit-and-reach test required the use of the sit-and-reach standardized box; the participant was required to sit with their knees straight and legs together, and their feet placed against the box, then they slowly reached forwards as far as possible and the furthest position the participant could reach (in centimetres) was recorded [32].

Hand grip was tested for the dominant hand only using a digital hand dynamometer (TKK 5101 Grip-D, Takey, Tokyo, Japan). The subjects looked forwards with their feet shoulder-width apart and were instructed not to touch the dynamometer with any part of the body except for the hand being measured. During the test, subjects stood with their arm straight down at their side, their shoulder slightly abducted (approximately 10°), their elbow in full extension, their forearm in a neutral position, and their wrist extended; the display of the dynamometer was aligned so it would face the examiner, providing blind measurements to the subject. Participants were instructed to squeeze gradually and continuously for at least 2 s and were encouraged to do their best when performing the tests [36].

For the standing broad jump for leg strength, the participant stood behind the starting line with their feet together and pushed vigorously in order to jump forwards as far as possible. The distance was measured with a 10 m line (echoENG, Cormano, Italy) from the take-off line to the point where the back of the heel was closest to the take-off line after landing on the mat or anti-slip floor [37,38].

Sit-ups were used to test abdominal strength and required the subjects to lie face-up on a mat in a supine position with their knees bent at 90-degree angles. The feet were placed flat on the mat and held in position by the examiner. The subjects' arms were crossed on their chest with the hands on the opposite shoulders. When the examiner signalled the start, a timer was started, and the subjects performed as many repetitions as they could within 30 s. To complete a full repetition, each subject flexed their trunk, allowing their lower back to come off the mat, until the subject's elbows contacted his or her thighs. This movement was reversed to the starting position, and the sequence was repeated until the 30 s had expired. The examiner counted the number of repetitions, and the passing of the 30 s was assessed with a stopwatch (Hanhart Delta E 200 1/100 sec., Hanhart, Gütenbach, Germany) [39,40].

For the flexed-arms hang tests that tested the arms' strength, participants were asked to hang for as long as possible on a horizontal bar with a flexed arm so that the chin was level with the horizontal bar [41]. The subject was assisted into position, and the bar was grasped using an overhand grip with the hands shoulder width apart; the timer started when the subject was released. The timer was stopped when the subject's chin fell below the level of the bar or the head tilted backwards to enable the chin to stay level with the bar. The time was recorded using a stopwatch (Hanhart Delta E 200 1/100 sec., Hanhart, Gütenbach, Germany).

In the 10 × 5 m shuttle test for speed and agility, marker cones were placed five metres apart, and participants were required to run back and forth between them for a total of 50 m. They started with a foot on one marker; when instructed by the timekeeper, the subject ran to the opposite marker, turned, and returned to the starting line. This was repeated five times without stopping. At each marker, both feet were required to fully cross the line, and the time it took to cover the 50 m was measured with a stopwatch (Hanhart Delta E 200 1/100 sec., Hanhart, Gütenbach, Germany) [42].

In the Cooper's 12-min run test for aerobic fitness, the distance travelled in this period was measured. The test was performed on an athletic track by counting the number of laps in the established perimeter with a known distance. The measurements of the perimeter and the distance of the incomplete turns were measured with a 50 m line (echoENG, Cormano, Italy) and the passing of the 12 min was assessed using a stopwatch (Hanhart Delta E 200 1/100 sec., Hanhart, Gütenbach, Germany) [43].

Tests were divided into two separate sessions. Session 1 comprised the Cooper's 12-min run, the sit-and-reach, the hand grip, and the standing broad jump tests. Session 2 comprised the 10 × 5 m shuttle, the flamingo, the sit-ups and the flexed-arms hang tests. The running test was completed at the end of the test session; the others were performed in a random order by each subject.

All tests were preceded by a 15 min warm-up consisting of running and stretching for both the upper and lower limbs as well as for core activation.

For each item, the best of 3 attempts was retained, except for the 10 × 5 m shuttle and the Cooper 12 min tests, which were performed once for the pre-test and once for the post-test. All the tests were administered by expert coach graduates in sports science; the same coach oversaw the tests both in the pre- and the post-pandemic periods.

2.3. Reference Fitness Test Values

Fitness test batteries have been applied in the school districts of our group of puberal and adolescent horse riders, ensuring that subjects may have come from similar ethnic, cultural, socio-economic, and socio-demographic groups. Physical education schoolteachers provided us with the results of their last collection of fitness values dated 2007. The results for the same 8 test items obtained from 1687 female high school non-athlete students were used. Since these values are age- and sex- matched (age: 11–18 years), they served as reference values to be compared with those of our subjects.

2.4. Statistical Analysis

For all data, descriptive statistics were calculated, and distributions were verified to identify potential outliers. We also checked the distribution to see if assumptions of normality had been violated by a Shapiro–Wilk test. In the case of skewed distribution, differences between the pre- and post-tests were analysed through a Mann–Whitney U as a non-parametric method. For variables that were normally distributed, we applied a repeated measure ANOVA and Bonferroni post hoc. This statistic model was chosen to evaluate the differences within the groups (pre and post phases) and the differences between the groups, specifically the three different equitation disciplines. Differences between endurance, pony games, and show jumping were tested through a Kruskal–Wallis test as a non-parametric method and by the Bonferroni post hoc test of repeated measure ANOVA in the case of normally distributed variables. To assess the differences between horse riders and age-matched reference values, an independent simple *t*-test was utilised. To understand possible relationships between riding experience and pre-test measured variables, Spearman rank correlation or Pearson correlation analyses were applied when proper. Significance was accepted at the level of $p < 0.05$.

3. Results

Height, BMI, flamingo test, abdominal strength, 5×10 m shuttle, and hip mobility presented a normal distribution of data, while age, riding experience, weight, hand grip, leg strength, arm strength, and the Copper 12 min test did not.

The comparison between pre and post anthropometrical measures revealed that the mean body weight and BMI significantly increased during the twelve weeks of training restrictions, by 3.9% and 8.5%, respectively, as shown in Table 1.

Table 1. Anthropometric measures collected before (pre-test) and after (post-test) the twelve weeks of training restrictions.

	Age (years)	Height (cm)	Weight (kg)	BMI
Pre-test	13.9 ± 2.7	159.4 ± 9.0	49.1 ± 7.9	19.1 ± 2.1
Post-test	13.9 ± 2.6	159.4 ± 8.9 *	51.0 ± 7.5	20.7 ± 3.4 *
F		29.779		9.918
Z	−1.732		−1.732	
p value	0.083	0.083	0.001	0.003
Effect size	−0.157	0.997	−0.157	0.146

* Significant differences between pre- and post-test results, $p < 0.05$.

As reported in Table 2, hand grip, abdominal strength, and hip mobility results significantly reduced after the training restrictions period—by −15.4%, −6.9%, and 82.9%, respectively. Furthermore, the 5×10 m shuttle, and Cooper 12 min test results also appeared significantly diminished in the post-test—by −3.5% and −11.5%, respectively.

Table 2. Motor fitness test battery results collected before (pre-test) and after (post-test) the twelve weeks of training restrictions.

	Hand Grip (kg)	Flamingo Test (s)	Legs Strength (cm)	Abdominal Strength (n)	Arms Strength (s)	5 × 10 m Shuttle (s)	Cooper 12 min (m)	Hip Mobility (cm)
Pre-test	29.3 ± 5.7	9.5 ± 4.2	146.0 ± 17.4	18.3 ± 3.8	10.2 ± 3.9	23.0 ± 1.9	1282.9 ± 196.8	1.1 ± 7.3
Post-test	24.8 ± 3.0 *	9.2 ± 4.7	144.2 ± 21.0	17.0 ± 3.1 *	9.5 ± 2.7	23.9 ± 2.2 *	1135.4 ± 149.3 *	2.1 ± 7.2 *
F		0.135		13.074		15.725		11.732
Z	−4.353		−0.779		−1.219		−4.816	
p value	0.000	0.714	0.436	0.001	0.223	0.000	0.000	0.001
Effect size	−0.384	0.002	−0.071	0.184	−0.110	0.213	−0.436	0.168

* Significant differences between pre and post-tests results, $p < 0.05$.

In Table 3, riders' results collected in the pre-tests are confronted with age- and sex-matched reference values obtained by a report on 1687 female middle and high school students (age: 11–18 years) of the same school district. Riders' body weight results were significantly lower (−5.6%) than age-matched non-athletes'. Pre-test fitness measurements were significantly lower except for handgrip, which was significantly higher (17%).

Table 3. Comparison of the fitness pre-test horse riders' results with reference values.

	Age (yrs)	Height (cm)	Weight (kg)	BMI	Hand Grip (kg)	Flamingo Test (s)	Legs Strength (cm)	Abdominal Strength (n)	Arms Strength (s)	5 × 10 m Shuttle (s)	Cooper 12 min (m)	Hip Mobility (cm)
Reference values	13.9 ± 2.7	158.2 ± 7.6	52.0 ± 7.4	19.1 ± 1.6	25.1 ± 4.0	10.7 ± 1.2	154.9 ± 7.6	19.3 ± 0.9	17.8 ± 2.8	21.0 ± 0.1	1743.1 ± 43.8	6.7 ± 1.9
% diff.	0.4	1.20	−5.6	−0.3	17.0	−11.2	−5.8	−5.3	−42.8	9.7	−26.4	−82.8
Z	0.000	−0.311	−2.636	−0.110	−4.236	−2.079	−3.857	−1.974	−8.399	−6.799	−9.547	−5.499
p values	1.000	0.756	0.008 *	0.912	0.000 *	0.038 *	0.000 *	0.048 *	0.000 *	0.000 *	0.000 *	0.000 *
Effect size	0.001	−0.028	−0.239	−0.010	−0.383	−0.188	−0.349	−0.179	−0.760	−0.616	−0.864	−0.498

* Significant differences between horse riders' results and age-matched reference values $p < 0.05$.

Riders of each discipline did not present significant differences in anthropometrical characteristics. The subjects were 14.3 ± 2.9, 13.2 ± 2.1, and 14.1 ± 3.0 years old; their heights (cm) were 161.1 ± 8.5, 155.3 ± 9.3, and 162.0 ± 8.1; their weights were (kg) 50.6 ± 9.3, 46.0 ± 7.0, and 50.8 ± 6.7; and their BMIs were 19.4 ± 2.5, 18.5 ± 2.2, and 19.3 ± 1.6 for endurance, pony games and show jumping, respectively.

Differences amongst equestrian disciplines highlighted that the endurance group (Table 4) presented the statistically lowest abdominal strength and the show jumping group showed the strongest hand grip values and the statistically highest arm strength in comparison to the other two disciplines.

Table 4. Fitness values of riders for each equestrian discipline.

	Handgrip (kg)	Flamingo Test (s)	Legs Strength (cm)	Abdominal Strength (n)	Arms Strength (s)	5 × 10 m Shuttle (s)	Cooper 12 min (m)	Hip Mobility (cm)
Endurance	28.2 ± 5.9 *	10.9 ± 32.	150.1 ± 9.0	16.1 ± 3.4 *	9.3 ± 3.7 *	23.9 ± 1.4	1301.7 ± 216.1	1.3 ± 8.7
Pony Games	28.3 ± 5.4 *	9.3 ± 5.5	144.0 ± 24.2	19.3 ± 3.6 *	8.8 ± 0.3 *	23.4 ± 2.6	1316.0 ± 170.5	2.3 ± 7.1
Show Jumping	31.6 ± 5.4 *	8.4 ± 3.0	144.0 ± 15.2	19.5 ± 3.5 *	12.6 ± 4.4 *	24.4 ± 2.4	1229.3 ± 201.1	−0.2 ± 6.1
p value	0.023			0.008	0.002			

* Significant differences amongst the riders' results of three equestrian disciplines, $p < 0.05$.

Correlation analysis revealed that riders' experience was significantly correlated with hand grip, leg strength, hip mobility, and with the 5 × 10 m shuttle and the Cooper 12 min test results, as reported in Table 5.

Table 5. Correlation coefficients of fitness values with months of equitation experience.

	Exp. (months)	Weight (kg)	Height (cm)	BMI	Handg. (kg)	Flamingo (s)	Abd. (n)	5 × 10 m (s)	Hip (cm)	Legs (cm)	Arms (s)	Cooper (m)
Age (y)	0.978 **											
Exp. (months)	1.000											
Weight (kg)	0.441 **	1.000										
Height (cm)	0.645 **	0.774 **	1.000									
BMI	−0.001	0.743 **	0.266 *	1.000								
Handg. (kg)	0.398 **	0.423 **	0.499 **	0.159	1.000							
Flamingo (s)	−0.093	−0.083	−0.098	−0.004	−0.364 **	1.000						
Abd. Str. (n)	0.075	−0.123	−0.109	−0.190	−0.068	−0.084	1.000					
5 × 10 m (s)	−0.343 **	0.013	−0.232	0.166	−0.226	0.209	−0.168	1.000				
Hip (cm)	−0.285 *	−0.141	−0.296 *	0.028	−0.259 *	0.211	0.013	0.194	1			
Legs (cm)	0.408 **	0.077	0.258 *	−0.085	0.126	0.025	0.219	−0.395 **	−0.083	1.000		
Arms (s)	0.139	0.108	0.234	−0.077	0.323 *	−0.187	0.229	−0.124	−0.304 *	0.256 *	1.000	
Cooper (m)	0.483 **	0.016	0.133	−0.181	−0.023	0.168	0.181	−0.429 **	−0.146	0.499 **	0.499 **	1.000

Age in years, Exp. (riding experience in months), Weight (in kilograms), Height (in centimetres), BMI, Handg. (hand grip in kg), Flamingo (balance test in seconds), Abd. Str. (abdominal strength test as number of repetitions), 5 × 10 m (10 × 5 m shuttle test in seconds), Hip (hip mobility tests in centimetres), Legs (legs strength in centimetres), Arms Str. (arm strength in seconds), Cooper (Cooper 12 min test in metres). * $p < 0.05$; ** $p < 0.01$.

4. Discussion

Results of the present study evidenced that twelve weeks of training restrictions due to the COVID-19 emergency and lockdown decreased the fitness level of young recreational horse riders. Even though pupils were instructed by coaches to practise home-based physical activities, it can be argued that either general and unguided exercise assignments of 45–50 min 2 days per week were insufficient to retain adolescent physical fitness or that assignments' compliance was not respected, if not both. It has been demonstrated that more experienced athletes of the same regional area (4 years of experience or more) who have had the opportunity to be remotely assisted, guided, and monitored by their coaches were more engaged in home training than their recreational counterparts, being able to keep high physical activity levels even in an extraordinary situation such as a nationwide lockdown [44]. It can be suggested that during training restriction periods, recreational athletes may need more thorough fitness programs with more detailed instructions and stricter surveillance than high-level athletes in order for home-based training to be effective. Moreover, due to the possibly more pronounced detraining effect on novice and recreational than on professional athletes, their training resumption should be even more carefully managed before returning to full training intensities and volumes.

Anthropometric measurements of our group of young riders showed no differences in height but significant increases in body weight and BMI. It can thus be argued that equitation training apparently allowed the subjects to keep weight and BMI under control before training restrictions intervened. Since BMI is generally related to an increased risk of various diseases such as type 2 diabetes and heart disease and can have an important influence on adults' health conditions, horse riding exercises can be suggested to be associated with people's health management [45].

It has also been put forward that, together with the athlete's physical fitness, their mental well-being can be affected by training restrictions [46–48]. The role of psychological components in equitation disciplines is considered vitally important and athletes are required to always be in control of both their body and mind [49–51]. The cooperative effort of two non-related species, horses and humans, is essential to continually adapt to various unpredictable situations. The horse's nature is governed by its instinctive reactions, by the different gait employed, and by the characteristics of the land where the practice is being carried out. Hence, a positive interaction between the horse and its rider when coping with the emotional and physical challenges of equestrian tasks is a prerequisite for success not only for competitions, but also for recreational activities [10,52]. Further supporting this, in competitive horse riders, 8 weeks of training restrictions decreased the performance outcome for up to six weeks following training resumption with a significant rise in anxiety and rate of perceived effort during competitions [17]. Athletes with higher levels of anxiety, such as those who do not respect sufficient recovery times, can suffer a higher risk of injuries [53,54]. When training restarts, great attention should be paid not only to the training workload but also to athletes' physical and mental conditions, perception of exertion, signs, and symptoms of anxiety [55]. For a safer and more efficient way to resume training, young novice riders can begin practising in conditions of reduced anxiety, such as on mechanical horse simulators [56,57]. Such simulators have been proven to be effective and sufficient indoor workout equipment for people with limited time and chances for outdoor activities and for enhancing neurologic functions in patients [6,58,59]. A study aimed to examine the energy expenditure and postural coordination of horse riders and non-riders on a mechanical horse indicates a change in the energy system from an aerobic mode at a low oscillation frequency to a lactic anaerobic mode at a high oscillation frequency for both groups [57]. Horse riding simulation training can thus be a fun and interesting alternative practice tool to resume equitation practice which allows the avoidance of the interference of emotional distress, which may increase the fitness level and the motivation to participate in exercise programmes.

Concerning horse riding training effects on physical fitness, medium-to-high training loads in various equitation disciplines have been reported for general competitive riders, for college females, for sedentary young female adults, and for healthy children, suggesting that it is possible to achieve health benefits through accumulated horseback riding exercise, particularly if riding is performed at the more intense gaits [6,52,60–65]. Olympic equestrian athletes have been reported to have high values of muscle strength and balance, good physical functions, and good maximal aerobic power [16]. Results of the present study on recreationally trained young horse riders indicated higher hip mobility (-82.8%) and hand grip (17%) with respect to age-matched reference values of the same geographical region. The latter could be expected since the greater effort in horse conduction relies on the upper limbs and hands, particularly in novice riders that depend on rough and taut controls of the horse, with the use of excessive muscular force of the arms and hands [63]. This is also confirmed by the significantly higher arm strength showed by the show jumping group, being the discipline that requires the most directional control by the riders as compared to endurance and pony games. High hip mobility can be explained by the fact that all coaches participating in the study included mobility exercises in their usual sessions, which is not a common practice of horse riding trainers.

On the other hand, our fitness test results indicated lower values, except for handgrip, than those obtained by teachers in the same school district from age- and sex-matched non-athlete students that we used as reference. However, it must be noted that reference values were collected fifteen years earlier and could be irrelevant for the present puberal and adolescent population [30]. Indeed, accelerometry data show that sedentary behaviours of adolescent girls (12–15 years old) are increasing over time from 2003, with higher rates reported in recent studies [66]. Consistently, in recent years, two thirds of European children and adolescents were categorized as not sufficiently physically active, with lower physical activity levels in Southern European countries and girls who are less active and more sedentary in all age categories [67]. Therefore, outdated values referring to a possibly more active population of the past may lead to an underestimation of the horse riding training effect on the contemporary young population. Indeed, values measured after the 12 weeks of forced restriction from equitation training indicated a significant loss of hand grip and abdominal strength and 5×10 m shuttle, and Copper 12 min test results and a significant increase in body weight and BMI. Moreover, our results showed that more experience in horse riding was significantly correlated with higher hand grip, leg strength, and hip mobility, and with the better results in the 5 × 10 m shuttle test and the Cooper 12 min test. Therefore, recreational equitation practice could be presumed to be a physical activity that offers some training effects suitable for improving the fitness level of young recreational riders.

With regards to the equestrian discipline that best suits fitness enhancement purposes, values of the three groups are consistent between them, indicating similar training effects. However, endurance riders appeared to achieve higher aerobic fitness involvement and lower abdominal strength, whilst show jumping riders showed the highest hand and arm strength. This could be ascribed to their opposite metabolic requests and different needs for precise guidance of the horse. It can thus be supposed that each of the two disciplines can be more suitable than the other if either cardiometabolic fitness or muscle strength is the main goal, whilst pony games could be envisioned as the least specialised equitation activity out of the three.

Limitations of the present study are represented by the lack of a control group, which does not allow us to determine if pre-test fitness levels were attributable solely to horse riding or if other aspects might have been involved. Additionally, during training restrictions, physical activity was entrusted to individual responsibility, giving rise to different sorts of fitness outcomes. Further limitations were the small number of subjects for each equitation discipline, the all-female subjects, and the sample of items chosen to be part of the test battery that could not represent the actual horse riders' training effects. It could certainly be useful to discriminate which physical attributes are most pertinent to equitation training and performance by broadening the motor fit test items and by correlating test results with performance outcomes.

5. Conclusions

Twelve weeks of training restrictions due to the COVID-19 sanitary emergency decreased the fitness level of puberal and adolescent female recreational horse riders. It could thus be suggested that home-based, unsupervised, and unattentively planned training can be insufficient to maintain their fitness level during home confinement.

Author Contributions: Conceptualization, S.D.; methodology, S.D.; formal analysis, E.C.; investigation, E.C.; data curation, E.C.; writing—original draft preparation, S.D.; writing—review and editing, C.C.; visualization, C.B.; supervision, S.D.; project administration, S.D. All authors have read and agreed to the published version of the manuscript.

Funding: This research received no external funding.

Institutional Review Board Statement: The study was conducted in accordance with the Declaration of Helsinki and approved by the Institutional Review Board of University of Rome "Foro Italico" (protocol code CAR-14/2019 and date of approval 21 October 2019).

Informed Consent Statement: Informed consent was obtained from all subjects involved in the study.

Data Availability Statement: Not applicable.

Conflicts of Interest: The authors declare no conflict of interest.

References

1. Kohl, H.W.; Fulton, J.E.; Caspersen, C.J. Assessment of physical activity among children and adolescents: A review and synthesis. *Prev. Med.* **2000**, *31*, 54–76. [CrossRef]
2. Verstraete, S.J.; Cardon, G.M.; De Clercq, D.L.; De Bourdeaudhuij, I.M. A comprehensive physical activity promotion programme at elementary school: The effects on physical activity, physical fitness and psychosocial correlates of physical activity. *Public Health Nutr.* **2007**, *10*, 477–484. [CrossRef] [PubMed]
3. Ortega, F.B.; Ruiz, J.R.; Castillo, M.J.; Sjöström, M. Physical fitness in childhood and adolescence: A powerful marker of health. *Int. J. Obes.* **2008**, *32*, 1–11. [CrossRef] [PubMed]

4. Ruiz, J.R.; Castro-Piñero, J.; Artero, E.G.; Ortega, F.B.; Sjöström, M.; Suni, J.; Castillo, M.J. Predictive validity of health-related fitness in youth: A systematic review. *Br. J. Sports Med.* **2009**, *43*, 909–923. [CrossRef]
5. Poitras, V.J.; Gray, C.E.; Borghese, M.M.; Carson, V.; Chaput, J.P.; Janssen, I.; Katzmarzyk, P.T.; Pate, R.R.; Connor Gorber, S.; Kho, M.E.; et al. Systematic review of the relationships between objectively measured physical activity and health indicators in school-aged children and youth. *Appl. Physiol. Nutr. Metab.* **2016**, *41* (Suppl. S3), 197–239. [CrossRef]
6. Wu, X.Y.; Han, L.H.; Zhang, J.H.; Luo, S.; Hu, J.W.; Sun, K. The influence of physical activity, sedentary behavior on health-related quality of life among the general population of children and adolescents: A systematic review. *PLoS ONE* **2017**, *12*, e0187668. [CrossRef]
7. Moeijes, J.; van Busschbach, J.T.; Bosscher, R.J.; Twisk, J.W.R. Sports participation and health-related quality of life: A longitudinal observational study in children. *Qual. Life Res.* **2019**, *28*, 2453–2469. [CrossRef]
8. Masanovic, B.; Gardasevic, J.; Marques, A.; Peralta, M.; Demetriou, Y.; Sturm, D.J.; Popovic, S. Trends in Physical Fitness Among School-Aged Children and Adolescents: A Systematic Review. *Front. Pediatr.* **2020**, *8*, 627529. [CrossRef]
9. Rigby, B.R.; Papadakis, Z.; Bane, A.A.; Park, J.K.; Grandjean, P.W. Cardiorespiratory and biomechanical responses to simulated recreational horseback riding in healthy children. *Res. Q. Exerc. Sport* **2015**, *86*, 63–70. [CrossRef]
10. von Lewinski, M.; Biau, S.; Erber, R.; Ille, N.; Aurich, J.; Faure, J.M.; Aurich, C. Cortisol release, heart rate and heart rate variability in the horse and its rider: Different responses to training and performance. *Vet. J.* **2013**, *197*, 229–232. [CrossRef]
11. Kim, Y.N.; Lee, D.K. Effects of horse-riding exercise on balance, gait, and activities of daily living in stroke patients. *J. Phys. Ther. Sci.* **2015**, *27*, 607–609. [CrossRef] [PubMed]
12. Lee, C.W.; Kim, S.G.; An, B.W. The effects of horseback riding on body mass index and gait in obese women. *J. Phys. Sci.* **2015**, *27*, 1169–1171. [CrossRef] [PubMed]
13. Sung, B.J.; Jeon, S.Y.; Lim, S.R.; Lee, K.E.; Jee, H. Equestrian expertise affecting physical fitness, body compositions, lactate, heart rate and calorie consumption of elite horse riding players. *J. Exerc. Rehabil.* **2015**, *11*, 175–181. [CrossRef] [PubMed]
14. Sainas, G.; Melis, S.; Corona, F.; Loi, A.; Ghiani, G.; Milia, R.; Tocco, F.; Marongiu, E.; Crisafulli, A. Cardio-metabolic responses during horse riding at three different speeds. *Eur. J. Appl. Physiol.* **2016**, *116*, 1985–1992. [CrossRef]
15. Dengel, O.H.; Raymond-Pope, C.J.; Bosch, T.A.; Oliver, J.M.; Dengel, D.R. Body Composition and Visceral Adipose Tissue in Female Collegiate Equestrian Athletes. *Int. J. Sports Med.* **2019**, *40*, 404–408. [CrossRef]
16. Demarie, S.; Galvani, C.; Donatucci, B.; Gianfelici, A. A Pilot Study on Italian Eventing Prospective Olympic Horse Riders: Physiological, Anthropometrical, Functional and Asymmetry Assessment. *Cent. Eur. J. Sport Sci. Med.* **2022**, *37*, 77–88. [CrossRef]
17. Demarie, S.; Galvani, C.; Billat, V.L. Horse-Riding Competitions Pre and Post COVID-19: Effect of Anxiety, sRPE and HR on Performance in Eventing. *Int. J. Environ. Res. Public Health* **2020**, *17*, 8648. [CrossRef]
18. Liu, I.Q. The impact of COVID-19 pandemic on high performance secondary school student-athletes. *Sport J.* **2020**, *41*, 1–11.
19. Fitzgerald, H.T.; Rubin, S.T.; Fitzgerald, D.A.; Rubin, B.K. COVID-19 and the impact on young athletes. *Paediatr. Respir. Rev.* **2021**, *39*, 9–15. [CrossRef]
20. Kelly, A.L.; Erickson, K.; Turnnidge, J. Youth sport in the time of COVID-19: Considerations for researchers and practitioners. *Manag. Sport Leis.* **2022**, *27*, 56–66. [CrossRef]
21. López-Bueno, R.; Calatayud, J.; Andersen, L.L.; Casaña, J.; Ezzatvar, Y.; Casajús, J.A.; López-Sánchez, G.F.; Smith, L. Cardiorespiratory fitness in adolescents before and after the COVID-19 confinement: A prospective cohort study. *Eur. J. Pediatr.* **2021**, *180*, 2287–2293. [CrossRef] [PubMed]
22. Audor González, M.H.; Lerma Castaño, P.R.; Roldán González, E. Effects of Physical Exercise on the Body Composition and Conditional Physical Capacities of School Children During Confinement by COVID-19. *Glob. Pediatr. Health* **2022**, *9*, 2333794X211062440. [CrossRef] [PubMed]
23. Tayech, A.; Mejri, M.A.; Makhlouf, I.; Mathlouthi, A.; Behm, D.G.; Chaouachi, A. Second Wave of COVID-19 Global Pandemic and Athletes' Confinement: Recommendations to Better Manage and Optimize the Modified Lifestyle. *Int. J. Environ. Res. Public Health* **2020**, *17*, 8385. [CrossRef] [PubMed]
24. Council of Europe. *EUROFIT: Handbook for the EUROFIT Tests of Physical Fitness*; Sports Division Strasbourg, Council of Europe Publishing and Documentation Service: Strasbourg, France, 1993.
25. Riso, E.M.; Toplaan, L.; Viira, P.; Vaiksaar, S.; Jürimäe, J. Physical fitness and physical activity of 6–7-year-old children according to weight status and sports participation. *PLoS ONE* **2019**, *14*, 0218901. [CrossRef] [PubMed]
26. Eid, L. *MOTORFIT: Monitoraggio Dello Stato di Benessere Fisico e Motorio Degli Studenti Della Lombardia*; Agenzia Nazionale per lo Sviluppo dell'Autonomia Scolastica: Milan, Italy, 2007.
27. Lee, J.T.; Soboleswki, E.J.; Story, C.E.; Shields, E.W.; Battaglini, C.L. The feasibility of an 8-week, home-based isometric strength-training program for improving dressage test performance in equestrian athletes. *Comp. Exerc. Physiol.* **2015**, *11*, 223–230. [CrossRef]
28. Nuttall, F.Q. Body Mass Index: Obesity, BMI, and Health: A Critical Review. *Nutr. Today* **2015**, *50*, 117–128. [CrossRef]
29. Ruiz, J.R.; Castro-Piñero, J.; España-Romero, V.; Artero, E.G.; Ortega, F.B.; Cuenca, M.M.; Jimenez-Pavón, D.; Chillón, P.; Girela-Rejón, M.J.; Mora, J.; et al. Field-based fitness assessment in young people: The ALPHA health-related fitness test battery for children and adolescents. *Br. J. Sports Med.* **2011**, *45*, 518–524. [CrossRef]
30. Tomkinson, G.R.; Olds, T.S.; Borms, J. Who are the Eurofittest? *Med. Sport Sci.* **2007**, *50*, 104–128. [CrossRef]

31. Smits-Engelsman, B.C.M.; Smit, E.; Doe-Asinyo, R.X.; Lawerteh, S.E.; Aertssen, W.; Ferguson, G.; Jelsma, D.L. Inter-rater reliability and test-retest reliability of the Performance and Fitness (PERF-FIT) test battery for children: A test for motor skill related fitness. *BMC Pediatr.* **2021**, *21*, 119. [CrossRef]
32. Chillón, P.; Castro-Piñero, J.; Ruiz, J.R.; Soto, V.M.; Carbonell-Baeza, A.; Dafos, J.; Vicente-Rodríguez, G.; Castillo, M.J.; Ortega, F.B. Hip flexibility is the main determinant of the back-saver sit-and-reach test in adolescents. *J. Sports Sci.* **2010**, *28*, 641–648. [CrossRef]
33. Tomkinson, G.R.; Carver, K.D.; Atkinson, F.; Daniell, N.D.; Lewis, L.K.; Fitzgerald, J.S.; Lang, J.J.; Ortega, F.B. European normative values for physical fitness in children and adolescents aged 9–17 years: Results from 2,779,165 Eurofit performances representing 30 countries. *Br. J. Sports Med.* **2018**, *52*, 1445–1456. [CrossRef] [PubMed]
34. Groselj, J.; Osredkar, D.; Sember, V.; Pajek, M. Associations between balance and other fundamental motor skills in pre-adolescents. *Med. Dello Sport* **2019**, *72*, 200–215. [CrossRef]
35. Sember, V.; Grošelj, J.; Pajek, M. Balance Tests in Pre-Adolescent Children: Retest Reliability, Construct Validity, and Relative Ability. *Int. J. Environ. Res. Public Health* **2020**, *17*, 5474. [CrossRef] [PubMed]
36. España-Romero, V.; Ortega, F.B.; Vicente-Rodríguez, G.; Artero, E.G.; Rey, J.P.; Ruiz, J.R. Elbow position affects handgrip strength in adolescents: Validity and reliability of Jamar, DynEx, and TKK dynamometers. *J. Strength Cond. Res.* **2010**, *24*, 272–277. [CrossRef] [PubMed]
37. Castro-Piñero, J.; Ortega, F.B.; Artero, E.G.; Girela-Rejón, M.J.; Mora, J.; Sjöström, M.; Ruiz, J.R. Assessing muscular strength in youth: Usefulness of standing long jump as a general index of muscular fitness. *J. Strength Cond. Res.* **2010**, *24*, 1810–1817. [CrossRef] [PubMed]
38. Pinoniemi, B.K.; Tomkinson, G.R.; Walch, T.J.; Roemmich, J.N.; Fitzgerald, J.S. Temporal Trends in the Standing Broad Jump Performance of United States Children and Adolescents. *Res. Q. Exerc. Sport* **2021**, *92*, 71–81. [CrossRef]
39. Esco, M.R.; Olson, M.S.; Williford, H. Relationship of push-ups and sit-ups tests to selected anthropometric variables and performance results: A multiple regression study. *J. Strength Cond. Res.* **2008**, *22*, 1862–1868. [CrossRef]
40. Kaster, T.; Dooley, F.L.; Fitzgerald, J.S.; Walch, T.J.; Annandale, M.; Ferrar, K.; Lang, J.J.; Smith, J.J.; Tomkinson, G.R. Temporal trends in the sit-ups performance of 9,939,289 children and adolescents between 1964 and 2017. *J. Sports Sci.* **2020**, *38*, 1913–1923. [CrossRef]
41. Anselma, M.; Altenburg, T.; Chinapaw, M. Kids in Action: The protocol of a Youth Participatory Action Research project to promote physical activity and dietary behaviour. *BMJ Open* **2019**, *9*, 025584. [CrossRef]
42. Altavilla, G.; D'Elia, F.; D'Isanto, T.; Manna, A. Tests for the evaluation of the improvement of physical fitness and health at the secondary school. *J. Phys. Educ. Sport* **2019**, *19*, 1784–1787. [CrossRef]
43. Calders, P.; Deforche, B.; Verschelde, S.; Bouckaert, J.; Chevalier, F.; Bassle, E.; Tanghe, A.; De Bode, P.; Franckx, H. Predictors of 6-minute walk test and 12-minute walk/run test in obese children and adolescents. *Eur. J. Pediatr.* **2008**, *167*, 563–568. [CrossRef] [PubMed]
44. Abate Daga, F.; Agostino, S.; Peretti, S.; Beratto, L. COVID-19 nationwide lockdown and physical activity profiles among North-western Italian population using the International Physical Activity Questionnaire (IPAQ). *Sport Sci. Health* **2021**, *17*, 459–464. [CrossRef] [PubMed]
45. Powell-Wiley, T.M.; Poirier, P.; Burke, L.E.; Després, J.P.; Gordon-Larsen, P.; Lavie, C.J.; Lear, S.A.; Ndumele, C.E.; Neeland, I.J.; Sanders, P.; et al. Obesity and cardiovascular disease: A scientific statement from the American Heart Association. *Circulation* **2021**, *143*, 984–1010. [CrossRef] [PubMed]
46. Brooks, S.K.; Webster, R.K.; Smith, L.E.; Woodland, L.; Wessely, S.; Greenberg, N.; Rubin, G.J. The psychological impact of quarantine and how to reduce it: Rapid review of the evidence. *Lancet* **2020**, *395*, 912–920. [CrossRef]
47. Gualano, M.R.; Lo Moro, G.; Voglino, G.; Bert, F.; Siliquini, R. Effects of COVID-19 Lockdown on Mental Health and Sleep Disturbances in Italy. *Int. J. Environ. Res. Public Health* **2020**, *17*, 4779. [CrossRef]
48. Stokes, K.A.; Jones, B.; Bennett, M.; Close, G.L.; Gill, N.; Hull, J.H.; Kasper, A.M.; Kemp, S.; Mellalieu, S.D.; Peirce, N.; et al. Returning to Play after Prolonged Training Restrictions in Professional Collision Sports. *Int. J. Sports Med.* **2020**, *41*, 895–911. [CrossRef]
49. Trotter, M.A.; Endler, N.S. An empirical test of the interaction model of anxiety in a competitive equestrian setting. *Personal. Individ. Differ.* **1999**, *27*, 861–875. [CrossRef]
50. Wolframm, I.A.; Micklewright, D. Effects of trait anxiety and direction of pre-competitive arousal on performance in the equestrian disciplines of dressage, showjumping and eventing. *Comp. Exerc. Physiol.* **2010**, *7*, 185–191. [CrossRef]
51. Wolframm, I.A.; Micklewright, D. Pre-competitive arousal, perception of equine temperament and riding performance: Do they interact? *Comp. Exerc. Physiol.* **2010**, *7*, 27. [CrossRef]
52. Dragoni, S. Sport Equestri. *Med. Dello Sport* **2002**, *55*, 313–324.
53. Johnson, U.; Ivarsson, A. Psychological predictors of sport injuries among junior soccer players. *Scand. J. Med. Sci. Sports* **2011**, *21*, 129–136. [CrossRef] [PubMed]
54. Trinh, L.N.; Brown, S.M.; Mulcahey, M.K. The Influence of Psychological Factors on the Incidence and Severity of Sports-Related Concussions: A Systematic Review. *Am. J. Sports Med.* **2020**, *48*, 1516–1525. [CrossRef] [PubMed]

55. Sarto, F.; Impellizzeri, F.M.; Spörri, J.; Porcelli, S.; Olmo, J.; Requena, B.; Suarez-Arrones, L.; Arundale, A.; Bilsborough, J.; Buchheit, M.; et al. Impact of Potential Physiological Changes due to COVID-19 Home Confinement on Athlete Health Protection in Elite Sports: A Call for Awareness in Sports Programming. *Sports Med.* **2020**, *50*, 1417–1419. [CrossRef] [PubMed]
56. Demarie, S.; Minganti, C.; Piacentini, M.F.; Parisi, A.; Cerulli, C.; Magini, V. Reducing anxiety in novel horse riders by a mechanical horse simulator. *Med. Sport* **2013**, *66*, 179–188.
57. Baillet, H.; Thouvarecq, R.; Vérin, E.; Tourny, C.; Benguigui, N.; Komar, J.; Leroy, D. Human Energy Expenditure and Postural Coordination on the Mechanical Horse. *J. Mot. Behav.* **2017**, *49*, 441–457. [CrossRef]
58. Baek, I.H.; Kim, B.J. The effects of horse riding simulation training on stroke patients' balance ability and abdominal muscle thickness changes. *J. Phys. Ther. Sci.* **2014**, *26*, 1293–1296. [CrossRef]
59. Yu, C.H.; Hong, C.U.; Kang, S.R.; Kwon, T.K. Analysis of basal physical fitness and lumbar muscle function according to indoor horse riding exercise. *Biomed. Mater. Eng.* **2014**, *24*, 2395–2405. [CrossRef]
60. Devienne, M.F.; Guezennec, C.Y. Energy expenditure of horse riding. *Eur. J. Appl. Physiol.* **2000**, *82*, 499–503. [CrossRef]
61. Meyers, M.C. Effect of equitation training on health and physical fitness of college females. *Eur. J. Appl. Physiol.* **2006**, *98*, 177–184. [CrossRef]
62. Roberts, M.; Shearman, J.; Marlin, D. A comparison of the metabolic cost of the three phases of the one-day event in female collegiate riders. *Comp. Exerc. Physiol.* **2009**, *6*, 129–135. [CrossRef]
63. Hobbs, S.J.; Baxter, J.; Broom, L.; Rossell, L.A.; Sinclair, J.; Clayton, H.M. Posture, flexibility and grip strength in horse riders. *J. Hum. Kinet.* **2014**, *42*, 113–125. [CrossRef] [PubMed]
64. Beale, L.; Maxwell, N.S.; Gibson, O.R.; Twomey, R.; Taylor, B.; Church, A. Oxygen Cost of Recreational Horse-Riding in Females. *J. Phys. Act. Health* **2015**, *12*, 808–813. [CrossRef] [PubMed]
65. O'Reilly, C.; Zoller, J.; Sigler, D.; Vogelsang, M.; Sawyer, J.; Fluckey, J. Rider Energy Expenditure During High Intensity Horse Activity. *J. Equine Vet. Sci.* **2021**, *102*, 103463. [CrossRef] [PubMed]
66. Bland, V.L.; Bea, J.W.; Roe, D.J.; Lee, V.R.; Blew, R.M.; Going, S.B. Physical activity, sedentary time, and longitudinal bone strength in adolescent girls. *Osteoporos. Int.* **2020**, *31*, 1943–1954. [CrossRef]
67. Steene-Johannessen, J.; Hansen, B.H.; Dalene, K.E.; Kolle, E.; Northstone, K.; Møller, N.C.; Grøntved, A.; Wedderkopp, N.; Kriemler, S.; Page, A.S.; et al. Variations in accelerometry measured physical activity and sedentary time across Europe—Harmonized analyses of 47,497 children and adolescents. *Int. J. Behav. Nutr. Phys. Act.* **2020**, *17*, 38. [CrossRef]

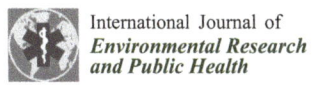

Article

Factors Influencing Use of Fitness Apps by Adults under Influence of COVID-19

Yanlong Guo [1,2,*], Xueqing Ma [1], Denghang Chen [3,4,*] and Han Zhang [5]

[1] Social Innovation Design Research Centre, Anhui University, Hefei 203106, China
[2] Anhui Institute of Contemporary Studies, Anhui Academy of Social Sciences, Hefei 203106, China
[3] Department of Science and Technology Communication, University of Science and Technology of China, Hefei 203106, China
[4] Research Center for Science Communication, Chinese Academy of Sciences, Hefei 203106, China
[5] College of Environmental Science and Engineering, Ocean University of China, Qingdao 266100, China
* Correspondence: 20106@ahu.edu.cn (Y.G.); hahn1122@mail.ustc.edu.cn (D.C.); Tel.: +86-15256556306 (Y.G.)

Abstract: During the coronavirus disease 2019 (COVID-19) pandemic, many countries imposed restrictions and quarantines on the population, which led to a decrease in people's physical activity (PA) and severely damaged their mental health. As a result, people engaged in fitness activities with the help of fitness apps, which improved their resistance to the virus and reduced the occurrence of psychological problems, such as anxiety and depression. However, the churn rate of fitness apps is high. As such, our purpose in this study was to analyze the factors that influence the use of fitness apps by adults aged 18–65 years in the context of COVID-19, with the aim of contributing to the analysis of mobile fitness user behavior and related product design practices. We constructed a decision target program model using the analytic hierarchy process (AHP), and we analyzed and inductively screened 11 evaluation indicators, which we combined with an indicator design questionnaire. We distributed 420 questionnaires; of the respondents, 347 knew about or used fitness apps. Among these 347, we recovered 310 valid questionnaires after removing invalid questionnaires with a short completion time, for an effective questionnaire recovery rate of 89.33%. We used the AHP and entropy method to calculate and evaluate the weight coefficient of each influencing factor and to determine an influencing factor index. Our conclusions were as follows: first, the effect of perceived usefulness on the use of fitness apps by the study groups was the most notable. Second, personal motivation and perceived ease of use considerably influenced the adult group's willingness to use fitness apps. Finally, the perceived cost had relatively little effect on the use of fitness apps by adults, and the study group was much more concerned with the privacy cost than the expense cost.

Keywords: COVID-19; adult group; fitness APP; influencing factors

Citation: Guo, Y.; Ma, X.; Chen, D.; Zhang, H. Factors Influencing Use of Fitness Apps by Adults under Influence of COVID-19. *Int. J. Environ. Res. Public Health* **2022**, *19*, 15460. https://doi.org/10.3390/ijerph192315460

Academic Editors: Clemens Drenowatz and Klaus Greier

Received: 31 October 2022
Accepted: 19 November 2022
Published: 22 November 2022

Publisher's Note: MDPI stays neutral with regard to jurisdictional claims in published maps and institutional affiliations.

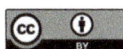

Copyright: © 2022 by the authors. Licensee MDPI, Basel, Switzerland. This article is an open access article distributed under the terms and conditions of the Creative Commons Attribution (CC BY) license (https://creativecommons.org/licenses/by/4.0/).

1. Introduction

The COVID-19 pandemic has hugely impacted people's ways of living, intellectual health, and quality of life worldwide [1]. The imposition of lockdown and quarantine measures on populations has been used to restrict the spread of COVID-19, but such measures have also had many serious consequences [2]. According to the results of multicountry surveys, measures such as restraint and seclusion have negatively impacted social participation, lifestyle pleasure, mental health, psychosocial and emotional disorders, sleep quality, and employment status [3–5]. Some authorities announced a stoppage of all services and activities except for a few basic services, which led to necessary adjustments in the lifestyles of the affected populations, which severely damaged their mental health. This was manifested by increased stress in the general population and an increase in the number of depressions [6,7]. These abrupt modifications in people's lives included, among others, physical activity and exercise. Ammer et al. stated that home confinement during

COVID-19 led to a reduction in physical activity (PA) and an increase of approximately 28% in the time spent sitting each day [8].

How humans coped and found approaches to being physically healthy in the face of pandemic-related restrictions (home isolation and closed gyms, parks, and gymnasiums) needs to be understood. Through health apps, users changed their traditional method of engaging in fitness imposed by time and geographical barriers and could choose to exercise anytime and anywhere, record their physical condition, and more flexibly control their exercise. People's intention to use fitness apps has substantially increased. However, the churn rate of these apps is high, with over 45% of customers stopping after the novelty wears off, so an in-depth perception of consumer motivation and the elements influencing the use of health apps is required [9,10]. To gain insight into these issues, in this study, we collected user data using a questionnaire and constructed a decision-goal scenario model based on TAM through the analytic hierarchy process (AHP). The questionnaire included questions about the user's basic information and what factors affected their use of fitness apps. We analyzed the user data to assess the factors that affected their continued use of fitness apps. Next, we reviewed the literature on the impact of the pandemic on physical health and described the factors influencing the use of fitness apps, and then presented the details of our analysis and the final findings.

2. Literature Review

Sports and physical exercise play a vital role in the physical and intellectual health of an individual [11]. The U.S. Physical Activity Guidelines suggest that all adults, even those with chronic conditions, should engage in at least 150 to 300 min of moderate-intensity exercise per week if they are capable [12]. Haider stated that decreased PA levels may negatively affect fitness and can be related to an increase in nervousness and despair [13]. The findings of a study in Austria showed an increase in the duration of predominant depressive signs and symptoms from 3% to 6% between pre- and post-pandemic [14]. Harleen et al. conducted semi-structured smartphone interviews in 2020 with 22 adults who had usually exercised at a fitness center before the COVID-19 pandemic but who stayed at home at some point during the countrywide lockdown. The results of the analysis showed that participants' situational perceptions at some stage during the lockdown were extremely negative, and they lacked the motivation to exercise at a gym. They exhibited mental health concerns and an over-reliance on social media. However, performing general health exercises indoors during lockdown remarkably helped them to overcome their psychological problems and fitness issues [15].

While experiencing a forced adaptation to new norms of maintaining social distancing, health apps can assist humans to manipulate a change in their dietary intake, engaging in both healthy and bodily activity, and promoting a wholesome lifestyle [16]. Based on the above advantages, humans from all groups seized the opportunities provided by the commercial online health industry, which vigorously improved their offerings of online fitness. This situation actively promoted the digital reform of the ordinary health industry. The Talking Data 2014 Mobile Internet Data Report showed that the number of users of mobile health management on both iOS and Android platforms reached 120 million, which was an increase of 113.4% from January to December 2014, and the growth rate was increasing. Users of apps such as Goudong and Le Power Running have exceeded 10 million in number, and the number of downloads of Nike Training and Super Diet King has increased by more than 300%. Sports and fitness apps have a wide range of people using them. In addition, the use of sports and health apps to assist in guiding exercise will change traditional sports and fitness methods, creating a shift in digital and scientific fitness.

In the context of the rapid development of mobile fitness apps, many scholars have focused on the factors influencing their use, engaging in theoretical research and practical studies. When studying the factors influencing college students' fitness app use, Yi considered fitness motivation, leisure, entertainment motivation, and structure rationality hardware requirements as antecedent variables of the perceived ease of use (PEOU) and perceived usefulness (PU) based on the technology acceptance model (TAM). Yi considered the perceived value variables as direct elements influencing university students' mindset toward health app use [17]. The empirical findings showed that PEOU, PU, and perceived price positively affected college students' attitudes toward using mobile fitness apps. PEOU was positively influenced by the ease of operation experienced when using the health software program and the rationality of the health software program design, whereas perceived price was influenced by cellular hardware requirement, the cost of the software program, and the value obtained in the course of its use. The factors that positively influenced PU were, in descending order, fitness motivation, PEOU, motivation to acquire fitness knowledge, perceived cost, and motivation to record fitness activities [18]. Cui investigated the willingness to use mHealth programs based on the technology readiness and acceptance model (TRAM) and extended the model by introducing health awareness. The constructed model was tested by surveying 639 mobile fitness app users and potential users using AMOS 22.0. The test results showed that optimism, revolutionary spirit, and health perception were necessary antecedent variables for the PEOU and PU of cell phone health apps, which indirectly influenced the intention to use. PU and usage mindset directly influenced cell phone health app users' intention to use them [19–22]. Ardion et al. conducted a technology acceptance model (TAM) test considering trust, social influence, and health valuation on 476 German fitness app users, examining the factors influencing the German users' intentions to continue using specific fitness software. The outcomes of the structural equation modeling showed that the respondents' intention to use a particular health app was primarily based on three factors: PEOU, PU, and prohibitive social norms [23].

In summary, in the context of the COVID-19 pandemic, country-wide fitness awareness has increased, and mobile phone fitness app use has become a commonly accepted new form of exercise [24]. Nowadays, the user and industry scales of mobile fitness apps are rapidly growing, and the mobile fitness industry has broad market prospects and is now an emerging area of general interest in the industry. In this context, we selected fitness apps as the research object and analyzed which factors affected the use of fitness apps through theoretical analysis and empirical testing. Our results benefit the analysis of mobile fitness user behavior and related product design practices.

3. Research Methodology

In this study, we first reviewed a large amount of the literature to determine the content of the study. We then summarized the relevant literature about the theoretical knowledge of technology acceptance, perceived cost, and self-determination theory and analyzed the relationship between them. Next, we selected reasonable judgment indicators to provide a theoretical basis for the subsequent study [25]. In determining the study population, according to the 2021 United Nations World Health Organization, the classification of age groups placed those aged 0–17, 18–65, 66–79, 80–99, and 100 years or more into the categories of minors, adults, middle-aged people, elderly people, and long-lived people, respectively. Among them, those who should pay the most attention to physical exercise and have a strong ability to make independent choices are adults aged 18–65 years. Therefore, in this study, we distributed a questionnaire to the study group and collected the data from the questionnaires. We screened the initially recovered data and then used SPSSAU for reliability and validity analysis. Finally, we used two assignment methods, AHP, and entropy weighting, to derive the comprehensive weighting results and analyze the relevant indicators affecting the weighting of the use of fitness apps by adults under 65 years old [26].

3.1. Hierarchical Analysis and Entropy Method

We needed to analyze the factors affecting the use of fitness apps by adults from multiple dimensions, and we selected the AHP method, which is used to combine the qualitative and quantitative aspects of multi-objective complex problems to calculate the decision weights and use the experience of decision makers to judge the relative importance of the weights between the criteria of whether each measurement goal can be achieved. The entropy weighting method is combined with the resynthesis of indicator weights to assign values, and the use of comprehensive weights makes the results more scientific, fair, and persuasive.

3.2. Indicator Construction

In our analysis of the factors influencing the use of fitness apps by adults aged 18–65 years, we needed to consider the current pandemic and policy guidance, the characteristics of health app use, and the relevant research results to build a scientific and reasonable indicator system. A wide range of elements may influence health app use: they may be multilevel, multifactor, and multi-indicator. For evaluation index selection, by collecting the opinions of relevant experts and designers, our final hierarchy of the fitness app-use influencing factors included one target layer, four guideline layers, and eleven program layers.

3.2.1. Establishing Guideline Level Indicators

The technology acceptance model (TAM), proposed by Davis et al. in 1989, is one of the most influential theories in the field of information systems research. In the preliminary TAM, PU, and PEOU are the elements that directly impact the usage attitude and user behavior through attitude intention [27]. Davis et al. reported that PEOU refers to the effort customers perceive as being required to operate a new technology; PU refers to how many customers accept as true that the technological device will enhance their overall work performance [27]. Karah anna et al. demonstrated that PEOU and PU affect the users' use behavior, and PEOU additionally impacts PU [28]. Bildad et al. found that the ease of using Internet technology plays a key role in improving user faith in software builders [29]. Therefore, in the specific construction of the corresponding indicators, we used PEOU (B1) and PU (B2) [30,31].

Despite the broad applicability of the TAM (Figure 1), the model can be modified by adding external premises and theoretically sound elements, which can expand the predictive power of the model [32]. The self-determination principle has been widely used to help encourage physical activity in individuals, and intrinsic motivation represents an archetype of independent activity, where people are motivated by intrinsic motivation and are free to engage in activities independent of external factors [33–35]. According to self-determination theory, consumer motivation (the reason why a person engages in an activity) and consumer-aim (the purpose for this activity) is intently associated [36]. In the field of advertising and customer behavior studies, researchers typically agree that customers perceive the cost as a necessary factor influencing purchase decisions: and the greater the perceived cost-utility of a product, the greater the motivation to buy it [37]. Regarding the elements affecting the perceived value, most researchers have considered the antecedent variables of the perceived cost for empirical analysis. Perceived immediate use advantages (i.e., perceived gains) and perceived sacrifices (i.e., perceived losses) are the antecedent variables of perceived cost [38]. Some scholars have also used factors such as perceived risk, cost of purchase, quality of service, and the quality of the product as antecedent variables affecting the consumers' perceived value (Wood and Scheer, 1996; Zhong, K., 2013) [39]. Regarding the elements impacting the customer's perceived value, we introduced two achievable variables to the technology acceptance model: perceived cost (B3) and personal motivation (B4) [40].

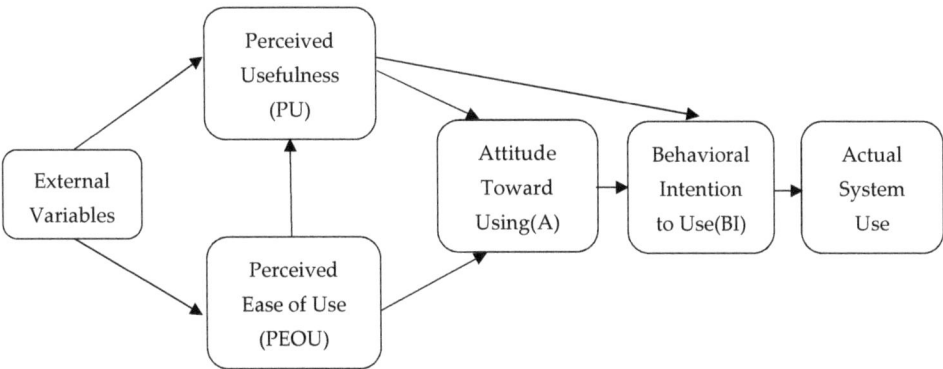

Figure 1. Technology acceptance model.

3.2.2. Determination of Program-Level Indicators

We analyzed and inductively screened 11 evaluation indicators from H1 to H11 according to the detailed division of the elements used for evaluating the first-level indicators (Table 1). To measure indicator B1 (PU), we used the scale developed by Yang et al. to set three measurement indicators: content adaptability (H1), content relevance (H2), and content quality (H3) [41]. To measure indicator B2 (PEOU), we used the scale developed by Gong et al.: the technology level (H4), interaction effectiveness (H5), and system compatibility (H6) [42–45]. For B3, the perceived value indicator, we measured the financial cost (H7) and privacy cost (H8) based totally on the evaluation by San et al., who focused on the effects of the perceived advantages and perceived dangers of people's transactional conduct [46–48]. To measure B4 (personal motivation indicator), we applied the scale developed by Park et al. and set three measures: health concerns (H9), outcome expectations (H10), and social influence (H11) [49–51].

Table 1. Index system used for analyzing factors influencing use of fitness apps by adults aged 18–65 years.

Target Layer	Guideline Layer	Program Level	References
A: Study factors influencing use of fitness app by adults under influence of COVID-19	B1: Perceived usefulness	H1: Content Adaptation H2: Content Targeting H3: Content Quality	Davis et al. (1989) [27] Karahanna et al. (1999) [28] Beldad et al. (2010) [29]
	B2: Perceived ease of use	H4: Technical Grade H5: Interaction Effectiveness H6: System Compatibility	Davis et al. (1989) [27] Chang et al. (2021) [31]
	B3: Perceived cost	H7: Financial Cost H8: Privacy Cost	Kwon et al. (2022) [47] Wang et al. (2022) [51] Park et al. (2018) [49]
	B4: Personal motivation	H9: Health Concerns H10: Outcome Expectations H11: Social Impact	Park et al. (2018) [49]

3.3. Questionnaire Design

Based on the literature review of the effect of the pandemic and health apps, we chose eleven attributes to examine the factors influencing the use of health apps amongst adults aged 18–65 years to determine the impact of COVID-19. We assessed these 11 attributes with a questionnaire (Table 2). We built the questionnaire with Questionnaire Star, and the first question required respondents to have used health apps or to have some knowledge of health apps. The questions could be answered on a scale, and every question consisted of a set of statements. Each statement had nine responses, ranging from 1 to 9 according to the evaluation of the degree of the effect, ranging from very unimportant to very important. The questionnaire included basic information (sex, age, education level, and whether they had used or known about fitness apps) and the evaluation of the importance of relevant factors influencing their use.

Table 2. Description of index conversion questionnaire.

Program-Level Indicator	Problem Description
H1: Content Adaptation	Fitness app can provide different exercise categories of fitness programs for you
H2: Content Targeting	Fitness app can meet your individual needs
H3: Content Quality	Fitness app can provide scientific and professional fitness guidance for you
H4: Technical Grade	Fitness app can be quickly opened on different types of devices
H5: Interaction Effectiveness	Fitness app interface design is clear, convenient, and easy for you to use
H6: System Compatibility	Fitness app can share data with all kinds of your wearable devices
H7: Financial Cost	Fitness app can save you money
H8: Privacy Cost	Fitness app can protect your personal privacy
H9: Health Concerns	Fitness apps can ease your health worries
H10: Outcome Expectations	Fitness app can achieve your expected results
H11: Social Impact	Fitness app has a high social impact on you

4. Statistics and Analysis

We distributed 420 questionnaires using Questionnaire Star to adults aged 18–65 years. The first part of the questionnaire asked the respondents whether they know about or have used a fitness app; if they responded yes, they continued to the second part containing influencing factor questions; if they responded no, the questionnaire ended. According to the data collected from the questionnaires, 347 out of 420 people had knowledge of or had used a fitness app. Among the 347 questionnaires, those with a shorter filling time and multiple scores of the same response were considered invalid questionnaires and deleted. Of the 347 questionnaires, 310 were valid, with an effective rate of 89.33%. Among them, men and women accounted for 50.32% and 49.68%, respectively, of the respondents, with most being 18–30 years old, followed by 31–40 years old (Table 3). Subsequently, we performed frequency analysis and AHP on the 310-sample data to derive the weight values for each index and perform the consistency test.

Table 3. Basic information of the questionnaire respondents.

Variable	Options	Frequency	Percentage (%)
Sex	Male	156	50.323
	Female	154	49.677
Age group (years)	18~30	225	72.581
	31~40	51	16.452
	Under 18	15	4.839
	41~50	12	3.871
	Over 50	7	2.258
Total		310	100.000

4.1. Confidence and Validity Analysis

Reliability research methods are often used when analyzing research projects to test whether they are reasonable and meaningful (Table 4). Validity analysis is performed using factor analysis methods to verify the validity level of the data with KMO values of commonality, variance explained values, factor loading coefficient values, and other indicators. KMO values are used to select the suitability of the fact extraction, and commonality values are used to eliminate unreasonable items (Table 5).

Table 4. Cronbach reliability analysis.

Cronbach's α	Standardized Cronbach's α	Number of Items	Number of Samples
0.917	0.918	11	310

Table 5. KMO and Bartlett test results.

	KMO Value	0.926
Bartlett's sphericity test	Approximate cardinality	1857.364
	df	55.000
	P	0.000 ***

Note: *** represents a significance level of 1%.

4.1.1. Questionnaire Reliability Test

The reliability coefficient, Cronbach's alpha, is used to measure the internal consistency or reliability of an instrument or questionnaire. This coefficient is often used for questionnaires developed using multiple Likert scales to determine whether the scale is reliable. We used Cronbach's alpha to determine the reliability using SPSSAU, resulting in a Cronbach's alpha value of 0.917 (Table 4), which indicated the good reliability and high internal consistency of this questionnaire for additional analysis.

4.1.2. Questionnaire Validity Test

Validity testing involves the measurement of the validity of the questionnaire research data: whether the results obtained through the questionnaire are true and whether the respondents' evaluations are objective. For questionnaire validity tests, structural validity is used, and the results reflect the accuracy of the questionnaire items. Structural validity reflects the relationship between the questionnaire measurement results and the measured items. The two indicators of structural validity are the KMO and Bartlett's sphericity test. The coefficients of the KMO range from 0 to 1; the closer the coefficient is to one, the higher the validity of the questionnaire. Bartlett's sphericity test result needs to be less than 0.01. We imported the questionnaire into SPSSAU for analysis, finding a KMO value of 0.926 and Bartlett's sphericity test result of 0.000, which indicated that the structural validity of the questionnaire was excellent and all the factors had a strong correlation (Table 5). According to Bartlett's sphericity check, the significance of this check is infinitely close to zero. Therefore, the questionnaire has appropriate validity and meets the conditions of applicability for factor analysis.

4.2. Determination of Index System Weights Based on Hierarchical Analysis

4.2.1. Establishing Comparison Judgment Matrix

Based on the evaluation scales in the AHP, the elements in the product hierarchy model are compared and assigned. To use mathematical methods for data processing, the data needs to be transformed into a matrix to quantify the results and determine the importance of the design elements. Supposing n influencing elements, b_1 ..., b_i ..., b_j ..., b_n, the project elements are compared with each other in pairs and transformed into a judgment matrix as follows:

$$B = \begin{bmatrix} 1 \cdots b_{1i} \cdots b_{1j} \cdots b_{1n} \\ b_{i1} \cdots 1 \cdots b_{ij} \cdots b_{in} \\ b_{j1} \cdots b_{ji} \cdots 1 \cdots b_{jn} \\ b_{nl} \cdots b_{ni} \cdots b_{nj} \cdots 1 \end{bmatrix} = (b_{ij})_{nxn} \quad (1)$$

The Perron–Fresenius theorem shows that matrix B has a unique nonzero eigenroot, i.e., the largest eigenroot (λ_{max}) corresponds to the eigenvector (w).

$$Bw = \lambda_{max} w \quad (2)$$

The specific steps for calculating the feature vectors using the sum-product method are as follows:

Normalize the data in b by column.

$$\overline{b_{ij}} = b_{ij} / \sum_{j=1}^{n} \overline{b_{ij}}(i,j,\ldots,n) \tag{3}$$

Sum the normalized matrix peers.

$$\widetilde{w}_i = \sum_{j=1}^{n} \overline{b_{ij}}(i=1,2,\ldots,n) \tag{4}$$

Divide the summed vector by n to obtain the weight vector.

$$\widetilde{w}_i = \widetilde{w}_i / n \tag{5}$$

Find the maximum characteristic root.

$$\lambda_{max} = \frac{1}{n}\sum_{i=1}^{n} \frac{n}{i=1} \frac{(B_w)_i}{w_i} \tag{6}$$

where $(B_w)_i$ denotes its component of the vector B_w.

Based on the above Equations (1)–(6), we calculated the weight values of the designed element objectives at the criterion and program levels and then ranked them in terms of importance to complete the decision on the influencing factors.

4.2.2. Calculating Weight Coefficients

Because the hierarchical structure model we constructed had more elements at the program level and the generated judgment matrix order was greater than nine, we used a combination of the AHP and entropy methods for data processing. We formed the evaluation indexes by decomposing the problem and comparing the judgment. We calculated the weightings to obtain the comprehensive weight values of the elements at the program level. We first calculated the AHP-based weight.

Check the consistency of matrix B. Calculate:

$$CR = CI/RI \tag{7}$$

where CI is the consistency index; CR is the consistency ratio; and RI is the common random consistency index.

$$CI = (\lambda_{max} - n)/(n-1) \tag{8}$$

From Equation (8), CR can be calculated. CR < 0.1 indicates that the calculation of matrix B is qualified and valid. If CR > 0.1, the matrix needs to be corrected [52].

Based on the above-mentioned ideas, we constructed the judgment matrix and calculated the weights of the impact factor (Tables 6–10).

From the outcomes in Tables 6–10, we found that the CR values of the judgment matrices were all <0.1, so we skipped the consistency test. From this, we calculated the weighting for the program-level elements to obtain the comprehensive weight values of the program-level elements (Table 11).

Table 6. Target layer judgment matrix and weight value of influencing factor.

A	B1	B2	B3	B4	w_i	λ_{max}	CI	CR
B1	1	0.990	0.972	1.005	0.2709			
B2	1.010	1	0.982	1.016	0.2737	4.000	0.000	0.000
B3	1.029	1.019	1	1.035	0.1858			
B4	0.995	0.984	0.967	1	0.2695			

Table 7. PU judgment matrix and weight values.

B1	H1	H2	H3	w_i	λ_{max}	CI	CR
H1	1	0.987	0.962	0.3276			
H2	1.013	1	0.974	0.3318	3.000	0.000	0.000
H3	1.040	1.027	1	0.3407			

Table 8. PEOU judgment matrix and weight values.

B2	H4	H5	H6	w_i	λ_{max}	CI	CR
H4	1	0.979	0.989	0.3297			
H5	1.022	1	1.010	0.3369	3.000	0.000	0.000
H6	1.012	0.990	1	0.3334			

Table 9. Perceived cost judgment matrix and weight values.

B3	H7	H8	w_i	λ_{max}	CI	CR
H7	1	0.970	0.4924	2.000	0.000	0.000
H8	1.031	1	0.5076			

Table 10. Personal motivation judgment matrix and weight values.

B4	H9	H10	H11	w_i	λ_{max}	CI	CR
H9	1	0.991	1.074	0.3401			
H10	1.009	1	1.083	0.3431	3.000	0.000	0.000
H11	0.932	0.923	1	0.3168			

Table 11. Comprehensive weight values of criterion-layer elements.

Guideline Layer	Guideline-Layer Weights	Program Level	Program-Level Weights
B1	0.2709	H1	0.0888
		H2	0.0899
		H3	0.0922
B2	0.2737	H4	0.0902
		H5	0.0922
		H6	0.0913
B3	0.1858	H7	0.0915
		H8	0.0943
B4	0.2695	H9	0.0917
		H10	0.0924
		H11	0.0854

4.2.3. Consistency Test

We performed consistency tests on the combined weight values of all the design elements in Table 11, and the operational procedure and results are shown:

$$CI = \sum_{j=1}^{m} b_j CI_j = (0.000\ 0.000\ 0.000\ 0.000) \begin{pmatrix} 0.2667 \\ 0.2759 \\ 0.1909 \\ 0.2663 \end{pmatrix} = 0 \quad (9)$$

$$CR = CI/RI = 0 \div 1.520 = 0 < 0.1 \quad (10)$$

Based on Equations (9) and (10), CR = 0 < 0.1. The hierarchical total ranking of matrix B was consistent with the consistency test principle, and we found that the calculations of the comprehensive weight values of the scheme-level elements in Table 9 were scientific and reasonable and so could effectively guide the practical analysis [53].

4.3. Entropy Method Weights

The entropy approach is a goal-undertaking method, and the weights determined with this method are more accurate than those obtained with the subjective challenge method. Entropy is a measure of the disorder of a system, and by measuring the degree of disorder in the variables, the weights of indicator variables can be obtained by comparing the amount of information possessed by the variables. However, the method is prone to imbalanced weights due to the large dispersion of a certain indicator.

In the entropy weight approach, the entropy weight of the index is first calculated by applying the record's entropy after standardizing the authentic data. The rank of item X, when the index is positive, is standardized with the following system.

$$Y_{ij} = \frac{X_{ij} - X_{i_{min}}}{X_{i_{max}} - X_{i_{min}}} \quad (11)$$

When the indicator is negative, its normalization treatment formula is:

$$Y_{ij} = \frac{X_{i_{max}} - X_{ij}}{X_{i_{max}} - X_{i_{min}}} \quad (12)$$

where $X_{i_{max}}$ and $X_{i_{min}}$ are the maximum and minimum values of the indices, respectively; Y_{ij} is the normalized result setting of the first impact factor affecting prevention and control. For a certain impact factor j, its information entropy calculation formula E_j is:

$$E_j = -\frac{1}{\ln m} \sum_{i=1}^{m} P_{ij} \ln P_{ij} \quad (13)$$

$$P_{ij} = \frac{Y_{ij}}{\sum_{i=1}^{m} Y_{ij}} \quad (14)$$

where P_{ij} is the proportion of the standardized value and Y_{ij} is the total standardized value. If the information entropy E_j of the factor influencing prevention and control is smaller, the degree of variability in the factor is smaller, the sample data are more orderly, the differentiation ability of the evaluation object is larger, and the information utility value provided by the factor is larger. The stronger the influence on border prevention and control, the higher the weight; conversely, the larger the information entropy E, the larger the degree of variability is for the influence factor, and the information utility value provided by the factor and the weight is smaller.

According to the calculated information entropy of each factor, $E_1, E_2, \cdots, E_k$, the weight formula W_j for each factor can be calculated as follows:

$$W_j = \frac{1 - E_j}{k - \sum_{j=1}^{k} E_j} \quad (15)$$

Based on Equations (11)–(15), we calculated the weights of each index (Tables 12 and 13).

Table 12. Weight results of each criterion layer based on entropy method.

Guideline Layer	Information Entropy Value E_j	Information Utility Value	Weighting Factor w_j
B1	0.9963	0.0037	0.2576
B2	0.9966	0.0034	0.2329
B3	0.9961	0.0039	0.2671
B4	0.9965	0.0035	0.2425

Table 13. Weight results of each index based on entropy method.

Guideline Layer	Information Entropy Value E_j	Information Utility Value	Weighting Factor w_j
H1	0.9946	0.0054	0.0968
H2	0.9951	0.0049	0.0882
H3	0.9957	0.0043	0.0782
H4	0.9952	0.0048	0.0861
H5	0.9951	0.0049	0.0885
H6	0.9952	0.0048	0.0861
H7	0.9953	0.0047	0.0851
H8	0.9947	0.0053	0.0962
H9	0.9952	0.0048	0.0857
H10	0.9953	0.0047	0.0846
H11	0.9931	0.0069	0.1244

4.4. Integrated Weight Calculation

In this study, based totally on the reliability and availability of the data, we used two strategies (subjective and goal weight replication) to resynthesize and assign the weights of the influencing factors affecting the use of health apps by adults. We continuously revised the influencing elements. The results indicated a large difference in the weighting of the indicators using the two methods, especially in the process of determining the weighted values of indicators H11 and H3. This difference was due to the difference between the weights calculated by the mathematical model and our understanding of the application of the indicators in practice, which led to the difference in the weight coefficients. Our finding also further confirmed the necessity of studying the assignment of subjective and objective integrated weights.

Based on the results of assigning weights to the indicators by the above two methods, we calculated the combined weight C_j:

$$C_j = \frac{w_i w_j}{\sum_{i=1}^{n} w_i w_j} \tag{16}$$

where w_i and w_j represent the weights of the evaluation indexes calculated by the hierarchical analysis and entropy value method, respectively. We synthesized and calculated the results of both the subjective and objective assignments (Tables 14 and 15).

Table 14. Comprehensive weight results (criterion layer) obtained using two weighting methods.

Guideline Layer	Hierarchical Analysis Weight w_i	Entropy Method Weight w_j	Combined Weight C_j
B1	0.2709	0.2576	0.2808
B2	0.2737	0.2329	0.2565
B3	0.1858	0.2671	0.1997
B4	0.2695	0.2425	0.2630

Table 15. Comprehensive weight results (scheme layer) obtained by two weighting methods.

Indicator	Hierarchical Analysis Weight w_i	Entropy Method Weight w_j	Combined Weight C_j
H1	0.0888	0.0968	0.0948
H2	0.0899	0.0882	0.0874
H3	0.0922	0.0782	0.0795
H4	0.0902	0.0861	0.0857
H5	0.0922	0.0885	0.0900

Table 15. Cont.

Indicator	Hierarchical Analysis Weight w_i	Entropy Method Weight w_j	Combined Weight C_j
H6	0.0913	0.0861	0.0867
H7	0.0915	0.0851	0.0859
H8	0.0943	0.0962	0.1000
H9	0.0917	0.0857	0.0867
H10	0.0924	0.0846	0.0862
H11	0.0854	0.1244	0.1172

4.5. Data Analysis

The weightings of B1 (PU), B2 (PEOU), B3 (perceived cost), and B4 (nonpublic motivation) for the assessment goal layer A were 0.2808, 0.2565, 0.1997, and 0.2630, respectively. The comprehensive weights of H1, H2, and H3 were 0.0948, 0.0874, and 0.0795, respectively. The weights of H4 (technical grade), H5 (interaction effectiveness), and H6 (system compatibility) for B2 PEOU were 0.0857, 0.0900, and 0.0867, respectively. The weight values of H7 (financial cost) and H8 (privacy cost) for B3 (perceived cost) were 0.0859 and 0.1000, respectively. The weight values of H9 (health concern), H10 (outcome expectations), and H11 (social influence) for B4 (personal motivation) had weight values of 0.0867, 0.0862, and 0.1172, respectively.

According to the criterion-stage weight values, we found that the ranking of the elements influencing the use of health apps by adults under the impact of COVID-19 were B1 (PU), B4 (nonpublic motivation), B2 (PEOU), and B3 (perceived cost) (Figure 2). That is, for this group, PU ranked first when people chose or used fitness apps, accompanied by private motivation, which was especially influential, and then the PEOU and perceived value. According to the weight values of the scheme layer, we found that these adults were more influenced by H11 (social), H8 (privacy cost), H1 (content adaptability), H5 (interaction effectiveness), and H2 (content relevance), and less influenced by H6 (system compatibility), H9 (health concerns), H10 (outcome expectation), H7 (financial cost), H4 (technical grade), and H3 (content quality) (Figure 3).

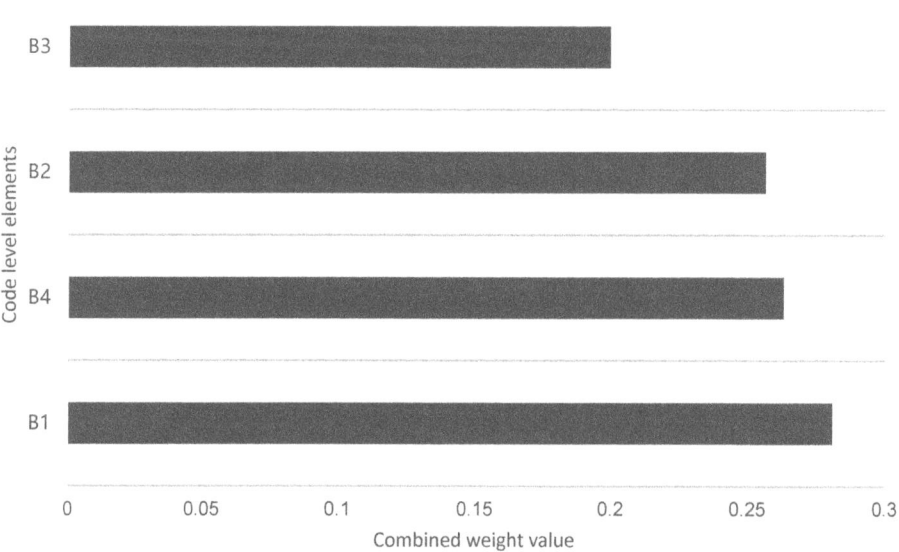

Figure 2. Statistical comprehensive weight values of criterion layer.

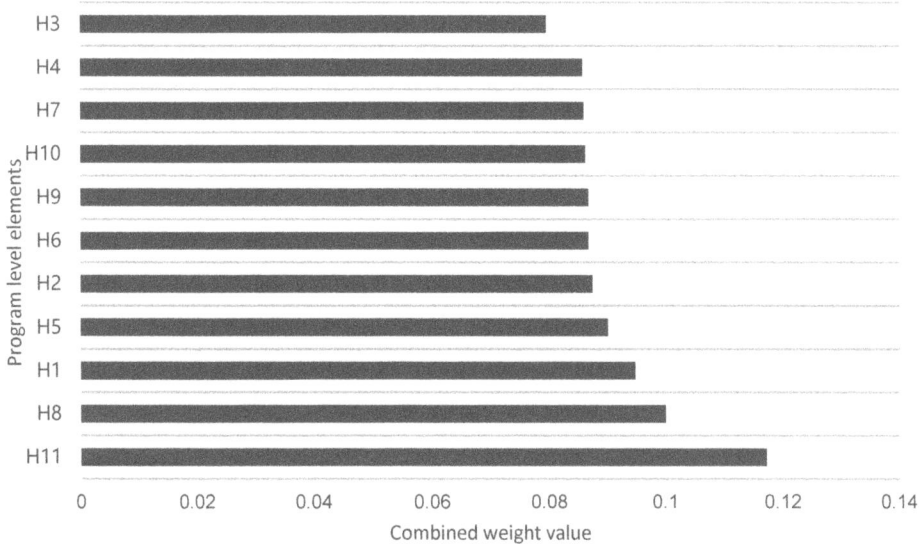

Figure 3. Statistical comprehensive weight values of scheme layer.

5. Discussion

First, PU had the most notable effect on the adult use of fitness apps. The indicators we used to measure B1 (PU) were the pair of H1 (content adaptability) and H2 (content relevance), as well as H3 (content quality). Among them, H1 was the influencing factor with the highest weight because the users of fitness apps are of different ages and have different exercise purposes, physical bases, and exercise programs, so users have different requirements for the content adaptability of fitness apps. If the app is not based on scientific and effective assessment data for personalized program settings, the user may perform improper or ineffective exercises. For example, some apps directly recommend HIIT exercise programs for primary training; such training is characterized by high exercise intensity, short duration, and high energy consumption, so is not suitable for most primary fitness, leading to the user feedback of exercise intensity being too high and the exercise program being difficult to implement. However, for people experienced with exercise, this kind of exercise may not meet their fitness needs. Exercise apps should also help users avoid injury due to exercise, allowing users to reduce the difficulty of the exercise and to choose low-risk and low-threshold programs to ensure the safety of exercise; however, this may prevent users from achieving the purpose of the exercise.

Second, personal motivation considerably influenced the study group's intention to use fitness apps. The indicators measuring B4 (personal motivation) were H9 (health concerns), H10 (outcome expectation), and H11 (social influence). Among them, H11 and H9 had higher weights. The higher weight of H11 indicated that people were more influenced by their community when using fitness apps. Social impact refers to the stress and impact that people experience from the humans around them when they perform a behavior [52]. The environment and people around an individual, such as family environment and members, friends, work environment, colleagues, etc., can substantially influence their specific behavior. Community influence is more important in Chinese culture. If companies want to improve their social influence, a long-term process is required; they should implement measures to proactively improve the quality of their products and services, improve customer experience, and assume their social role. H9 had a stronger impact on personal motivation, indicating that the study group was aware of the importance of physical health; therefore, concerns about their health will increase their autonomy in fitness. Given the effect of COVID-19, people's fitness awareness has increased, and their intention to engage in PA is stronger, increasing their motivation to use health apps.

Third, B2 (PEOU) strongly impacted the study participants' use of fitness apps. PEOU was influenced in decreasing order by interaction effectiveness, system compatibility, and technical level. This indicated that this group preferred software that was easy to operate, appropriate, with a reasonable design, and that had a user-friendly software interface, which could provide a good user experience. The discovery, installation, and login of the software, the use, recording, and uploading of results and sharing in the fitness process should be easy and not require time or effort to learn. In addition, the interface of the software should be reasonably designed, and the content should be relevant so that the user feels that this product is suitable for them. In the design of mobile fitness apps, user-friendliness should be considered.

Fourth, B3 (perceived cost) had relatively little impact on the use of fitness apps by the study group; however, adults of this age were considerably more worried about H8 (privacy cost) than financial cost according to the weights of the scheme-level indicators. Users face many risks in the process of using the mobile Internet; private information may be leaked, and the perception of privacy risks negatively affects the perceived value. Privacy price has a sizable poor impact on the perceived price. Fitness APPsapps should have a clear, effective, and easy-to-understand security privacy policy. Expense cost also affects the users' experience of perceived cost during use. The perceived economic cost is the users' perception of objective costs with a certain subjectivity, and the higher the perceived cost, the lower the perceived value. Therefore, enhancing the best of merchandise and offerings and enhancing the value effectiveness is one of the core aggressive benefits of sports activities and health apps. The degree of satisfaction with the merchandise and offerings immediately determines whether or not customers are inclined to use them continuously, and companies should focus on providing users with high-quality products and services.

6. Conclusions

Our results showed that, first, in the criterion layer, the weight of PU was 0.2808, which was much larger than that of the other indicators, indicating that PU most strongly influenced the study group's use of fitness apps under the influence of COVID-19. Among the criteria that we used for measuring PU, the study group was more concerned about content adaptability. Therefore, developers of health apps need to pay attention to the special traits of users, provide more customized and scientific strategies and content, and select reasonable and scientific fitness programs tailored to users according to their age, occupation, height, weight, personal preferences, etc. Second, the weights of personal motivation and PEOU were 0.2630 and 0.2565, respectively, indicating their stronger impact on the willingness of the study groups to use fitness apps. We recommend that fitness APP developers pay attention to the different characteristics of users and provide more personalized service methods and content, improve the fun of exercise, and reduce the fatigue experienced when users exercise. Third, the perceived cost had the lowest weight of 0.1997, indicating a weaker influence on the group's use of fitness apps. The data of the indicators measuring the perceived cost showed that the study group was much more worried about privacy than the financial cost, indicating that the group had a strong sense of privacy. Security and privacy policies imply a commitment to users' personal information. Due to the small operating interface of cell phones and portable devices, companies should proactively and prominently display protection policies so that users can feel the company's commitment to security and privacy.

Currently, the COVID-19 pandemic is still ongoing. Increasing people's physical activity during the pandemic to ensure physical and mental health and to improve the well-being of the population remains a difficult task. The data from this study can help subsequent fitness app developers understand user needs and provide an empirical basis for subsequent fitness app development or iterations.

Author Contributions: Conceptualization, Y.G. and D.C.; methodology, Y.G. and H.Z.; software, X.M.; validation, Y.G. and D.C.; formal analysis, Y.G.; investigation, Y.G. and X.M.; resources, Y.G.; data curation, X.M.; writing—original draft preparation, Y.G. and H.Z.; writing—review and editing, Y.G.; visualization, X.M.; supervision, Y.G.; project administration, Y.G. All authors have read and agreed to the published version of the manuscript.

Funding: This study was conducted by the Anhui University 2020 Talent Introduction Scientific Research Start-up Fund Project (Project No. S020318019/001).

Institutional Review Board Statement: Not applicable.

Informed Consent Statement: Informed consent was obtained from all subjects involved in the study.

Data Availability Statement: The experimental data used to support the findings of this study are included in the article.

Conflicts of Interest: The authors declare no conflict of interest.

References

1. Azzouzi, S.; Stratton, C.; Muñoz-Velasco, L.P.; Wang, K.; Fourtassi, M.; Hong, B.-Y.; Cooper, R.; Balikuddembe, J.K.; Palomba, A.; Peterson, M.; et al. The Impact of the COVID-19 Pandemic on Healthy Lifestyle Behaviors and Perceived Mental and Physical Health of People Living with Non-Communicable Diseases: An International Cross-Sectional Survey. *Int. J. Environ. Res. Public Health* **2022**, *19*, 8023. [CrossRef] [PubMed]
2. Kaur, H.; Singh, T.; Arya, Y.K.; Mittal, S. Physical Fitness and Exercise during the COVID-19 Pandemic: A Qualitative Enquiry. *Front. Psychol.* **2020**, *11*, 590172. [CrossRef] [PubMed]
3. Ammar, A.; Chtourou, H.; Boukhris, O.; Trabelsi, K.; Masmoudi, L.; Brach, M.; Bouaziz, B.; Bentlage, E.; How, D.; Ahmed, M.; et al. On Behalf of the Eclb-Covid Consortium. COVID-19 Home Confinement Negatively Impacts Social Participation and Life Satisfaction: A Worldwide Multicenter Study. *Int. J. Environ. Res. Public Health* **2020**, *17*, 6237. [CrossRef] [PubMed]
4. Xiao, H.; Zhang, Y.; Kong, D.; Li, S.; Yang, N. Social Capital and Sleep Quality in Individuals Who Self-Isolated for 14 Days during the Coronavirus Disease 2019 (COVID-19) Outbreak in January 2020 in China. *Med. Sci. Monit.* **2020**, *26*, e923921. [CrossRef] [PubMed]
5. Ammar, A.; Trabelsi, K.; Brach, M.; Chtourou, H.; Boukhris, O.; Masmoudi, L.; Bouaziz, B.; Bentlage, E.; How, D.; Ahmed, M.; et al. Effects of home confinement on mental health and lifestyle behaviours during the COVID-19 outbreak: Insights from the ECLB-COVID19 multicentre study. *Biol. Sport* **2021**, *38*, 9–21. [CrossRef]
6. Chtourou, H.; Trabelsi, K.; H'mida, C.; Boukhris, O.; Glenn, J.M.; Brach, M.; Bentlage, E.; Bott, N.; Shephard, R.J.; Ammar, A.; et al. Staying Physically Active during the Quarantine and Self-Isolation Period for Controlling and Mitigating the COVID-19 Pandemic: A Systematic Overview of the Literature. *Front. Psychol.* **2020**, *11*, 1708. [CrossRef]
7. Sui, W.; Rush, J.; Rhodes, R.E. Engagement with Web-Based Fitness Videos on YouTube and Instagram during the COVID-19 Pandemic: Longitudinal Study. *JMIR Form. Res.* **2022**, *6*, e25055. [CrossRef]
8. Ammar, A.; Brach, M.; Trabelsi, K.; Chtourou, H.; Boukhris, O.; Masmoudi, L.; Bouaziz, B.; Bentlage, E.; How, D.; Ahmed, M.; et al. Effects of COVID-19 Home Confinement on Eating Behaviour and Physical Activity: Results of the ECLB-COVID19 International Online Survey. *Nutrients* **2020**, *12*, 1583. [CrossRef]
9. Krebs, P.; Duncan, D.T. Health App Use among US Mobile Phone Owners: A National Survey. *JMIR MHealth UHealth* **2015**, *3*, e101. [CrossRef]
10. Vairavasundaram, S.; Varadarajan, V.; Srinivasan, D.; Balaganesh, V.; Damerla, S.B.; Swaminathan, B.; Ravi, L. Dynamic Physical Activity Recommendation Delivered through a Mobile Fitness App: A Deep Learning Approach. *Axioms* **2022**, *11*, 346. [CrossRef]
11. Yan, Z.; Spaulding, H.R. Extracellular Superoxide Dismutase, a Molecular Transducer of Health Benefits of Exercise. *Redox Biol.* **2020**, *32*, 101508. [CrossRef] [PubMed]
12. Powell, K.E.; King, A.C.; Buchner, D.M.; Campbell, W.W.; DiPietro, L.; Erickson, K.I.; Hillman, C.H.; Jakicic, J.M.; Janz, K.F.; Katzmarzyk, P.T.; et al. The Scientific Foundation for the Physical Activity Guidelines for Americans, 2nd Edition. *J. Phys. Act. Health* **2018**, *16*, 1–11. [CrossRef] [PubMed]
13. Haider, S.; Smith, L.; Markovic, L.; Schuch, F.B.; Sadarangani, K.P.; Lopez Sanchez, G.F.; Lopez-Bueno, R.; Gil-Salmerón, A.; Rieder, J.; Tully, M.A.; et al. Associations between Physical Activity, Sitting Time, and Time Spent Outdoors with Mental Health during the First COVID-19 Lock down in Austria. *Int. J. Environ. Res. Public Health* **2021**, *18*, 9168. [CrossRef] [PubMed]
14. Budimir, S.; Pieh, C.; Dale, R.; Probst, T. Severe Mental Health Symptoms during COVID-19: A Comparison of the United Kingdom and Austria. *Healthcare* **2021**, *9*, 191. [CrossRef] [PubMed]
15. Chen, X.; Zhu, Z.; Chen, M.; Li, Y. Large-Scale Mobile Fitness App Usage Analysis for Smart Health. *IEEE Commun. Mag.* **2018**, *56*, 46–52. [CrossRef]
16. Liu, Y.; Avello, M. Status of the Research in Fitness Apps: A Bibliometric Analysis. *Telemat. Inform.* **2021**, *57*, 101506. [CrossRef]
17. Ranjbarnia, B.; Kamelifar, M.J.; Masoumi, H. The Association between Active Mobility and Subjective Wellbeing during COVID-19 in MENA Countries. *Healthcare* **2022**, *10*, 1603. [CrossRef]

18. Lin, S.-Y.; Juan, P.-J.; Lin, S.-W. A TAM Framework to Evaluate the Effect of Smartphone Application on Tourism Information Search Behavior of Foreign Independent Travelers. *Sustainability* **2020**, *12*, 9366. [CrossRef]
19. Kusonwattana, P.; Prasetyo, Y.T.; Vincent, S.; Christofelix, J.; Amudra, A.; Montgomery, H.J.; Young, M.N.; Nadlifatin, R.; Persada, S.F. Determining Factors Affecting Behavioral Intention to Organize an Online Event during the COVID-19 Pandemic. *Sustainability* **2022**, *14*, 12964. [CrossRef]
20. Hammann, T.; Schwartze, M.M.; Zentel, P.; Schlomann, A.; Even, C.; Wahl, H.-W.; Rietz, C. The Challenge of Emotions—An Experimental Approach to Assess the Emotional Competence of People with Intellectual Disabilities. *Disabilities* **2022**, *2*, 611–625. [CrossRef]
21. Cho, J.; Quinlan, M.M.; Park, D.; Noh, G.-Y. Determinants of Adoption of Smartphone Health Apps among College Students. *Am. J. Health Behav.* **2014**, *38*, 860–870. [CrossRef] [PubMed]
22. Chen, Y.; Zhao, S. Understanding Chinese EFL Learners' Acceptance of Gamified Vocabulary Learning Apps: An Integration of Self-Determination Theory and Technology Acceptance Model. *Sustainability* **2022**, *14*, 11288. [CrossRef]
23. Beldad, A.D.; Hegner, S.M. Expanding the Technology Acceptance Model with the Inclusion of Trust, Social Influence, and Health Valuation to Determine the Predictors of German Users' Willingness to Continue Using a Fitness App: A Structural Equation Modeling Approach. *Int. J. Hum. Comput. Interact.* **2018**, *34*, 882–893. [CrossRef]
24. Page Glave, A.; Di Brezzo, R.; Applegate, D.K.; Olson, J.M. The Effects of Obesity Classification Method on Select Kinematic Gait Variables in Adult Females. *J. Sports Med. Phys. Fitness* **2014**, *54*, 197–202.
25. Mola, L.; Berger, Q.; Haavisto, K.; Soscia, I. Mobility as a Service: An Exploratory Study of Consumer Mobility Behaviour. *Sustainability* **2020**, *12*, 8210. [CrossRef]
26. de Jesus França, L.C.; Lopes, L.F.; de Morais, M.S.; dos Santos Lisboa, G.; da Rocha, S.J.S.S.; de Morais Junior, V.T.M.; Santana, R.C.; Mucida, D.P. Environmental Fragility Zoning Using GIS and AHP Modeling: Perspectives for the Conservation of Natural Ecosystems in Brazil. *Conservation* **2022**, *2*, 349–366. [CrossRef]
27. Davis, F.D.; Bagozzi, R.P.; Warshaw, P.R. User Acceptance of Computer Technology: A Comparison of Two Theoretical Models. *Manage. Sci.* **1989**, *35*, 982–1003. [CrossRef]
28. Karahanna, E.; Straub, D.W. The Psychological Origins of Perceived Usefulness and Ease-of-Use. *Inf. Manag.* **1999**, *35*, 237–250. [CrossRef]
29. Beldad, A.; de Jong, M.; Steehouder, M. How Shall I Trust the Faceless and the Intangible? A Literature Review on the Antecedents of Online Trust. *Comput. Human Behav.* **2010**, *26*, 857–869. [CrossRef]
30. bin Wan Abu, W.H.R.; binti Misaridin, N.A.F.; bin Mokhtar, M.Z. Determinant of Users' Intention to Adopt Pahang Mart on-Line Portal in Malaysia: The Role of Perceived Ease of Use. *J. Phys. Conf. Ser.* **2021**, *1874*, 012049. [CrossRef]
31. Chang, C.-J.; Hsu, B.C.-Y.; Chen, M.-Y. Viewing Sports Online during the COVID-19 Pandemic: The Antecedent Effects of Social Presence on the Technology Acceptance Model. *Sustainability* **2021**, *14*, 341. [CrossRef]
32. Chillakanti, P.; Ekwaro-Osire, S.; Ertas, A. Evaluation of Technology Platforms for Use in Transdisciplinary Research. *Educ. Sci.* **2021**, *11*, 23. [CrossRef]
33. Jung, S.-H.; Kim, J.-H.; Cho, H.-N.; Lee, H.-W.; Choi, H.-J. Brand Personality of Korean Dance and Sustainable Behavioral Intention of Global Consumers in Four Countries: Focusing on the Technological Acceptance Model. *Sustainability* **2021**, *13*, 11160. [CrossRef]
34. Ong, A.K.S.; Prasetyo, Y.T.; Bagon, G.M.; Dadulo, C.H.S.; Hortillosa, N.O.; Mercado, M.A.; Chuenyindee, T.; Nadlifatin, R.; Persada, S.F. Investigating Factors Affecting Behavioral Intention among Gym-Goers to Visit Fitness Centers during the COVID-19 Pandemic: Integrating Physical Activity Maintenance Theory and Social Cognitive Theory. *Sustainability* **2022**, *14*, 12020. [CrossRef]
35. Hohmann, L.A.; Garza, K.B. The Moderating Power of Impulsivity: A Systematic Literature Review Examining the Theory of Planned Behavior. *Pharmacy* **2022**, *10*, 85. [CrossRef] [PubMed]
36. Molina, M.D.; Myrick, J.G. The 'How' and 'Why' of Fitness App Use: Investigating User Motivations to Gain Insights into the Nexus of Technology and Fitness. *Sport Soc.* **2021**, *24*, 1233–1248. [CrossRef]
37. Zang, W.; Qian, Y.; Song, H. The Effect of Perceived Value on Consumers' Repurchase Intention of Commercial Ice Stadium: The Mediating Role of Community Interactions. *Int. J. Environ. Res. Public Health* **2022**, *19*, 3043. [CrossRef]
38. Markiewicz, Ł.; Muda, R.; Kubińska, E.; Augustynowicz, P. An Explanatory Analysis of Perceived Risk Decision Weights (Perceived-Risk Attitudes) and Perceived Benefit Decision Weights (Perceived-Benefit Attitudes) in Risk-Value Models. *J. Risk Res.* **2020**, *23*, 739–761. [CrossRef]
39. Ghani, E.K.; Ali, M.M.; Musa, M.N.R.; Omonov, A.A. The Effect of Perceived Usefulness, Reliability, and COVID-19 Pandemic on Digital Banking Effectiveness: Analysis Using Technology Acceptance Model. *Sustainability* **2022**, *14*, 11248. [CrossRef]
40. Fenton, A.; Cooper-Ryan, A.M.; Hardey, M.M.; Ahmed, W. Football Fandom as a Platform for Digital Health Promotion and Behaviour Change: A Mobile App Case Study. *Int. J. Environ. Res. Public Health* **2022**, *19*, 8417. [CrossRef]
41. Alkhwaldi, A.F.; Alharasis, E.E.; Shehadeh, M.; Abu-AlSondos, I.A.; Oudat, M.S.; Bani Atta, A.A. Towards an Understanding of FinTech Users' Adoption: Intention and e-Loyalty Post-COVID-19 from a Developing Country Perspective. *Sustainability* **2022**, *14*, 12616. [CrossRef]
42. Humer, E.; Probst, T.; Wagner-Skacel, J.; Pieh, C. Association of Health Behaviors with Mental Health Problems in More than 7000 Adolescents during COVID-19. *Int. J. Environ. Res. Public Health* **2022**, *19*, 9072. [CrossRef] [PubMed]

43. Gupta, P.; Prashar, S.; Vijay, T.S.; Parsad, C. Examining the Influence of Antecedents of Continuous Intention to Use an Informational App: The Role of Perceived Usefulness and Perceived Ease of Use. *Int. J. Bus. Inf. Syst.* **2021**, *36*, 270. [CrossRef]
44. Jiang, L.C.; Sun, M.; Huang, G. Uncovering the Heterogeneity in Fitness App Use: A Latent Class Analysis of Chinese Users. *Int. J. Environ. Res. Public Health* **2022**, *19*, 10679. [CrossRef]
45. Hutchinson, S.; Mirza, M.M.; West, N.; Karabiyik, U.; Rogers, M.K.; Mukherjee, T.; Aggarwal, S.; Chung, H.; Pettus-Davis, C. Investigating Wearable Fitness Applications: Data Privacy and Digital Forensics Analysis on Android. *Appl. Sci.* **2022**, *12*, 9747. [CrossRef]
46. San-Martín, S.; Prodanova, J.; Jiménez, N. The Impact of Age in the Generation of Satisfaction and WOM in Mobile Shopping. *J. Retail. Consum. Serv.* **2015**, *23*, 1–8. [CrossRef]
47. Kwon, J.-Y.; Lee, J.-S.; Park, T.-S. Analysis of Strategies to Increase User Retention of Fitness Mobile Apps during and after the COVID-19 Pandemic. *Int. J. Environ. Res. Public Health* **2022**, *19*, 10814. [CrossRef]
48. Abu Bakar, A.; Mahinderjit Singh, M.; Mohd Shariff, A.R. A Privacy Preservation Quality of Service (QoS) Model for Data Exposure in Android Smartphone Usage. *Sensors* **2021**, *21*, 1667. [CrossRef]
49. Park, M.; Yoo, H.; Kim, J.; Lee, J. Why Do Young People Use Fitness Apps? Cognitive Characteristics and App Quality. *Electron. Commer. Res.* **2018**, *18*, 755–761. [CrossRef]
50. Cai, J.; Zhao, Y.; Sun, J. Factors Influencing Fitness App Users' Behavior in China. *Int. J. Hum. Comput. Interact.* **2022**, *38*, 53–63. [CrossRef]
51. Wang, C.; Wu, G.; Zhou, X.; Lv, Y. An Empirical Study of the Factors Influencing User Behavior of Fitness Software in College Students Based on UTAUT. *Sustainability* **2022**, *14*, 9720. [CrossRef]
52. Venkatesh, V.; Morris, M.G.; Davis, G.B.; Davis, F.D. User Acceptance of Information Technology: Toward a Unified View. *MIS Q.* **2003**, *27*, 425. [CrossRef]
53. Cheunkamon, E.; Jomnonkwao, S.; Ratanavaraha, V. Determinant Factors Influencing Thai Tourists' Intentions to Use social media for Travel Planning. *Sustainability* **2020**, *12*, 7252. [CrossRef]

MDPI
St. Alban-Anlage 66
4052 Basel
Switzerland
Tel. +41 61 683 77 34
Fax +41 61 302 89 18
www.mdpi.com

International Journal of Environmental Research and Public Health Editorial Office
E-mail: ijerph@mdpi.com
www.mdpi.com/journal/ijerph

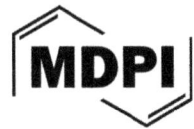

www.ingramcontent.com/pod-product-compliance
Lightning Source LLC
LaVergne TN
LVHW070617100526
838202LV00012B/663